A Dictionary of Pharmacology and Allied Topics

D.R. Laurence MD FRCP
*Professor Emeritus of Pharmacology and Therapeutics,
University College London, UK*

with contributions from
J.R. Carpenter BSc PhD
*Honorary Fellow, and lately Lecturer in Pharmacology,
University of Manchester.
Senior Medical Editor, Gardiner-Caldwell Communications Ltd,
Macclesfield, UK*

"If language is not correct, what is said is not what is meant"
(Confucius: Chinese philosopher, 551–479 BCE)

1998
ELSEVIER
Amsterdam – Lausanne – New York – Oxford – Shannon – Singapore – Tokyo

ELSEVIER SCIENCE B.V.
Sara Burgerhartstraat 25
P.O. Box 211, 1000 AE Amsterdam, The Netherlands

Library of Congress Cataloging in Publication Data
A catalog record from the Library of Congress has been applied for.

ISBN Hardbound: 0 444 82591 6
ISBN Paperback: 0 444 50050 2

Printed in The Netherlands.

PREFACE

- Please read this preface; it is an important part of the book.

  Pharmacology is a science with its own distinctive attitudes and practices.

  It is also a science that links many others in the massive enterprise of developing chemicals that affect living tissues to the benefit of humankind. The most prominent of these activities is the development of new medicines, but there are many others.

  It is important that pharmacologists understand these other disciplines with which they are involved, and that the latter understand pharmacology, for all are engaged in enterprises fundamental to human happiness and to the good of society.

  Hence the discursive title of this book.

- **Who this book is intended for:**
- Pharmacologists, basic and clinical,
- All people engaged in clinical drug evaluation, whether or not they would describe themselves as pharmacologists,
- Those who write about drugs, medicines and clinical drug evaluation,
- Other people whose interests require that they have access to the world of drugs and medicines.

  We invite them all to *browse* in it as well as to use it for *reference*, for "A dictionary [is not] a bad book to read. There is no cant in it, no excess of explanation, and it is full of suggestion" (*Ralph Waldo Emerson*, 1803–1882, poet and essayist, USA).

- **The scope of pharmacology** (see main entry in the text).

  Pharmacology is a discipline that, although having its own territory and terminology, also 'trespasses' extensively into virtually all branches of medicine, as well as into allied sciences, such as physiology and biochemistry, and into law and social policy. It is the basis for an efficient and powerful research-based industry.

  Pharmacologists need to understand each other and other scientists, and to be themselves understood by scientific, medical and social policy-makers.

  Because pharmacology is such a highly diverse discipline we have kept browsers particularly in mind throughout, for leisurely browsing is a comfortable way of assimilating information.

- **The need for clarity.**

  "Most men think indistinctly and therefore cannot speak with exactness", and "Language is only the instrument of science, and words are but the signs of ideas". Thus, in 1755, wrote Dr Samuel Johnson in the preface to his great work, the first comprehensive Dictionary of the English Language; and his statements remain true today.

The need for lucidity in speech and writing has never been greater than it is now. On a practical personal level, failure to communicate effectively can be a major barrier to career success. If words are not used with precision and in accordance with their currently accepted meaning, "what is said is not what is meant" (*Confucius*).

- **The meaning of words.**

The meaning of words changes with time (*semantic change*), and the pedant's belief that the first recorded use of a word must remain its correct meaning is erroneous (*etymological fallacy*). Language alteration with time may be abrupt or gradual. Change cannot be successfully resisted *except* for some scientific jargon (terminology) where it is in the interest of practitioners of the science and of its application to social purposes that certain meanings remain constant (lawyers in particular are familiar with this necessity); or changed only by intellectual consensus; or by regulation in the cases of statutory authorities, e.g. official medicines regulation. Similar considerations apply to the invention of new terms.

- **Definitions are needed.**

We find support for our enterprise from philosophers and scientists, for example:
- *Voltaire* (1694–1778): "If you wish to converse with me, define your terms."
- *RW Emerson* (1803–1882): "He that can define ... is the best man."
- *L Wittgenstein* (1880–1951): "If language is to be a means of communication there must be agreement not only in definitions but also (queer as this may sound) in judgements."
- *U Trendelenburg* (1983): "The clarity of our nomenclature should concern us deeply, and not only from the point of view of pedantic linguistics. After all, scientists have to rely on language to formulate their hypotheses and theories, express their view and describe their insights into the workings of nature. Moreover, a considerable percentage of them have to rely on a foreign language (known as basic English, scientific English or simply poor English). Without a precisely defined nomenclature, all our attempts to master this foreign language are doomed to failure, and we are quite unable to convey to others our own insights and thoughts."

We also find support from politicians, who, it is no surprise to learn, have never favoured precision of language:
- *B Disraeli* (1804–1881): "I hate definitions."
- *E Burke* (1724–1779): "I have no great opinion of a definition, the celebrated remedy of [uncertainty and confusion]."

Some philosophers, however, can seem ambivalent. *Karl Popper* (1902–1994) (see **science in pharmacology**) said that any special interest in definitions leads to 'empty verbalism' and that he had tried for decades to combat the 'superstition' [his word] that if we want to be precise we have to define our terms. However, he appears not to have been referring to practising scientists seeking data that may be put to use in the relief of real disease in real people in the real world, but rather to armchair philosophers of the Humpty

Dumpty persuasion, "'When I use a word,' Humpty Dumpty said in a rather scornful tone, 'it means just what I choose it to mean – neither more nor less'" (*Lewis Carroll*, 1832–1898). But Popper also said that *nothing is so important as language*.

Yet there are scientists (often ultra-specialists working at the growing edge of knowledge in their field) who disapprove of attempts to generate standard or model nomenclature as adversely restricting their intellectual and scientific freedom. Their restricted view is comprehensible, but it shows lack of understanding, of consideration, and even of compassion for the broader community of scientists in which they themselves live; and, in particular, for students (as all of them once were), who need to know what is being said as precisely as possible. We agree with the *International Union of Pharmacology (IUPHAR) Committee on Receptor Nomenclature and Drug Classification* that: "The literature of pharmacology presents many inconsistencies in the use of nomenclature and symbols. These are particularly common in operational studies in which receptors are characterized by quantitative measurements of receptor-mediated function and of ligand binding. The problem is compounded by the fact that sometimes a given term is used in quite different senses. For these reasons, it would, we believe, be helpful to adhere to (as far as is practicable and reasonable) a common terminology, set of definitions, and symbol usage. These issues have been addressed in most other biological and physical sciences ..." The committee consulted widely and, "These consultations notwithstanding, the recommendations ... are to be regarded as provisional in nature. Their aim is to aid communication and ease of comprehension without being rigidly prescriptive, and they will certainly require periodic revision and updating as new ideas and information arise."

"It should be added that variations from the suggested notation and usage may well be desirable under particular circumstances..."

"*The only essential is that the new terms are clearly defined*" (*Pharmacological Reviews* 1995;47:255). We consider this good advice.

- **The lexicographer.**

Dr Johnson (in 1755) described the *lexicographer* or "writer of dictionaries" as "the slave of science" and as "a harmless drudge that busies himself in tracing the original, and detailing the significance of words". He added that although "Every other authour may aspire to praise, a lexicographer can only hope to escape reproach, and even this negative recompence has been yet granted to very few". In concluding his preface he addresses his critics with a little less than his customary self-assurance: "In this work, when it shall be found that much is omitted, let it not be forgotten that much likewise is performed." We, after our so much more modest endeavours, know how he felt.

- **The reasons why this book has been compiled.**

We have undertaken this enterprise because we think the need for it is increasingly apparent. We include words and terms that are met and used by pharmacologists beyond the strictly technical terms of the discipline. Our decades of joint experience of practice and teaching have taught us the desirability of thus broadening the scope of the book. We invite anyone who dissents to question students about the meaning of the words they use. Indeed, we recommend questioning professional colleagues – by those willing to risk the unpopularity and resentment that is apt to ensue. But, "... philosophical problems arise when *language goes on holiday*" (*L Wittgenstein*). "To say that a word has meaning is not to say that those who use the word correctly have ever thought out what the meaning is" (*B Russell*, 1872–1970). We all get by thus in daily talk, but a more rigorous approach is necessary in scientific communication and debate.

- **The benefits of a broad view of pharmacology.**

The reasons why we emphasize that we treat 'allied topics' and offer this book for browsing as well as for reference are that we think that current circumstances of education, training and practice of pharmacology, plus the increasingly competitive scramble for resources, create conditions that inevitably have a narrowing intellectual effect at all levels; and this is enhanced by exploding technological advance and information overload.

Practice of individuals must unavoidably be circumscribed, but a broad view remains important if pharmacology is to flourish and so to be enabled to fulfil its potential for massive relief of suffering and for practical gains to society (including the economy), everywhere.

- **Choice of entries.**

Our choice of entries from the enormous range of appropriate topics is necessarily idiosyncratic and we make no apology for this. Also, the space allotted to each has no inherent validity – we have been guided by the general accessibility of other sources of information. For example, the legions of individual drugs and classes of drugs are accessibly and comprehensively listed in innumerable textbooks, pharmacopoeias and formularies, and we include only those relatively few that seem to have a special claim for one reason or another, sadly, sometimes, for the harm they have done. *This book is not a dictionary of drugs.* Because relevant aspects of the publications of official and semi-official bodies, such as regulatory authorities, the World Health Organization, World Medical Association, European Community/Union, International Committee of Medical Journal Editors and the International Union of Pharmacology, never seem to be at hand when wanted, we quote selectively from these.

D.R. LAURENCE   J.R. CARPENTER

NOTES

1. **Bold type** in an entry signifies a separate entry for the emboldened term.
2. **Etymology** (Gr. *etumon*, basic meaning; *logos*, word, study) is provided for most technical terms, and for other words where it seems to us to benefit understanding and facilitate the use of language. The majority of words derive from *Greek* (Gr.) and *Latin* (L.); other languages are indicated by (self-evident) abbreviations. The definition of some words bears little relation to etymology. This is because the meaning of a word develops over time and may depart from its origins. The criterion for meaning has to be *currently accepted* usage, however much we may sometimes dislike this.* "For a *large* class of cases ... the meaning of a word is its use in the language" (*L Wittgenstein*).

    We do not always repeat the etymology when there are multiple entries of a word in sequence.
3. **The use of hyphens** is an issue of which Fowler (*A dictionary of modern English usage*, 1965) writes that "its infinite variety defies description". We have found ourselves in good company in practising Fowler's advice that "The hyphen is not an ornament but an aid to being understood and should be employed only when it is needed for that purpose"; although "There are no hard and fast rules" (*Oxford companion to the English language*). Hyphen (Gr. *huphen*, from *hupo-*, under; *hen*, one).

*****Lexiconjugally speaking**. France's greatest lexicographer, [and physician] Emile Littré (1801–1881), was once found by his wife *in flagrante* [*delicto*] [in blazing crime], and in their conjugal bedroom, with their housemaid. "Emile," cried Mrs Littré, "I am surprised!" "No, my dear," replied the erring lexicographer calmly, "You are astonished. It is we who are surprised."

His precision was right, certainly in his own language, and at least arguably in English: the original sense of *surprise* is indeed 'to take unawares'. But Mrs Littré, had she been speaking English, could have replied that her usage went back at least to the 18th century. The question is whether Mr Littré was right, in any but a lexicographer's sense, in his attitude to language. Is the more precise word always to be preferred? And how rigorously, if at all, is a derived or secondary usage to be rejected?

Such issues arise with thousands of sliding words and usages. They are part of the endless debate between – to caricature both – the pedantic view of language and the 'anyfink-goes' one. The wise man expects no resolution of this debate. Dr Samuel Johnson's heart is with the pedants; his head tells him that what is 'right' really is often relative. It depends who is talking to whom, where, why, about what (*The Economist*).

Note: lexiconjugally (Gr. *lexis*, word; L. *coniux*, a spouse) is a word invented by *The Economist* to tell this story more entertainingly. It is a *neologism* (Gr. *neos*, new; *logos*, word) which is unlikely to enter the language because of the extremely limited circumstances in which its use would be appropriate. But it illustrates how readily new compound words can be coined in English, rooted as it is in Greek and Latin. This has great advantages for science, though it can encourage the invention of obfuscating **jargon**. In some languages, the invention of technical terms to meet new needs in science is difficult, if not impossible.

4. **References**. It would be impossible, even if it were desirable, to provide a reference to every important statement. In general, full references are given for a few highly technical concepts, and acknowledgement only by name where we have quoted, or followed closely, an individual author.

5. **Terms used by official regulatory authorities**. Medicines regulation is a massive worldwide bureaucratic operation which inevitably develops its own language of convenience, or jargon; but this has yet to be effectively internationally harmonized. Some knowledge of this language beyond immediate professional circles is desirable. We either quote from an individual agency or blend the definitions of more than one.

ACKNOWLEDGEMENTS

In about 1980 one of us (DRL) resolved to attempt a dictionary for pharmacologists. The initial modest outcome was printed privately at University College London. In 1984 a second informal edition was produced in collaboration with Dr (now Professor) Ian Shaw. In 1994 an edition was formally published (UCL Press) by DR Laurence and JR Carpenter (the above under slightly differing titles). In 1998 a second formal edition (Elsevier Science) is published.

We frankly acknowledge that this compilation is founded on the scholarship and assistance of others who we here thank for their scientific, editorial and computer expertise.

"Every book is a quotation", wrote Ralph Waldo Emerson (1803–1882, essayist, USA), and this is particularly true of a dictionary. But we have tried to avoid *plagiarism* (see entry in this book). Of those who have made contributions over the years we are particularly beholden to (in alphabetical order):

Dr JK Aronson	Dr D Girdlestone
Mrs T Bashford	Professor DH Jenkinson
Professor D Colquhoun	Dr S Jones
Ms R Comish	Professor HP Rang
Dr RW Foster	The late Dr JMH Rees

We are deeply grateful for permission to quote from many sources. In particular, Professor Malcolm Rowland has given us permission to quote from his authoritative work, with Thomas N Tozer: *Clinical Pharmacokinetics: Concepts and applications* (Lea and Febiger, 1989), and the International Union of Pharmacology (IUPHAR) has permitted us to reprint some definitions of its Committee on Receptor Nomenclature and Drug Classification published in *Pharmacological Reviews* (permission of the American Society for Pharmacology and Experimental Therapeutics). *IUPHAR is not responsible for any material that is not directly attributed to it in the text.*

We have scoured, and are deeply indebted to, journals, reports and books too numerous to mention and glossaries of official drug regulatory bodies, without all of which this book could not have been made. We hope that this collective acknowledgement will be acceptable.

If we have omitted any individual acknowledgement that ought to have been made we will, on being told, make such amends as we can as soon as we can.

Errors are our responsibility

DRL   JRC

A

α   See **maximal agonist effect (α)**

abbreviations   (L. *ab,* away from; *brevis,* brief, short)
                                               See alphabetic entries, **acronym**

abortifacient   (L. *ab,* away, from; *oriri,* to appear; *faciens,* doing)
- Substance that causes abortion. Some contraceptives act by preventing implantation or by causing early abortion rather than by preventing conception
  (fertilization).   See **teratothanasia**

ABPI
- Association of the British Pharmaceutical Industry.

abridged application (for a licence/marketing application)
                                               (L. *abbreviare,* to shorten)
- Plainly, the full research and development procedures for **new active substances** are inappropriate in the case of **medicinal products** of **well established medicinal use**, e.g. insulin, **aspirin**. But regulatory authorities have a
  legitimate concern for pharmaceutical quality including **bioequivalence**. They
  provide for this situation by allowing appropriately shortened (abridged) applications.

absorption   (L. *ab,* away, from; *sorbere,* to suck)
- The process by which one substance penetrates or enters another. In relation
  to drugs, the process by which a drug is taken up from its site of administration.   See **adsorption**

abstinence syndrome   (L. *ab,* away, from; *tenere,* to hold;
                                               Gr. *sun,* with; *drome,* run)
                                               See **withdrawal syndrome**

abuse and misuse of drugs   (L. *ab,* away; *uti,* to use; *missa,* divergen)
- A distinction may be made between the two words:
  - *Abuse* is non-medical use without therapeutic intent, e.g. to get intoxi-
    cated. Also, the use of a drug to an extent that seriously interferes with
    health and social or economic functioning of the individual.
                                               See **recreational (use) drugs**
  - *Misuse* is over-prescribing by a doctor, i.e. for too many people or of too
    much or for too long; or inappropriate choice, i.e. the wrong drug or a drug
    when no drug would be better. Also excessive self-medication.
                                               See **substance abuse**

abuse liability (of drugs)
- An imprecise concept concerning the proclivity of a drug or class of drugs to
  induce drug-seeking behaviour.
- The events that precede or accompany strong drug-seeking behaviour as it

relates to the social context in clinical studies and to the operant schedule in animal studies (*Scott E Lukas*).

academic (academy)   (etymol, see **academic freedom**)
- The original (16th century) use of the term implies guardianship of standards in reasoning, including a questioning (sceptical) attitude to facts and the soundness of inferences, that forms the basis of the intellectual attitudes of a university.
- Since 1886 the term has acquired an added derogatory (or pejorative) overtone meaning: unpractical, merely theoretical, having no practical application. Academics understandably don't like this, but they are probably going to have to live with it.
- USA English does not distinguish between academic (as a noun) and academician (member of an Academy)
                                    See **academic usage/English, academic freedom**

academic freedom   (Gr. *academe*, from Academus, an ancient Greek hero
                            who made himself useful to the captured daughter of Jupiter)
- Plato (d 348 BCE) set up his school of philosophy in Academus' pleasure garden. The school concentrated so solemnly on literature that laughter was forbidden – so much for freedom.
- "One of the problems in writing about academic freedom is that the phrase is much misused, sometimes out of sheer woolly-mindedness but more often by those who wish to conceal dubious actions under a high-minded disguise.
- "Academic freedom is the right of any scholar, within his field of expertise, to think about and do research on any problem that interests him, to make public his conclusions, and to teach what he sincerely believes to be true." [But it does not mean that the community has a duty to pay for the implementation of all academics' research interests].
- To this may be added, "without placing themselves in jeopardy of losing their jobs and any privileges they may have at their institutions."
- But academic freedom has an 'enemy within', i.e. "those who say that academic freedom is an unchallengeable right and deduce from this that they are not answerable to anyone for the way in which they carry out their duties – or even for their failure to carry them out at all" (after *P Swinnerton-Dyer*, The importance of academic freedom. *Nature* 1995;373:186).

academic usage/English
- An elevated and often complex style associated with concern for accuracy, objectivity and dispassionate comment and characterized by:
    - *Qualifying expressions*, e.g. may, usually.
    - *Parenthetical asides*, e.g. as far as can be determined at this point in time.
    - *Passive constructions*, serving to minimize or remove personality, e.g. 'it' was found that, instead of 'we' found, or (horror!) 'I' found (after *Oxford Companion to the English Language 1992*). The result of this 'stultifying convention' is that reading most scientific papers has become 'tedious drudgery' (*ND Mermin, ibidem*) (L. *ibidem*, in the same place).
                                                        See **academic**

acceptable daily intake (ADI)   (L. *ac, ad*, before, to; *capere*, to take)
- A term used in evaluation of an environmental chemical to which the human population is expected to be exposed. It is expressed in mg kg^{-1} day^{-1}. "It has proved the most practicable approach for establishing the acceptable levels of intentional and unintentional food additives, pesticide residues, food and environmental contaminants" (Risk assessment; *Royal Society of London,* 1983).

acceptance range   See **area under the curve (AUC)**

acceptor site   (L. *ac, ad*, before, to; *capere*, to take; *situs*, placed)
- A **binding site** for a molecule that does not mediate a biological effect directly via that site.

accident   (L. *ac, ad*, before, to; *cidere*, to fall)
- Unexpected event.
- Unintended misfortune.
- In discussing whether or not the victim of a drug accident during routine therapy should be compensated by society or by the person or organization responsible for the injury or not at all, it is relevant to distinguish whether or not there has been fault.
- Drug accidents affecting thousands of people include **thalidomide, stilbestrol, practolol** and **clioquinol**.   See **compensation, liability, injury**

accumulation/cumulation (of drugs)   (L. *accumulare,* to heap up; *cumulus,* a heap)
- A progressive increase in the amount of drug in the body due to the rate of administration (intake) exceeding the rate of *metabolism* or *elimination.*
- *In isolated tissue preparations*: serial additions of drug without the usual washouts between doses – hence *cumulative* dose–response curves.

accuracy   (L. *ac, ad*, before, to; *cura*, care)
- The closeness of agreement of a determined value with a true (or accepted) reference value.   See **precision**

ACE
- **Angiotensin-converting enzyme.** (Gr. *angeion*, vessel; L. *tensio*, stretched)

acetylcholine   (L. *acetum*, vinegar; Gr. *khole*, bile)
- A **neurotransmitter,** the effects of which are classically divided into:
  - *Nicotinic effects*: actions of acetylcholine (mimicked by **nicotine)** at acetylcholine **receptors** (previously known as *cholinoceptors*) on the postsynaptic membrane of the following structures:
    - *autonomic ganglion cells*, causing **depolarization** of the postsynaptic nerve (fast excitatory postsynaptic potential). These effects are blocked by hexamethonium (**ion channel block**), tetraethylammonium, mecamylamine.

- *skeletal muscle (endplates)*, causing depolarization of the postsynaptic muscle fibre (endplate potential). These effects are blocked by suxamethonium (**depolarizing block**), **curare**, gallamine (**competition block**).
- *adrenal medulla*, causing release of stored **catecholamine**.
  See **fast receptors**
- *Muscarinic effects*: actions of acetylcholine (mimicked by **muscarine**) at acetylcholine receptors on effector organs receiving postganglionic **cholinergic** innervation, including:
  - *heart*, causing bradycardia and decreased force of contraction. These effects are blocked by atropine, methoctramine.
  - *smooth muscle*, e.g. ileum, causing contraction. This effect is blocked by atropine, **4-DAMP**
  - *exocrine glands*, causing secretion. This effect is blocked by atropine, **4-DAMP**   See **slow receptors**
- Acetylcholine is also a **neurotransmitter** in the CNS, with major **cholinergic nerve** pathways arising in the basal forebrain and septum to innervate the cortex, thalamus and hippocampus.   See **anticholinergic drug, muscarinic acetylcholine receptors, nicotinic acetylcholine receptors**

acid   (L. *acidus,* sour, sharp)
- A proton donor.
- A substance which liberates hydrogen fully in solution, yielding hydrogen ions. A weak acid is one that dissociates only partially in solution.
  See **dissociation constant, Henderson–Hasselbalch equation, pK$_a$**

acronym   (Gr. *akros*, beginning, end; *onoma*, name)
- A *pronounceable* word formed from the initial letters of other words, e.g. DOPA (dihydroxyphenylalanine), **WHO** (World Health Organization), WYSIWYG (what you see is what you get), ARMI (age related memory impairment). Many disciplines have their private abbreviations which amount to a secret language. The reasons for using acronyms are obvious, but they have got out of control in scientific literature. Examples from a single issue of a pharmacological journal current when this entry was written include: ANT, OHAMT, OHNT, NAL, NOSIE, AMO, COH, GOT, TRIS, AUCO. In mitigation it should be added that most are explained at the first use in any article. This is obligatory except for those thought to be universally known.

acupuncture, moxibustion   (L. *acus*, needle; *punctura*, a pricking; Jap. *mokusa*, burning herb; L. *burere*, to burn)
- Acupuncture involves treatment of disease by stimulation, with needles, of special locations of the body (acupuncture points: 360+) chosen according to the "system of anatomy and pathophysiology inherent in Chinese traditional medicine", i.e. according to channels (12+8) and collaterals (12) believed to permeate the body. There is evidence that acupuncture induces release of **endorphins**, etc. in the central nervous system; this may account for relief of pain, and add to any **placebo** effect. An alternative mode of stimulation at the

acupuncture point is to apply heat by burning a piece of the Chinese plant *Artemisia moxa* on the skin or on the acupuncture needle; this is known as *moxibustion*.

acute   (L. *acus*, needle)
— Sharp, quick onset; of short duration; the antonym of **chronic**. Use of *acute* to mean *severe* is misuse.

adaptive clinical trial designs/allocation (L. *ad*, to; *aptus*, fit; *allocare*, to place)
— The standard basic formal therapeutic trial design may be adapted for special circumstances, e.g. unequal groups, and especially where it is desired on scientific or ethical grounds to take multiple looks at the outcomes as the trial proceeds, or where it is essential for ethical reasons to allow patients a degree of self-selection.
— A treatment assignment process in **clinical trials** in which the treatment allocation ratio is allowed to change as a function of the number of patients enrolled, baseline data or observed outcomes (after **FDA**).
        See **sequential analysis, interim analysis, play-the-winner allocation (in clinical trials), random, therapeutic trial (***Zelen randomization***)**

addiction/addict   (L. *addicere*, to give one's assent to; *ad*, to; *dicere*, to say)
— Addiction is a state in which a drug is taken compulsively. The term **dependence** is preferred. The noun *addict* (for a person) continues in use for lack of a convenient alternative.

additive responses/addition   (L. *ad*, to; *addere*, to put)
— The situation where administration of two drugs with similar action produces neither **synergism** nor **antagonism**, i.e. if drugs *x* and *y* in concentrations X and Y, produce equal effects, $X + Y$ will produce an effect equal to that produced by $2X$ or $2Y$. But if $2X$ and $2Y$ do not themselves produce equal responses, then no unambiguous definition of additivity can be given.
                                                                        See **summation**

add-on therapy/trial
— A drug, the sole or principal role of which is in addition to another drug that has provided incomplete (therapeutic) **efficacy**.
— An **adjuvant** drug.
— A trial in which the test drug is added-on to existing therapy for safety and ethical reasons.

adenylate cyclase   See **adenylyl cyclase**

ADE   See **adverse drug experience**

adenylyl cyclase
— Enzyme responsible for producing **cyclic-AMP** from **ATP**. In older literature it is called adenylate cyclase, and before that adenyl cyclase. Both are chemically inaccurate.

ADEPT
– Antibody-directed enzyme prodrug therapy. This therapeutic technique involves the injection of a tumour-seeking antibody which has been linked to a specific enzyme not elsewhere present in the body. After an interval a **prodrug** is given and this is converted to a cytotoxic drug by the enzyme. The concept is to deliver the active drug only to the tumour cells targeted by the antibody. This both reduces adverse effects and allows higher doses to be given. The term 'letterbox bomb' has been coined – it is inert until opened.

adherence (patient) to prescribed treatment   See **compliance**

adhesion molecules/adhesins   (L. *adhaerere*, to stick to)
– 'Sticky' proteins that cause cells to adhere either to one another or to other cell types. In inflammation, for example, production of adhesion molecules by leucocytes and endothelial cells is part of the process that helps leucocytes to adhere to the site of an inflammatory lesion, promoting cellular accumulation.
                    See **integrins**

adjuvant   (L. *ad*, to; *juvare*, to help)
– In immunology, an adjuvant is an agent that enhances antigenicity.
– A drug used in addition to another drug to increase the effectiveness of the latter; **add-on therapy**.

ADME studies
– **Acronym** for absorption, distribution, metabolism and elimination, i.e. **pharmacokinetic** studies.

administration   (L. *ad*, to; *minister*, serve)
                    See **bureaucracy, management**

ADP
– Adenosine diphosphate.

ADR
– **Adverse drug reaction**.

adrenaline (epinephrine)   (L. *ad*, at; *renes*, kidneys)
– Transmitter/hormone produced by the adrenal medulla. JJ Abel isolated, purified and determined the structure of the main constituent of an extract of adrenal medulla in 1899 or 1900 with the help of J Takamine, a visitor to his laboratory in Baltimore, USA. Takamine immediately patented the process for isolating the pure substance and sold it to Parke–Davis and Company, who in turn registered the trade name "Adrenalin". Henceforth another name had to be used to refer to the transmitter in general literature in the USA. **Epinephrine** was chosen (and it is now the recommended **INN** in medicine). In the rest of the world, however, the name adrenaline persists in physiology, pharmacology and medicine. Interestingly, in demotic (Gr. *demotikos,* one of the

people) American speech, the term "adrenaline" is used as the word to describe the substance responsible for the surge of excitement that occurs after a shock or during athletic exertion. Somehow "a surge of epinephrine" seems odd. The term "epinephric gland" is not used. The journalistic misspelling without the final 'e' is common and derives from the **proprietary name** (Adrenalin) and the general illiteracy of journalists.   See **epinephrine**

adrenergic   (L. *ad*, to; *renes*, kidneys; Gr. *ergos*, to work)
– Working by means of **adrenaline**. An adjective used for classifying nerves, synapses and transmission processes in terms of the neurotransmitter involved. In American English, **-ergic** is used to describe **receptors** (see **adrenoceptors**). The term was coined when adrenaline was thought to be the postganglionic sympathetic neurotransmitter. Now that **noradrenaline** is known to be the neurotransmitter, **noradrenergic** is more appropriate, allowing *adrenergic* to be used for transmission involving nerves that release adrenaline, e.g. in the CNS.

adrenergic-blocking agent   See **adrenoceptor-blocking agent**

adrenergic/noradrenergic-neuron-blocking agent/drug
– A drug which inhibits the physiological release of transmitter from adrenergic nerves. This definition includes not only drugs acting like guanethidine but also reserpine and methyldopa, although some prefer these latter to fall outside the class. More accurately these drugs should now be called *noradrenergic-neuron-blocking agents* as postganglionic sympathetic nerves are *nor*adrenergic, not **adrenergic**.   See **blockade, -ergic**

adrenergic receptor   See **adrenergic, adrenoceptor, -ergic**

adrenoceptor/adrenoreceptor   (L. *ad*, to; *renes*, kidneys; *capere*, to take)
– A **receptor** responsible for mediating the physiological/pharmacological actions of **adrenaline** and noradrenaline. The general class is subdivided into:
   – α-adrenoceptors (subtypes 1 and 2, further subdivided)
   – β-adrenoceptors (subtypes 1, 2 and 3, further subdivided).
   – Adrenergic receptor is USA usage.

adrenoceptor-blocking agent
– A substance that selectively inhibits responses to adrenergic nerve activity and to injected catecholamines and other **sympathomimetic** amines by combining with the **adrenoceptor** on the effector organ, i.e. adrenoceptor **antagonists**, including **syntopic** antagonists of adrenaline, noradrenaline, isoprenaline (isoproterenol) and their **analogues.**
– *Adrenergic blocking agent* is widely used as synonymous, but it is less precise. This is because the use of the **-ergic** suffix implies blockade of transmission at **adrenergic** synapses, either by antagonism of the released neurotransmitter *or* by inhibition of the release of the neurotransmitter.
                See **adrenergic/noradrenergic-neuron blocking agent,**
                block, beta-(β)-adrenoceptor antagonists

adrenolytic   (L. *ad*, to; *renes*, kidneys; Gr. *lusis*, release)
- Agent that blocks the effect of catecholamines secreted by the adrenal medulla (adrenaline, noradrenaline). Conventionally it does not include block of the effects of stimulation of postganglionic sympathetic nerves, for which the term **sympatholytic** is used.

ADROIT
- Adverse Drug Reactions On-line Information Tracking.   See **COSTART**

adsorption   (L. *ad*, to; *sorbere*, to suck)
- The binding of a substance on a solid surface, whether by strong or weak bonds.   See **absorption, Langmuir adsorption isotherm**

adverse drug experience   See **adverse event**

adverse drug reaction   (L. *adversus*, hostile)
- A harmful or significantly unpleasant effect caused by a drug at doses intended for therapeutic effect (or prophylaxis or diagnosis) which warrants reduction of dose or withdrawal of the drug and/or foretells hazard from future administration.
- There are no harmless substances, only harmless ways of using substances. "All things are poisons and there is nothing that is harmless: *the dose alone decides that something is no poison*" (*Paracelsus,* 1493–1541, physician and alchemist, Switzerland) (see **alchemy**).
- Minor unwanted effects, e.g. slight dry mouth, are not dignified with the designation adverse reaction; to record them all would clog surveillance systems.
    See **side-effect**
- Adverse reactions may be classified:
  - *Type A (augmented)*: dose-related; occur in all subjects.
  - *Type B (bizarre)*: occur only in some subjects, e.g. **allergy**.
  - *Type C (continuous)*: due to chronic use, e.g. **tardive dyskinesia**.
  - *Type D (delayed)*: e.g. teratogenesis, carcinogenesis.
  - *Type E (ending of use)*: e.g. rebound or withdrawal effects.
    See **discontinuation syndrome**
- *Causation.* Reliable attribution of a cause-effect relationship provides the biggest problem in this field. Karch and Lasagna proposed the following degrees of certainty for attributing adverse *events* to drugs:
  - *Definite*: time sequence from taking the drug is reasonable; event corresponds to what is known of the drug; event ceases on stopping the drug; event returns on restarting the drug (rarely advisable).
  - *Probable*: time sequence is reasonable; event corresponds to what is known of the drug; event ceases on stopping the drug; event not reasonably explained by patient's disease.
  - *Possible*: time sequence is reasonable; event corresponds to what is known of the drug; event could readily have been result of the patient's disease or other therapy.

- *Conditional*: time sequence is reasonable; event does not correspond to what is known of the drug; event could not reasonably be explained by the patient's disease.
- *Doubtful*: event not meeting the above criteria.
- The term *disabling* adverse reaction/effect has led to public controversy because people travelling for pleasure feel 'disabled' (and resentful) if they are not enjoying themselves all the time, whereas manufacturers are inclined to restrict the term to effects that warrant admission to hospital.
- *Severity* may be classified:
    - *Trivial*:   nuisance value only.
    - *Mild*:   some interference with patient function: dose may be altered.
    - *Serious*:   treatment necessarily discontinued.
    - *Disabling*:   usual daily activities prevented.
- The **EC/EU** considers a *serious* adverse event/reaction to mean an adverse experience that is fatal, life-threatening, disabling or which results in in-patient hospitalization or prolongation of hospitalization. Congenital anomaly and occurrence of malignancy are always considered serious. An unpredicted adverse event/reaction is classed as *unexpected* if it has not been previously reported.   See **pharmacovigilance**

adverse drug reaction terminology (international)
- The **WHO** Programme for International Monitoring of Adverse Reactions to Drugs fulfils an evident need for which a prime requirement is an agreed terminology. This is not easy.
- The WHO structure uses:
    - *Preferred terms*: These are terms used to describe drug adverse reactions reported to the WHO system. They are the terms mainly used at the input side. Each preferred term is designated a record number.
    - *High level terms*: These are group preferred terms for qualitatively similar, but quantitatively different conditions. They may be used at the output side, e.g. thrombophlebitis leg and thrombophlebitis arm represent two different *preferred terms* but are grouped under thrombophlebitis as a *high level term*.
    - *System–organ classes*: These are groups of adverse reaction preferred terms pertaining to the same system–organ, and are for some purposes used at the output side. A preferred term can be allocated to a maximum of three different system–organ classes [WHO publishes a complete list of the classes and their codes].
    - *Included terms*: These are synonyms to preferred terms and have been provided by reporting countries. They are only used to assist in finding the corresponding preferred term for proper coding of the adverse reaction reported.
    - *Input to the computer files is usually made at the preferred term level, although included terms can also be used*. At the output side preferred terms, high level terms or system–organ classes can be used, depending on the objectives of the printout. For example:

High level terms	Record number	Preferred term	Included term
Heart block	0436	Bundle branch block	QRS prolonged
Myocardial ischaemia	0422	Angina pectoris	Coronary insufficiency.

adverse events (in clinical trials) (L. *ad*, towards; *vertere*, to turn; *eventus*, happening)
– Any undesirable experience occurring to a subject during a **clinical trial**, whether or not considered related to the investigational product(s) (European Commission definition). The objective is to avoid reliance on the fallible contemporary opinion of the investigator as to whether the event is or is not caused by the drug. See **adverse drug reaction**

advertorial
– A blend word of advertisement and editorial applied to an advertisement (for a drug) masquerading as impartial editorial opinion.

aequorin See **drugs as tools**

aerosol (Gr. *aer*, air; *sol*, colloid)
– Colloidal particles (liquid or solid) dispersed in a gas. The particles are small enough to remain in suspension for a long time.
– Metered-dose aerosol formulations for delivering drugs to the mouth or the lower respiratory tract for absorption employ halogenated hydrocarbons (chlorofluorocarbons) as propellants. Alternative propellants (hydrofluoroalkanes) less harmful to the environment replace them.
  See **inhalation of drugs**

aetiology (Gr. *aitia*, cause; *logos*, word, reason, discourse)
– The cause of a disease, symptom etc.

affinity chromatography See **chromatography**

affinity/affinity constant (L. *affinis*, related; *constans*, standing firm)
– *Affinity*: the proclivity of a **drug** to form a complex with a **receptor** or a **binding site**.
– *Affinity constant*: a numerical quantity describing the relative proportions of drug (D), receptor or binding site (R), and drug–receptor/binding site complex at equilibrium. The larger the *affinity constant*, the greater is the *affinity* of the drug for its receptors/binding sites:

$$D + R \underset{k_{-1}}{\overset{k_1}{\rightleftarrows}} DR$$

– The (equilibrium) association or affinity constant, $K_A = k_1/k_{-1}$, where k and k_{-1} are the rate constants for association and dissociation respectively. K_A is a **dilution**, i.e. it has the dimensions of concentration^{-1}, and it is the reciprocal of the **dissociation equilibrium constant.**

- The **association equilibrium constant** is often represented by K_a or K_A when applied to **agonists**, and as K_b or K_B when applied to antagonists (**ligand** B). This creates some confusion because these same forms are used for their reciprocals, the *dissociation* equilibrium constants. It is therefore wise to define whether association or dissociation constants are meant whenever K_a, K_A, K_b or K_B is used. In an alternative nomenclature, K_a and K_d represent the association and dissociation constants respectively for a single ligand (usually an agonist), and K_a' and K_d' represent the association and dissociation constants for the second, competing ligand (or antagonist).

affinity fingerprinting   (L. *affinis*, related)
- A technique for rapidly identifying substances with potentially interesting pharmacodynamic activity. The technique consists of determining the **affinity** with which a potential new drug binds to a 'panel' of target proteins that have widely diverse binding characteristics. In practice, statistical tests are used to show that the binding characteristics of the proteins selected for the panel are unrelated to one another. None of these target proteins need be itself a pharmacodynamic target. The pattern of binding of the potential new drug is its affinity fingerprint and by reference to the affinity fingerprint of a library of reference drugs, the potential pharmacodynamic activity of the new molecule can be predicted. The assay can be automated and very large numbers of new substances can be screened in a short period of time (*high throughput* **screen**). The technique can be combined with **combinatorial chemistry**.

aflatoxins   (Etymol. from the name of the fungus that produces them)
- Poisonous substances from the fungus *Aspergillus flavus* growing in stored crops, e.g. groundnuts. Aflatoxins are hepatotoxic and carcinogenic.

agenda   (L. the gerundive of *agere*, to do)
- List of items of business to be considered at a meeting.
- Although *agenda* is a plural word, it is pedantry to object to the common and convenient practice of treating it as singular. If a singular is needed for *one item of the agenda* there seems no escape from that rather cumbrous phrase; *agendum* (singular) is pedantic (*Fowler's Modern English Usage*).
- Users of this Dictionary underestimate at their peril the value of acquiring **committee** skills, including preparing and debating agendas, and detecting *hidden agendas*. Agendas are subject to manipulation, e.g. placing controversial matters at the end when many members will have left the meeting, after boring them by prolonging discussion of bland items placed at the beginning; deliberately inaccurate summaries of discussion by the chairman; delaying sending out minutes of the meeting for weeks so that members will have forgotten.

agonist   (Gr. *agon*, a struggle)
- A **ligand** that binds to **receptors** and thereby increases the proportion of them that are in an active form, resulting in a biological response. Conven-

tional agonists increase this proportion, whereas **inverse agonists** reduce it (**IUPHAR**, with permission; *Pharmacological Reviews* 1995;47:255–266).

– A drug, hormone or neurotransmitter which, on combining with a receptor, induces in the receptor a change which leads to a biological response.

– **Full agonist**: originally, a drug that can elicit the maximal response that the tissue is capable of. This is unsatisfactory as the classification depends as much on the nature of the response and tissues as on the drug. Now usually defined as an agonist that has high **efficacy**, in the sense that each drug–receptor interaction causes a strong-enough **stimulus** to the tissue that a full response is possible. If the receptor density is high (i.e. there are *spare receptors* or a **receptor reserve**), then a maximal response is possible when only a fraction of the receptors is occupied. This definition is not entirely empirical but depends to some extent on ideas that are hypothetical. It may therefore be ambiguous or inapplicable in the case of some drugs, tissues or responses.

– **Partial agonist**: a drug with low **efficacy**, so that even when all the receptors are occupied, the *stimulus* to the tissue is insufficient to generate a maximal response. Consequently, when partial agonist and full agonist molecules compete for the same receptors the response will be less than when the full agonist alone occupies the same fraction of receptors. This is because the total *stimulus* to the tissue is reduced (it is the algebraic sum of that from the partial and the full agonist). Partial agonists are therefore also **antagonists**.

See **captive agonist, inverse agonist, primary agonist, receptor**

agonist-trafficking hypothesis (Gr. *agon*, a struggle; Old Fr. *traffique*, trade, commerce)

– Theoretical explanation for the process that can occur when a receptor type is coupled (*promiscuously*) to two or more effector systems, as a result of which a series of agonists at a single receptor type can have different rank orders of **potency** according to the system to which the receptor is coupled. According to this hypothesis the different patterns of **efficacy** arise because each agonist promotes its own specific receptor conformational state.

See **promiscuous receptors, receptor** (*Three-state model*)

agranulocytosis (Gr. *a*, without; *granulum*, small grain; *kutos*, container, body, and so cell)

– Absence of polymorphonuclear leucocytes (granulocytes) from blood. Allergic reaction to drugs is one cause. See **allergy, granulocytopenia**

AIM

– Active ingredient manufacturer (regulatory term).

alchemy (Arabic *al*, the; *khimia*, "the Egyptian art" of transmutation)

– Owing to confusion between the derived Greek word for Egypt and the similar Greek word for pouring and infusion, alchemy became the word for pharmaceutical chemistry. Eventually it became applied to the chemistry of the Middle Ages which was particularly concerned with the conversion (transmutation) of base metals into gold, and the search for a 'universal remedy' (**panacea**) that could confer immortality. The alchemists believed that there was a fundamental particle out of which all matter was made. They have been ridiculed for this, as well as for wearing robes and funny hats, until modern physicists began to think the same.

alcohol (ethanol) units (drinks)
- Consumption studies employ arbitrary *units* based on the volume of a social drink measure (beer, wine, spirits) that contains a designated amount of alcohol. The UK unit contains 8 g (10 ml); the USA unit is 50% greater; Austria is less and Japan is more: efforts are being made (1997) to agree an international standard.
- Doctors taking an alcohol intake history from patients are accustomed to ask them if they pour their own drinks and, if they do, to double the patients' estimates.

aleatory   (L. *alea*, game of chance, dice)
- Dependent on chance, random, stochastic.

algogen   (Gr. *algesis*, sense of pain; *gen*, produced)
- A substance which induces pain, for example endogenous mediators released during inflammatory processes.

ALGOL
- Algorithmic Oriented Language; a **computer** programing language.

algorithm   (L. *algorismus*, from Arabic, *al-Khwarazmi*,
                                        from *Abu-Ja'far Mohammed ibn-Musa*,
                                        9th century Persian mathematician)
- A set of instructions involving finite routine steps for solving a problem.
                                                        See **heuristic**

alkaloid   (L. from Arabic, *al-quili*, ashes [of a plant])
- Organic nitrogenous **base** of plant origin; names end in *-ine*.

alkylating agent   (Ger. *alk(ohol)*; Gr. *-yl*, from *hule*, wood, matter)
- A drug that reacts with constituents of the body by alkylation, leading to a stable, **covalent bonded** complex. The site of attachment may be one of the bases present in DNA (in the case of **cytotoxic** alkylating agents) or a **receptor** site (in the case of irreversible antagonists of catecholamines or acetylcholine).   See **alkylation, non-equilibrium antagonist**

alkylation   (Ger. *alk(ohol)*; Gr. *-yl*, from *hule*, wood, matter)
- Replacement of a hydrogen atom in a compound by an alkyl group (group related to a paraffin hydrocarbon).

allele   (Gr. *allel*, one another)
- Alternative forms of a **gene** at a given locus.

- In diploid organisms, both parents contribute genetic material to each gene, one for each member of the chromosome pair. Each half is an *allele*. Alleles are either of the normal (*wild*) type, or *mutants* which means that they encode an unusual form of the protein. If one allele is normal and the other mutant, whether the mutant characteristic is expressed depends upon the type of allele and the inheritance pattern:
    - *Additive* or *autosomal autonomous*: Neither allele predominates over the other and the inherited characteristic is the algebraic sum of the contributions from each parent. This is the common inheritance pattern for most enzymes.
    - *Autosomal recessive*: The normal allele predominates over the mutant form. For the characteristic to be expressed, two mutant alleles must be inherited, one from each parent.
    - *Autosomal dominant*: The mutant allele predominates over the normal form. The characteristic is expressed when only one mutant allele is inherited (from either parent).
    - *Sex-linked* (either *recessive* or *dominant*): The allele is located on the X-chromosome. In recessive X-linked inheritance, the female will only show the mutant characteristic if she inherits the mutant allele from both parents (one on each X-chromosome). If she has only one mutant allele, she will not express the characteristic but will be a *carrier* of the *trait*. On the other hand, a male inheriting a single mutant allele on his X-chromosome (from his mother, the carrier) will exhibit the mutant characteristic. (This is the usual form of transmission of colour-deficient vision and haemophilia.)

allergy/allergic/allergen   (Gr. *allos*, other, different; *ergon*, activity, work)
- An immunologically-mediated reaction, usually harmful, to a foreign substance.
- *Allergy to drugs* is classified in four *types* according to the immunological mechanism involved (*Coombs and Gell classification, 1975*).
- A substance provoking allergy is an *allergen*, e.g. pollen, drug or metabolite covalently bound to protein.   See **covalent bond**.
- Colloquially used to mean anything or anyone disliked.
                              See **anaphylaxis, hypersensitivity**

allometric scaling   (Gr. *allos*, other, different;
                         metrikos, relating to measuring; L. *scala*, a ladder)
- Techniques for assessing the relationship of pharmacokinetic analyses between different species.

allopathy   (Gr. *allos*, different; *pathos* or *patheia*, suffering)
- A system of medicine based on the belief that induction of a new disease (or symptoms) would drive out an existing disease (or symptoms). It was largely practised by making the patient ill with purging, sweating, bleeding and vomiting. Under such treatment patients often did cease to complain of their original illness. Many even recovered. *It is not correct to use the term to mean conventional scientific medicine.*   See **homoeopathy**

all-or-none response
- A response to a drug that is either present or absent is said to be an all-or-none or a **quantal response**, e.g. death or survival.   See **graded response**

allosteric activator   See **allosteric agonist**

allosteric agonist   (Gr. *allos*, other, different; *stereos*, solid; *agon*, a struggle)
- **Agonist** that produces its effect by combining with a region of the **receptor** different from that at which the endogenous agonist acts. Sometimes referred to as *allosteric activator*. (After **IUPHAR**; *Pharmacological Reviews* 1995;47: 255–266).

allosteric interaction   (Gr. *allos*, other, different; *stereos*, solid)
- An interaction in which one molecule binding to one site on a macromolecule (e.g. a **receptor** or **enzyme**) alters the characteristics of the interaction between another molecule and a different site on the same macromolecule. The two interacting molecules may be structurally identical or different. Where the macromolecule consists of several subunits, allosteric interactions can occur between the subunits – a molecule binding to a site on one subunit may cause a change in the characteristics of interactions at a site on another subunit.
- Commonly the interaction causes a change in the **affinity** of binding at the second site. If affinity at the second site is increased, the interaction is said to show positive **cooperativity**. Negative cooperativity is rare.
- Where one substance acting at one site alters the characteristics of its own interaction at another site on the macromolecule, the process is known as *autotrophic* interaction. Where one substance alters the characteristics of the interaction between another substance and a different site on the macromolecule, the process is known as *heterotrophic* interaction.
- Examples of *positive heterotrophic allosteric interactions* include benzodiazepines acting at a site on the **GABA**$_A$ receptor, and zinc acting at a site on non-**NMDA** receptors and **purinoceptors**.
- *Negative heterotrophic allosteric interactions* include zinc acting at a site on NMDA receptors and GABA$_A$ receptors.   See **cross-talk**

allotopic   (Gr. *allos*, other, different; *topos*, place)
- Acting at different sites. True competitive antagonism is a **syntopic** interaction, i.e. the two drugs interact with the same site on the receptor. **Allosteric interactions** and **uncompetitive antagonism** are examples of *allotopic* interactions.   See **antagonist/ism**

alloxan   See **drugs as tools**

alternative medicine   (L. *alter*, other, another)
                                        See **complementary medicine**

altruistic vaccine   (L. *alteri huic*, to this other; *vacca*, cow,
                           a reference to the origin of the first product from cowpox virus)

– A vaccine (or other medicine) that does not benefit the taker but stops a disease being transmitted to others, e.g. progress has been reported on development of a vaccine that may prevent malaria parasite *transmission* from an infected to a healthy individual. **See societal drug**

amblyopia (Gr. *amblus*, dim, dull; *ops,* eye)
– Impaired vision, e.g. tobacco amblyopia.

Ames test (*Bruce Ames*, a microbial geneticist, USA)
– A method for identifying substances with mutagenic properties.
– The method involves the use of specially selected strains of *Salmonella typhimurium*. The strains have been selectively bred to have a single mutation which renders the organism incapable of surviving in a medium lacking a particular nutrient (usually histidine). The bacteria are cultured in a medium which has a concentration of histidine that limits their growth. The potentially mutagenic chemical is added to the medium. If it causes mutations in the organism, some bacteria will become capable of thriving without histidine (i.e. will *revert* to the wild type). Samples taken from the culture and plated onto culture dishes will therefore produce more colonies capable of growing readily in a histidine-deficient environment than control samples.
– The method has been further refined to test for mutagenicity in both the parent chemical and its metabolites by adding homogenized rat liver to the culture medium to provide the necessary drug-metabolizing enzymes.
– The test is very sensitive – only nanograms of mutagen can give a positive result.

amino acids
– *Excitatory:* certain amino acids, particularly **glutamate** and aspartate, and possibly homocysteate, which are the principal and ubiquitous transmitters mediating fast excitatory synaptic responses in the CNS (see **kainate**).
– *Inhibitory:* the principle inhibitory amino acid transmitters in the CNS are GABA (γ-aminobutyric acid) and glycine. GABA is the main inhibitory transmitter in the brain and there are high concentrations of glycine in the spinal cord.

amoebicide/amebicide (Gr. *amoibe*, change, referring to the
perpetually changing shape of the unicellular organism; L. *cidium*, kill)
– Agent that kills amoebae, especially *Entamoeba histolytica*.

AMPA
– α-Amino-3-hydroxy-5-methyl-4-isoxazole propionic acid; selective agonist used to classify excitatory **amino acid** receptors; AMPA receptors mediate fast excitatory transmission at many CNS synapses. Formerly called *quisqualate* receptors.

ampakines (**AMPA** plus Gr. *kinein*, to move)
– Family of drugs developed as **cognition enhancers** that act by binding to an

accessory site on the **AMPA**-type glutamate receptor and enhance the gluta-mate-mediated signal.

amphipathic (Gr. *amphi*, both sides/kinds; *pathikos*, passive)
– Molecules having both **hydrophilic** and **hydrophobic** regions are described as amphipathic. See **liposomes**

anabolic steroids (Gr. *ana*, up; *ballo*, throw; see **steroid**)
– Androgenic (male sex) steroid hormones also have anabolic effects, i.e. they cause tissue growth, forming complex molecules from simple molecules, e.g. protein from amino acids. It has been possible to synthesize **congeners** with minimal androgenic (sex) action but which retain their anabolic effect. The use of these to improve success in sport is illicit, unethical, unfair and widely practised; it is pursued by sporting authorities with sophisticated chemical testing.

anabolize (Gr. *ana*, up; *ballo*, throw)
– The complement of **catabolize**, i.e. an enzymatically mediated process in which a chemical group (or groups) is (or are) added to a molecule, e.g. 5-fluorouracil is converted to fluorouridine triphosphate and fluorodeoxyuridylate (false nucleotides). The former is incorporated into a functionless RNA and the latter inhibits the enzyme thymidylate synthase.

anaemia (Gr. *an*, without; *haima*, blood)
– Diminution in the number of blood erythrocytes, the amount of haemoglobin per 100 ml blood and the volume of packed (by centrifugation) erythrocytes per 100 ml blood. Drugs can cause anaemia and can cure anaemia.

anaesthesia/etic (Gr. *an,* without; *aisthesis*, feeling)
– A reversible state of insensibility, which may be *local* or *general*, induced by drugs (see following entries). The American man of letters and physician *Oliver Wendell Holmes* (1846) wrote after the demonstration of the effect of ether: "The state should, I think, be called 'anaesthesia'. This signifies insen-sibility...The adjective will be 'anaesthetic'. Thus we might say the 'state of anaesthesia', or 'the anaesthetic state'."

anaesthetic (basal) (Gr. *an,* without; *aisthesis*, feeling; *basis*, stepping)
– A drug used to provide sedation short of loss of consciousness.

anaesthetic (general) (Gr. *an,* without; *aisthesis*, feeling;
genus, birth, race, stock and so almost universal)
– General anaesthetics induce loss or impairment of consciousness. They are administered by inhalation or intravenously.
See **dissociative anaesthesia, neuroleptanalgesia**

anaesthetic (local) (Gr. *an,* without; *aisthesis*, feeling; L. *locus*, place)
– A drug which prevents the generation and conduction of nerve impulses, both

sensory and motor (sometimes called, misleadingly, local **analgesic**). Local anaesthetics may be administered by:
- Surface (**topical**) application, e.g. cornea.
- Local infiltration.
- Selective nerve block.
- Injection into the vein of a limb 'drained' of blood (by posture) and isolated from the general circulation by a tourniquet (*regional anaesthesia*).
- Injection into the epidural or subarachnoid space.

analeptic/sis   (Gr. *analambanein*, to revive; *analeptikos*, stimulating)
- 'Restorative' medicine.
- A drug that stimulates the central nervous system, especially in subjects with depressed respiration or consciousness. High doses may cause convulsions.
- To restore to health and strength, to come to one's senses (now obsolete).

analgesic   (Gr. *an*, without; *algesis,* sense of pain)
- Drug that relieves pain; in popular speech a 'pain-killer'.

analgesic nephropathy   (Gr. *an*, without; *algesis,* pain;
                                                        nephros, kidney; *patheia,* suffering)
- Renal damage due to prolonged overdose of nonsteroidal anti-inflammatory and analgesic drugs, especially phenacetin (perhaps) and combined formulations.

analogue/analog   (Gr. *analogos*, proportionate)
- Having resemblance in form or function, but not identical.
- *In pharmacology:* compounds which are structurally similar.
- *Of display devices*, in which the variable displayed is indicated by a moving cursor or pointer as in a traditional clock. This is in contrast to displays in which the variable is displayed as numbers – *digital* displays.

analogy/ous   (Gr. *analogia*, proportion, correspondence)
- Agreement or similarity in a limited number of aspects of features; process of reasoning from parallel or similar cases.

analysis of variance (ANOVA) and of covariance (ANCOVA)
        (Gr. *ana*, up, again, back; *luein*, to loosen; L. *co*, together; *varius*, changing)
- The principle behind ANOVA is to partition the total variability of a set of **data** into components due to sources of variation (*D Altman*). ANOVA has a number of forms, one-way, two-way, etc., according to the number of sets of data (groups); and variations by **Mann–Whitney**, **Wilcoxon** and others. ANCOVA is an extension of ANOVA that permits elimination of variables that are not to be studied.

analytical dilution assay
- A type of **biological assay** in which the relative **potency** of a drug (the 'unknown') is measured by determining the dilution of the unknown that must be

made from a stock solution in order that responses to the unknown exactly match responses to a known concentration of 'standard' drug of known potency. Before the development of chemical assays the analytical dilution assay was also the principal technique for measuring the concentrations of drugs and biological **mediators**.   See **Latin square design**

anamnestic response   (Gr. *anamnesis*, recollection, memory)
 – A second dose of an **antigen** producing a larger response than the first.

anandamines   (Sanskrit *ananda*, bliss)
 – Endogenous ligands for cannabinoid receptors.

anaphylactoid   (Gr. *ana*, up; *phulaxis*, guarding)
 – Resembling **anaphylaxis**, but where the mechanism is uncertain or does not involve the immune system, e.g. rapid intravenous injection of enzymes, colloids, which may cause explosive release of **autacoids**.
                                   See **pseudo-allergic reaction**

anaphylatoxin   (Gr. *ana*, up; *phulaxis*, guarding; *toxicon*, arrow poison)
 – Substances generated from **complement**, which release histamine and other mediators of **anaphylaxis**. They are of low molecular weight (10 000) and comprise fragments of complement proteins known as C5a and C3a.

anaphylaxis   (Gr. *ana*, up; *phulaxis*, guarding)
 – An immediate-type immunological reaction on the cell membrane of mast cells and basophil leucocytes which results in release of histamine and other biologically active molecules from these cells. In extreme cases severe hypotension and bronchoconstriction occur (*anaphylactic shock*). The term was originally coined to mean lack of protection, referring to the situation in which prior inoculation of an animal with a poisonous protein (from a sea anemone) had the unexpected effect of rendering a second injection more, rather than less, lethal. Unfortunately the author's Greek was shaky and he used the inappropriate prefix 'ana-' – instead of 'a-' (Gr. not).   See **anaphylactoid**

ancillary study/trial   (L. *ancilla*, handmaid)
 – An investigation, stimulated by a **clinical trial** and intended to generate information of interest to the trial. The ancillary trial is designed and carried out by the investigators from one or more of the centres in the main trial and utilises resources of the trial, but is not a required part of the design or data collection procedures of the trial (after **FDA**).

ANDA (regulatory term)
 – Abbreviated new drug application.   See **abridged application**

anecdotal studies   (Gr. *anekdota*, thing unpublished)
 – Case reports of individuals or a few patients tell what *may* happen and should not be despised for they may allow **hypotheses** that lead to formal research studies.

angel dust
– Idiom or **jargon**. Colloquial or 'street' name for phencyclidine, a hallucinogen.

angiotensin-converting enzyme (ACE) (Gr. *angeion*, vessel; L. *tensio*, stretched)
– The plasma enzyme responsible for the conversion of angiotensin I (inactive) to angiotensin II (potent vasoconstrictor and releaser of aldosterone). ACE-inhibitors have an important role in treating cardiovascular disease.

anhedonia (Gr. *an*, not, without; *hedone*, pleasure)
– A diminished capacity to experience pleasure, e.g. in schizophrenia, depression or as a consequence of cocaine use.

animals in research (L. *anima*, breath, life)
– Scientists are under increasing pressure to use fewer animals in their research.
– A **EU** directive instructs researchers to choose non-animal methods if they are scientifically satisfactory [and] reasonably and practically available. It provides for the control and use of animals in research including authorization of premises, personnel and procedures. The framework of the directive ensures that the number of animals used for experimental purposes is reduced to a minimum, that the animals are properly housed and cared for, and that no pain, suffering, distress or lasting harm is inflicted unnecessarily. As far as possible, pain, suffering or distress where unavoidable are kept to the minimum. Similar provision is applied to breeding and supply of laboratory animals, and special controls exist for experiments involving anaesthesia and for certain species deemed to require special protection.
– Scientists, businessmen and policy-makers have been developing alternatives to the use of live animals for biomedical research and toxicology testing. They have made impressive progress.
Their approach can be summed up in three words: reduce, refine and replace (the three Rs). That is, use fewer animals in tests and experiments; make the tests that remain necessary both more informative and more humane; and develop procedures in which animals no longer have to be used at all (*The Economist*).
– For debate see: Forum: The benefits and ethics of animals research (*Scientific American* 1997;276:63–77). **See FRAME**

anion (Gr. *ana*, up, negative; *ion*, going)
– Ion bearing a negative charge, i.e. moves towards the anode.

anorectic/anorexiant (Gr. *an*, not, without; *orexis*, appetite)
– Drug that reduces appetite.

anorexia (Gr. *an*, not, without; *orexis*, appetite)
– Lack of appetite. In *anorexia nervosa* the subject has a distorted self-image and seeks to maintain an abnormally low body-weight.

ANOVA See **analysis of variance**

antacid, gastric   (Gr. *anti*, against; L. *acidus*, sour, sharp; Gr. *gaster*, stomach)
- Substances that neutralize gastric acid. They are said to be *systemic* if they alter the acid–base balance of the body (e.g. sodium bicarbonate), and *non-systemic* if they do not (e.g. magnesium trisilicate).

antagonist/-ism   (Gr. *anti*, against; *agon*, to struggle)
- A drug that reduces the action of another drug, generally an **agonist**. Many act at the same **receptor** macromolecule as the agonist. Antagonism of this kind may be *surmountable* or *insurmountable*, depending on the experimental conditions. Antagonism may also result from combination with the substance being antagonized (*chemical antagonism*), or the production of an opposite effect through a different receptor (*functional* [or *physiological*] *antagonism*) or as a consequence of competition for the binding site of an intermediate that links receptor activation to the effect observed (*indirect antagonism*). The term *functional antagonism* is also used to describe a less well-defined category in which the antagonist interferes with other events that follow receptor activation (**IUPHAR**, with permission; *Pharmacological Reviews* 1995;47:255–266).
- Drug that reduces or neutralizes (blocks) the effect of an (**agonist**) drug (whether *reversibly* or *irreversibly*).
- Antagonists may also be classified as follows:
  - *Pharmacokinetic*: one drug decreases the concentration of the other at the latter's site of action.
  - Pharmacodynamic:
    - **allotopic**: the antagonist binds to a site distinct from the agonist-binding site, but intimately associated with the receptor. This is also known as **noncompetitive** antagonism. This kind of antagonism can be reversible or irreversible
    - **syntopic**: the antagonist can bind at the same site as the agonist (mutually exclusive binding) so that binding is **competitive**. Syntopic antagonism can be either reversible or irreversible over a practicable time course. If the binding is essentially irreversible, classical kinetic treatments cannot be used because the system never reaches equilibrium – hence the term **non-equilibrium antagonism**. (*Note*: in older texts, non-equilibrium antagonism was often referred to as *non-competitive antagonism*). Although both agonist and irreversible antagonist compete for binding sites, it is confusing to describe this as 'competitive (irreversible) antagonism'. In pharmacological **jargon**, competitive antagonism means reversible **syntopic** antagonism to which classical kinetic treatments can be applied. (*Note*: *Reversible* syntopic antagonism is *surmountable* whereas *irreversible* syntopic antagonism is *insurmountable*. See **competition** for a fuller account).
  - *Nonspecific*: a type of antagonism in which the antagonist causes a general depression of cellular activity, or alteration of the physicochemical state of cell membranes, e.g. general anaesthetics. This is sometimes classed as a type of *functional antagonism*.

- The correct way to use the verb *to antagonize* is 'drug *x* antagonizes drug *y*' (not 'drug *x* antagonizes *the effect of* drug *y*').
  See **mass action, surmountable antagonism, uncompetitive antagonism**

anthelmintic (or -thic)   (Gr. *anti*, against; *helmins*, parasitic worm)
- Agent that destroys or expels parasitic worms.

anthroposophic medicine   (Gr. *anthropos*, mankind; *sophistes*, a wise man)
- Medical practice based on the mystical spiritual teaching of Rudolf Steiner (1861–1925), Austrian philosopher.

anti-   (Gr. *anti*, against)
- Used as a prefix in many situations, especially of competitive antagonist drugs (e.g. antihistamine, antiadrenaline) and in therapeutics (e.g. antiepileptic, antihypertensive). It would be impracticable as well as unnecessary to attempt to list all such terms: "all the examples cannot be accumulated, because the use of these [prefixes], if not wholly arbitrary, is so little limited that they are hourly affixed to new words as occasion requires, or is imagined to require them" (*Samuel Johnson*, preface to his *Dictionary*, 1755). Nevertheless, some examples follow.

antiallergic drug   (Gr. *anti*, against; *allos*, other, different; *ergon*, activity)
- Any drug used in treatment of allergic disease.
- More limited: a substance used prophylactically against allergic diseases and whose principal mode of action is to prevent the release of chemical mediators of allergic reactions from mast cells or other cells, i.e. **autacoids**.

antiarrhythmic/antidysrhythmic (cardiac) drug   (Gr. *anti*, against; *a*, not; *dus*, bad; *rhuthmos*, flowing)
- Drug effective in preventing, controlling or terminating cardiac dysrhythmias; but some can also cause dysrhythmias.   See **dysrhythmia**

antibiotic   (Gr. *anti*, against; *bios*, life)
- Substance produced by a microorganism that, in high dilution*, kills or prevents multiplication of other microorganisms. Conventionally the term also includes substances made by chemical syntheses, and also semisynthetic variants. Increasingly, this limited meaning of the word is being lost as users cease to find it helpful to know whether an *antimicrobial drug* is or is not produced by a microorganism, and so employ it for useful antimicrobial drugs in general, such as sulphonamides. It may seem pedantic to insist on the more limited definition when this use itself displaced a previous meaning. The word antibiotic was first used in 1860. It is described (**OED**) as a rare adjective meaning "opposed to a belief in the presence or possibility of life", as in, "I incline to the antibiotic hypothesis", and, "the antibiotic prejudice".
(*This proviso is necessary to exclude various metabolic products such as ethanol and hydrogen peroxide, which are generally agreed not to be antibiotics).

antibody   (Gr. *anti*, against; Old Eng. *bodig*, corpse)
- Protein produced by cells of the immune system in response to exposure to a foreign (i.e. 'nonself' protein or other substance), the **antigen**. The antibody has a structure complementary to part of the antigen molecule and so can bind to the antigen, thereby allowing the immune system to recognize and react with the foreign protein.
- *Catalytic antibodies* bind to selected target molecules, mediating chemical reactions that break them down; they themselves emerge unchanged, ready to bind again, and again. Thus a small amount of antibody can inactivate a large amount of drug (*DW Landry*). The therapeutic potential of developing such antibodies (that will persist in the body for weeks) is being explored, e.g. as an adjuvant to managing cocaine dependence.

anticholinergic drug   (Gr. *anti*, against; *khole*, bile; *ergon*, work)
- A drug that inhibits **acetylcholine**-mediated synaptic transmission
    - Selective antagonists acting at:
      muscarinic acetylcholine receptors
      nicotinic acetylcholine receptors
    - Acetylcholine synthesis inhibitors, e.g. hemicholinium.
- The term is so unspecific as to be of very little use. It is better to use a term that describes more precisely what is meant, e.g. muscarinic antagonist or depolarizing neuromuscular blocking agent.
- The use of anticholinergic to mean only muscarinic antagonists is of long standing, but it is imprecise and the term antimuscarinic is now preferred.
                                                                    See **-ergic**

anticholinesterase   (Gr. *anti*, against; *khole*, bile;
                                -ase, suffix denoting an enzyme, from *diastasis*, separation)
- A substance that inactivates, reversibly or irreversibly, the enzyme acetylcholinesterase. This enzyme hydrolyses the neurotransmitter **acetylcholine**. Inhibition allows the acetylcholine to survive longer, with multitudinous effects in the many physiological systems where it is a transmitter.

antidote   (Gr. *anti*, against; *dotes*, one who gives)
- Medicine that counteracts a poison. Antidotes may be specific (e.g. naloxone) or non-specific (e.g. activated charcoal).   See **specificity**

antidysrhythmic drug (cardiac)   See **antiarrhythmic drug, dysrhythmia**

antigen   (Gr. *anti*, against; *genes*, born)
- A molecule that is capable of stimulating the production of an **antibody** which has specific binding sites for the antigen itself.

antimetabolite   (Gr. *anti*, against; *meta*, change, going before or after;
                                                            ballein, to throw)
- **Analogue** of a normal metabolite that acts as an effective counterfeit and so disrupts normal metabolic processes, e.g. folic acid and purine antagonists

used as **cytotoxic** drugs. Also known as **counterfeit incorporation mechanism**

antimicrobial drug   (Gr. *anti*, against; *mikros,* small; *bios*, life)
See **antibiotic**

antimuscarinic   (Gr. *anti*, against)
- **Antagonist** at **muscarinic acetylcholine receptors**. There are two major classes of acetylcholine receptors named after the two alkaloids originally used to distinguish between them, namely **nicotine**, hence **nicotinic acetylcholine receptors**, and **muscarine**, hence **muscarinic acetylcholine receptors**.   See **acetylcholine**

antineoplastic   (Gr. *anti*, against; *neos*, new; *plasma*, formation)
- Directed against (malignant) neoplasms (tumours), i.e. anticancer.

antiplatelet drugs   (Gr. *anti*, against)
- Drugs (e.g. **aspirin**, sulphinpyrazone) that modify blood platelet function (e.g. stickiness, thromboxane production) and so reduce the likelihood of thromboembolic disease.

antipruritic drug   (Gr. *anti*, against; L. *prurire*, to itch or lust after)
- Drug that diminishes itching.

antipsychotic   (Gr. *anti*, against; *psukhe*, breath, soul)
- Agent useful in the treatment of psychoses, most commonly applied to drugs effective against schizophrenia.   See **neuroleptic, tranquillizer**

antipyretic drug   (Gr. *anti*, against; *pura*, fire)
- Agent that reduces **pyrexia** (fever).

antipyrine (phenazone)   See **drugs as tools**

antiriot agent   See **harassing agent**

antisense oligonucleotides   (Gr. *anti*, against; L. *sentire*, to feel; Gr. *oligo*, few; L. *nucleus*, a little nut, kernel)
- Antisense **oligonucleotides** are short lengths of single-stranded DNA made by **biotechnology** to have a sequence of **bases** complementary to the bases in the target segment of a gene or the RNA message produced by that gene. Antisense oligonucleotides bind to their target (by Watson–Crick base pairing) with exquisite **specificity** and prevent the **expression** of that piece of genetic information. They provide a precise means of inhibiting the function of a **gene** or **gene product**. The commonest target is mRNA so that **translation** is blocked. Potential uses include the inactivation of **oncogenes** and genes responsible for drug resistance in cancer treatment and antiviral therapy.
- Antisense molecules are also used to inactivate specified genes, for example,

receptor genes, in order to investigate the function of the expressed protein – a technique analogous to the production of **knockout mutants**.

antiseptic   (Gr. *anti*, against; *septikos*, rotten)
– Substance that kills or prevents growth of microorganisms and which is suitable for **topical** use on living tissue (skin, eye) but not for internal use (e.g. hypochlorites, **povidone**-iodine, chlorhexidine).

antitussive drug   (Gr. *anti*, against; L. *tussis*, cough)
– Agent that suppresses cough (e.g. dextromethorphan).

'Anton Piller order'
– An order (UK law) that allows application by a plaintiff to a court sitting *in camera* (L., in a private room, and so, privately, not in public), to make an order requiring defendants to permit access to their premises. The defendant is *not told* that the application has been made. The purpose is to prevent removal of evidence before the order is served on the defendant. The order has been used in the pursuit of **counterfeit drugs**. The term derives from a legal case in the UK (*Anton Piller KG v. Manufacturing Processes Ltd [1976] Court of Appeal, UK*).

anxiolytic   (L. *angere*, to torment; Gr. *luein*, to release)
– Reducing anxiety.
– *Anxiolytic sedative*: antianxiety drug, or 'minor' **tranquillizer**, such as a benzodiazepine.

apamin   See **drugs as tools**

aperient   (L. *aperire*, to open)
                                                                                      See **purgative**

aphrodisiac   (Gr. *aphrodisios*, belonging to Aphrodite,
                                               goddess of love and beauty, daughter of Zeus. Her festivals,
                                               the aphrodisia, 'were very much frequented' (*Lemprière*))
– A drug that increases sexual drive and/or performance. Ideally (presumably) an aphrodisiac would in a single dose, reliably, selectively, quickly, reversibly, in a dose-related fashion, increase sexual drive and performance of either sex over a period of, say, 55 minutes. It would be rapidly absorbed across the buccal mucous membrane or from the stomach. An elimination $t_{1/2}$ of about 30 minutes would seem to be about right. There should be available a reliable competitive antagonist. It should have a low apparent volume of distribution, it should be acidic and have a **pK$_a$** in the range that would allow alkaline diuresis (more convenient than acid diuresis) to multiply the rate of renal elimination in the event of serious overdose. It should be instantly inactivated by alcohol *in vitro* or *in vivo*. It should have a distinctive taste and other properties so that it could not be administered without knowledge of the recipient. It should certainly not be a potent odourless vapour. Happily for society no such drug exists.

aplastic anaemia   (Gr. *a*, without; *plassein*, form; *an*, without; *haima*, blood)
- Deficiency of haemoglobin associated with reduced numbers of *all* cellular elements of the blood, resulting from depression of function of the bone marrow. It occurs as a frequently fatal rare adverse drug reaction, most notoriously from chloramphenicol.

apoptosis   (Gr. *apo*, off; *ptosis*, a falling)
- Programmed cell death.
- Physiological cell death, characterized by chromatin condensation, cytoplasmic blebbing and DNA fragmentation. The process is an integral part of normal tissue maintenance and repair, and development. It often depends on RNA and protein synthesis by the dying cell, i.e. the instructions for the process are built into the cell's genetic material.
- Selective drug-induced apoptosis has therapeutic possibilities, e.g. in cancer, chronic inflammation.

a posteriori   (L. *a*, from; *posterus*, coming next or after)
- Phrase describing the process of reasoning from known effects (or outcomes) to causes, i.e. inductive reasoning.
     See **Bayes' theorem, induction, *a priori***

apparent volume of distribution   See **volume of distribution**

approved drug names   See **names of drugs**

a priori   (L. *a*, from; *prior*, previous, before)
- An *a priori* proposition can be known to be true or false without reference to experience (*O'Grady*), i.e. it is self-evident.
- Reasoning from causes to effects (deductive reasoning), e.g. the decision to test a drug for therapeutic efficacy.
     See **Bayes' theorem, deduction, *a posteriori***

APUD cells
- Amine-precursor-uptake-decarboxylation. An **acronym** introduced by AGE Pearse to describe the common cytochemical characteristics of a series of cells, having a common origin in neural or specialized ectoderm, the majority of which have as their primary function the production of peptide or amine hormones. There are five functional groups of these cells:
  - *Endocrine*: cell system that secretes **hormone** directly into the bloodstream.
  - *Exocrine*: cell system that secretes into the gut lumen or to the exterior.
  - *Neuroendocrine*: cell system that secretes via axons into the bloodstream.
  - *Neurocrine*: cell system that secretes hormone, directly or indirectly, on/ into neurons.
  - *Paracrine*: cell system that secretes hormone directly to neighbouring cells.
- Included in this group (of APUD cells) are SIF (small intensely fluorescent) cells which contain high concentrations of catecholamines (hence the intense

fluorescence induced by formaldehyde) and which are present in sympathetic ganglia, but which are distinct from sympathetic nerve cells.

aquaretic/-sis (L. *aqua*, water)
− A drug that promotes the excretion of solute-free water rather than, for example, Na^+. See **diuretic**

arachidonic acid (Acid derivative of oil from the peanut, *Arachis hypogaea*)
− 5,8,11,14-eicosatetraenoic acid. A 20-carbon unsaturated fatty acid with four double bonds, the starting material for the synthesis of the **prostaglandins, thromboxanes** and **leukotrienes**. Arachidonic acid is one of the common fatty acids incorporated into the phospholipids of the cell membrane.

arbitrary (L. *arbitrare*, to give judgement)
− Dependent on will or pleasure; discretionary, not fixed; based on mere opinion or preference.

archive/-ing (Gr. *archeia*, public office)
− The place where public records or historic documents are kept (in the plural).
− Collected documents bearing historical or otherwise important information.
− In the pharmaceutical industry all experiments or trials of new drugs that are to be quoted in the new drug application (to the regulatory authority) must now be recorded ('archived') in such a way that they can be checked, as there have been instances of fraud.
 See **audit trail, GCP, GLP, regulation (official) of medicines**

area under the curve (AUC)
− The area under the plasma concentration v. time curve. If calculated from the time of administration of the drug to infinity, it represents the total amount of drug eliminated, and hence the total amount of drug absorbed. The ratio of the AUC after oral administration to the AUC after intravenous bolus administration (of the same dose) is an expression of **bioavailability**.
− AUC is used in **bioequivalence** studies for regulatory purposes. In general the 90% **confidence limits** should be within the chosen *acceptance range* of 80–125%; but for drugs of a particularly narrow therapeutic range (see **therapeutic index**) the acceptance range may need to be smaller (**WHO**).
 See **trapezoid rule (linear)**

area under the (first) moment curve (AUMC)
− Quantity used in the calculation of **mean residence time** in **pharmacokinetics**. If the product of time since injection (t) and plasma concentration at time t (C_t) is plotted v. time, the curve increases to a peak and then declines. The area under this curve, extrapolated to infinity, is *the area under the (first) moment versus time curve*. See **first moment (of the concentration)**

argentaffin/-oma (L. *argentum*, silver; *affinis*, neighbouring)
− Pertaining to tissues that stain black with silver. Tumours of argentaffin cells (argentaffinoma, carcinoid) secrete **serotonin** (5-hydroxytryptamine, 5-HT).
 See **carcinoid tumour**

ARMI
- Age-Related Memory Impairment.

aromatherapy   (Gr. *aromat*, spice; *therapeueo*, cure)
- A form of **complementary medicine** in which the so-called 'essential' aromatic oils obtained from plants are used to treat patients in the belief either
that sickness results from deficiencies of these essential oils, or that stimulation of the olfactory mechanism with specially selective odours can aid the
body's recuperative powers, whether by **placebo**, by conditioning or by
pharmacodynamic action.

arrhythmia (cardiac)   (Gr. *a, an*, without; *rhuthmos*, rhythm, flow)
- Any variation from the normal rhythm. Synonymous with **dysrhythmia** (which
is etymologically preferable).

artefact   (L. *ars*, art; *facere*, to make)
- A thing that is not naturally present.
- An event in an experiment that is unintended, incidental, extraneous, caused
by the experimental intervention itself or by defective technique.

Arunlakshana & Schild method
- Graphical method for determining the K_B (**dissociation equilibrium constant**) of an **antagonist**. This is a **null method** first described by Arunlakshana (pharmacologist, India) and Schild, but is commonly attributed to
Schild alone (*HO Schild*, 1906–1984, pharmacologist, UK). (See K_A, K_B, K_d)
- If the **Gaddum–Schild equation** is expressed in logarithmic form it becomes
the equation for a straight line with unit slope:

$$\log(r - 1) = \log[B] - \log K_B$$

where r = the equieffective **concentration ratio** (the dose ratio), $[B]$ is the
concentration of drug B (the antagonist), and K_B is the dissociation equilibrium constant for drug B (the antagonist).
Log$(r - 1)$ is plotted against $\log[B]$. When the concentration ratio, represented
by r, is 2, the value of the expression $\log(r - 1)$ is zero. The intercept on the
$\log[B]$ axis is therefore the log of the antagonist dissociation equilibrium constant, K_B. In other words, the dissociation equilibrium constant for a **competitive antagonist** is the concentration of the antagonist that produces a concentration ratio of 2 (i.e. shifts the agonist concentration–response curve two-
fold to the right). If the slope of the regression line differs significantly from 1,
or the line has significant curvature, one or more of the following may apply:
  - The antagonism is not competitive.
  - There is an interfering factor (e.g. dispositional) so that the concentration
    of either agonist or antagonist in the bulk phase of the tissue bath differs
    from that at the receptors.
  - Equilibrium conditions have not been reached.
  - There is **cooperativity** (positive or negative) in the system.
- In many older texts, the concentration ratio was referred to as the *dose ratio*

and represented by the symbol *x*. The terminology used here is that recommended by **IUPHAR**.   See **competition/competitive antagonism/inhibition, disposition (of drugs)**

AS-ODN
– **Antisense**-oligodeoxynucleotide.

aspirin (acetylsalicylic acid)
– Reputedly the most frequently consumed medicine in history.
– Derived from salicin that occurs naturally in willow trees (*Salix alba*) and meadowsweet (*Spiraea*, now *Filipendula, ulmaria*). The name is made from *a* for *acetyl,* and *spirin* from *Spiraea.* It was the first nonsteroidal anti-inflammatory drug. Synthesized and introduced into medicine in 1899, it has had a major place in therapeutics ever since; first as an analgesic/anti-inflammatory/antipyretic, and latterly in the prevention of coronary heart disease (antiplatelet effect). All its actions are due to inhibition of the prostaglandin-forming enzyme **clyclooxygenase**.   See **Reye's syndrome**

ASPP
– Anonymized single patient print: part of **ADROIT**.

assay   (L. *exagium*, weighing)
– The process of estimating an unknown concentration or potency. The unknown is compared with a standard of known concentration or potency.
                    See **biological assay**

association (causal/noncausal)   See **science in pharmacology**

association constant   See **association equilibrium constant**

association equilibrium constant   (L. *associare*, to join together; *constare*, to stand firm)
– The reciprocal of the **dissociation equilibrium constant**. It expresses the relative proportions of the free and of the associated species of the reactant (e.g. drug molecules reacting with **receptors**) when the system has come to equilibrium. The association equilibrium constant is also known as the *affinity constant* or **affinity**.   See K_A, K_B, K_d

assumption   (L. *assumere*, to take up)
– Something that is taken for granted; as true for the purpose of argument or action; as true in the absence of evidence.   See **axiom**

astringent   (L. *astringens*, a drawing together)
– Substance having a weak and limited protein coagulant effect so that a relatively impermeable film is formed on the epithelial surface treated (e.g. zinc and aluminium salts and dilute acids, tannic a., etc.). Used in dermatology. Known as **styptic** when used to stop capillary bleeding.

asymptote/-otic (Gr. *a*, not; *syn*, together; *ptotos*, inclined to fall)
— Approaching more and more closely but never quite meeting (except at infinity). For example an **exponential curve** (e.g. plotting the course of drug elimination) approaches zero asymptotically; the **Langmuir adsorption isotherm/equation** approaches an asymptote of unity as the concentration of ligand is increased.

ataractic drug (Gr. *a*, without; *tarassein*, to trouble)
— A loose term meaning an antianxiety agent. See **anxiolytic, tranquillizer**

attention bias (L. *ad*, to; *tendere*, to stretch)
See **bias, Hawthorne effect**

ATP
— Adenosine triphosphate. The principal biochemical supplier of energy in cell metabolism. "ATP is an intracellular storehouse of energy" (*Guyton*).
— ATP is also a transmitter in **purinergic** neurons, as well as a **co-transmitter** with **noradrenaline, acetylcholine** and **substance P** in postganglionic sympathetic, postganglionic parasympathetic and sensory neurons, respectively.

AUC
— **Area under the curve.** See **trapezoid rule (linear)**

audiogenic seizures (L. *audire*, to hear; Gr. *gen*, to be produced)
— Epileptiform convulsions induced by loud noise. Certain strains of mice are particularly susceptible. Audiogenic seizures have been used in **screens** for anticonvulsant drugs.

audit (L. *audire*, to hear, hence *auditus*, a hearing)
— The systematic and scientific process of determining the extent to which an action or set of actions was successful in the achievement of predetermined objectives.
— Audit and research: "*Research* is finding out what you ought to be doing; *audit* is seeing whether what you are doing is what you ought to be doing" (*A Hopkins*).
— The World Health Organization (WHO) recognizes seven stages of audit:
  1. Problem identification.
  2. Setting priorities.
  3. Determining methodology.
  4. Setting criteria and standards.
  5. Comparing performance with standards.
  6. Designing and implementing remedial action.
  7. Re-evaluating the quality of care.
— Verification of financial accounts by a professional accountant.

audit trail (L. *audire*, to hear, hence *auditus*, a hearing; *tragula*, trawl net)
— In **regulation (official) of medicines**, all tests and trials which form part of

the submission for a *product licence* (*new drug application*) must be recorded (**archived**) in such a way that all the data can be found, checked and cross-checked. This is to deter unscrupulous pharmaceutical companies from falsifying their records. It also expedites the follow-up of events that were not anticipated when the trials or experiments were begun.

augmentation (L. *augere*, to increase)
- An interaction between two drugs such that the response to a given dose of one drug is increased by the second drug, which does not usually itself cause a response. It is a common mistake for augmentation to be described as **potentiation** where there is no evidence to distinguish between the two phenomena. Although potentiation will cause an increase in response (at submaximal doses), other phenomena can also do so, notably an increase in **responsiveness** of the target. Before a mechanism can be described as potentiation there must be clear evidence that the **dose–response curve** has been shifted to the left; without this it is prudent to describe any increased response as augmentation.

AUMC
- **Area under the (first) moment curve.** See **mean residence time**

autacoid (Gr. *autos*, self; *akos*, remedy)
- "A motley collection of substances of intense pharmacological activity that are normally present in the body or may be formed there, and that cannot conveniently be classed with other members of this broad group, such as neurohumors [neurotransmitters] and hormones. These different substances have been variously described as local hormones, autopharmacological agents and the like: but a generic term that is at once shorter, more accurate and euphonious, is autacoid, a word derived from the Greek autos ('self') and akos ('medicinal agent' or 'remedy'). This term was devised by Sir Edward Schafer (1916), later Sharpey-Schafer, as a substitute for Starling's word hormone, which, being derived from the Greek *hormaein* meaning 'to stir up', is a misnomer for the inhibitory substances that also came to be embraced by this designation. However, Starling's term hormone, albeit unsatisfactory from the etymological standpoint, has won the day, and Schafer's has passed into limbo. Such a good word deserves a better fate...". (*WW Douglas*, in *The pharmacological basis of therapeutics*, LS Goodman & A Gilman (eds) 1965). Autacoids act close to the site of their release (unlike classical hormones which are transported via the blood circulation). They include **histamine, serotonin** (5-HT), angiotensin, **kinins, prostaglandins**. Despite this persuasive plea, the word has not fully entered general currency, although it is gaining ground.
- *Spelling: a diversion into etymology.* Autacoid is often misspelt, autocoid. To make this convenient classical compound word it is necessary to adapt two Ancient Greek words (see above): *auto-* and *-acoid*. For the word to be easily pronounceable, either the *o* (of auto) or the *a* (of acoid) has to be dropped. The *o* is chosen because to drop the *a* renders the second Greek word

meaningless. The word is *aut-acoid* (not *auto-coid*). There are only about five words in English where this o/a juxtaposition occurs and they are all seldom used. But there are more than forty words beginning *auto-*, many of which are in colloquial use. Thus societies, no longer educated in the niceties of classical languages, feel at ease with *auto* and uncomfortable with *auta*. Consequently incorrect spelling drives out correct spelling (just as bad money drives out good; *Gresham's Law, 1588*). Some people think such concerns as these are mere pedantry, but those who consider them to be important will find much of interest in the *Oxford Companion to the English Language*, *T McArthur* (ed) (Oxford University Press).

authorship (scientific) (L. *auctor*, originator)

– Research is increasingly performed by teams and the result is a proliferation of authors and acknowledgements and the inclusion of names for nonscientific contributions. The **International Committee of Medical Journal Editors** has recommended the following:

"All persons designated as authors should qualify for authorships. Each author should have participated sufficiently in the work to take public responsibility for the content.

"Authorship credit should be based only on substantial contributions to 1) conception and design, or analysis and interpretation of data; and to 2) drafting the article or revising it critically for important intellectual content; and on 3) final approval of the version to be published. Conditions 1, 2, and 3 must all be met. Participation solely in the acquisition of funding or the collection of data does not justify authorship. General supervision of the research group is not sufficient for authorship. Any part of an article critical to its main conclusions must be the responsibility of at least one author.

"Editors may ask authors to describe what each contributed; this information may be published.

"Increasingly, multicenter trials are attributed to a corporate author. All members of the group who are named as authors, either in the authorship position below the title or in a footnote, should fully meet the above criteria for authorship. Group members who do not meet these criteria should be listed, with their permission, in the acknowledgments or in the appendix.

"The order of authorship should be a joint decision of the co-authors. Because the order is assigned in different ways, its meaning cannot be inferred accurately unless it is stated by the authors. Authors may wish to explain the order of authorship in a footnote. In deciding on the order, authors should be aware that many journals limit the number of authors listed in the table of contents and that the U.S. National Library of Medicine (NLM) lists in MEDLINE only the first 24 plus the last author when there are more than 25 authors" (*Annals of Internal Medicine* 1997;126:36–47).

– The problems of authorship are wider than the above. They have been addressed in an important paper; (*D Rennie, V Yank, L Emanuel*. When authorship fails. A proposal to make contributors accountable. *Journal of the American Medical Association* 1997;278:579–585), as follows:

"A published article is the primary means whereby new work is communicated, priority is established, and academic promotion is determined. Publication depends on trust and requires that authors be held to standards of honesty, completeness, and fairness in their reporting, and to accountability for their statements. The system of authorship, while appropriate for articles with only 1 author, has become inappropriate as the average number of authors of an article has increased; as the work of coauthors has become more specialized and relationships between them have become more complex, and as both credit and, even more, responsibility have become obscured and diluted. Credit and accountability cannot be assessed unless the contributions of those named as authors are disclosed to readers, so the system is flawed. We argue for a radical conceptual and systematic change, to reflect the realities of multiple authorship and to buttress accountability. We propose dropping the outmoded notion of authors in favor of the more useful and realistic one of contributors. This requires disclosure to readers of the contributions made to the research and to the manuscript by the contributors, so that they can accept both credit and responsibility. In addition, certain named contributors take on the role of guarantor for the integrity of the entire work. The requirement that all participants be named as contributors will eliminate the artificial distinction between authors and acknowledgees and will enhance the integrity of publications."

These ideas have gained significant support, and progress can be monitored in the practice of current biomedical journals.

See **International Committee of Medical Journal Editors.**

– In large, hierarchically structured institutes, the head of research may have his/her name on all publications The world record (1981–1990) seems to be held by a crystallographer with one paper every 4 days, followed by an endocrinologist (one every 5 days).

– The practice of naming as authors people who do not qualify as authors is objectionable; it is known as *gift-authorship* or *hitch-hiking*.

– "Every listed author should at least be able to give a brief talk at a public meeting on the substance of what has been reported in writing" (*J Maddox*).

– "In a scientific article, only those who can rewrite the text if the original is lost can be considered as co-authors" (*A Kaldor*): a stern criterion.

– *Books*: Pharmacologists should be cautious regarding publishers' contracts. It is important that they do not undervalue their worth and/or accept inappropriate restrictions.   See **copyright, publication**

– *Ghost writing*: There are specialist companies who will prepare (review) articles to the satisfaction of commercial sponsors and then find a prominent/ respected doctor to be 'guest author' (for an **honorarium**). The final version, when submitted to the journal, may contain no clues about its origins.

  – A widespread practice is for a potential author to be asked to collaborate in the preparation of an article which will be written mainly by a ghost writer, but with 'full' control by the 'author'. Many ghost-written reviews start life as an outline and list of references prepared by the 'author'. Several stages of drafts may be sent to the 'author' for correction and the final version will

only be submitted to the journal when written approval has been provided by the 'author'. Ghost writers are sometimes acknowledged, but this usually only happens if the 'author' insists upon doing so.
- In today's world ghost writing is legitimate and probably necessary but it is open to abuse.   See **interest (conflict of)**

autocrine   (Gr. *autos*, self; *krinein*, separate)
- A word derived from **endocrine**. In autocrine secretion the **mediator** acts upon the cell from which it is released, e.g. some **cytokines**.
                    See **autoreceptor, endocrine, exocrine, paracrine**

autoinduction   (Gr. *autos*, self; L. *in*, in; *ducere*, to lead)
                                                      See **enzyme induction**

automaticity   (Gr. *automatos*, acting independently)
- Tendency of an excitable tissue to initiate impulses spontaneously. Usually applied to the myocardium.

autonomic   (Gr. *autos*, self; *nomos*, law)
- Term coined by Langley (physiologist, UK) in 1898 and meaning *occurring spontaneously or involuntarily*. The *autonomic nervous system* functions without the individual's awareness or will, although it is subject to some voluntary control, e.g. micturition, defaecation, ocular accommodation; it is a target for numerous therapeutic drugs.

autoradiograph/-y   (Gr. *autos*, self; L. *radius*, ray; Gr. *graphos*, written)
- A technique for locating precisely a **radioactive label** in a tissue. The process involves the close application of photographic film to the labelled tissue, usually by dipping a slide carrying the tissue directly into melted photographic emulsion (in the dark). After a suitable time, usually weeks or months, the emulsion is developed and fixed. Where radioactive decay has occurred in the tissue, ionizing particles or rays will have been generated and these will show up as grains of reduced silver. If the tissue is also stained, the silver grains show the location of the label in relation to cell or tissue structures. The technique can also be combined with electron microscopy in order to locate the grains more precisely.

autoreceptor   (Gr. *autos*, self; L. *re*, again; *capere*, to take)
- Presynaptic receptor involved in the **modulation** of transmitter release; it responds to the transmitter released by the nerve upon which it is located. It usually mediates negative **feedback**, e.g. presynaptic α_2-adrenoceptors on noradrenergic neurons.   See **heteroreceptor**

autotrophic regulation   See **allosteric interaction**

auxometry   (Gr. *auxein*, to increase; *metron*, measure)
- Measurement of rate of growth, e.g. in cancers.

auxotonic   (Gr. *auxein*, to increase; *tonos*, tension)
- Method of recording responses from isolated muscles in which the resistance to contraction (tension) increases as the muscle contracts. It is more usual to make **isometric** or **isotonic** measurements.

average   (Arabic: *awar*, damage, blemish)
- Equitable distribution of costs of damage to a ship or cargo amongst the owners, and so by 'transferred use', the *arithmetic mean*.   See **mean**

axiom/-atic   (L. *axioma*, a principle)
- Self-evident statement that is universally accepted; a generally accepted proposition.

Ayurvedic medicine   (Sanskrit: *ayur*, life; *veda*, knowledge; L. *memere*, to heal)
- Ancient Hindu medical system. It is *kaya-chikitea* or *body-treatment* and is based on a philosophy of maintaining equilibrium within the body, of *air* (which influences the nervous system), *fire* (which influences metabolism and the digestive system) and *water* (which influences cellular function). Treatment is by drugs (largely based on mercury, sulphur and herbs), diet and exercise.

'backtracking booze'   (Middle Dutch, *busen*, drink to excess)
- *Back-estimation of blood alcohol concentration* from the time of sampling to the time of an incident under investigation, e.g. road-traffic accident. "In the absence of continuing absorption reasonably robust estimates of blood ethanol concentrations at preceding times can be made. However, when absorption continues after drinking, especially when at a slow rate, backtracking calculations may become markedly inaccurate" (*PR Jackson et al.* 1991).
- *Back-estimation* after death is of importance for forensic reasons. It presents problems additional to alcohol diffusion from the stomach. There is often alcohol absorption from vomitus in the lungs. Within a few hours of death bacterial production of alcohol (from blood glucose and lactate) can be enough to generate concentrations that, in life, would be enough to affect behaviour and performance. The ocular vitreous humour and the urine in the bladder are for pathophysiological reasons relatively excluded from this artefact and are used cautiously as controls for assessing the likely ante-mortem blood alcohol concentration.   See **hip-flask defence**

barbiturate   (Named by the original synthesizer
                                        after "a charming lady named Barbara")
- A derivative of barbituric acid.
- A class of drug used principally as an intravenous anaesthetic and previously as a sedative–hypnotic and antiepileptic.

β-blocker   See **beta-(β-)adrenoceptor antagonists**

base   (L. *basis*, pedestal)
- A proton acceptor.
- A substance that liberates hydroxyl ions when dissolved in water.
- A strong base is one that dissociates fully in solution, yielding 1 **mole** of hydroxyl ions per mole of base: a weak base is one that dissociates only partially in solution.
- A 'free' base (see **crack**) exists in its basic form without a neutralizing acid moiety.
- The *basic* groups attached to each sugar **moiety** in RNA and DNA are referred to as *bases*. Each base is either a *purine* or a *pyrimidine*. In DNA the bases are *adenine* and *guanine* (purines), *cytosine* and *thymine* (pyrimidines). In RNA *uracil* replaces *thymine*. Conventional abbreviations are A, G, C and T (or U). The sequence of bases in a nucleic acid is expressed using these abbreviations, reading from the phosphorylated 5´ end (on the left) to the hydroxylated 3´ end (on the right).
                    See **dissociation equilibrium constant, nucleotide, pK$_a$**

BASIC
- Beginners' all-purpose sequential instruction code; a **computer** programming language.

batrachotoxin   See **drugs as tools**

Bayes' theorem (L. *theorema*, something to be viewed)
- This provides an inductive (see **induction**) statement of the probability of a hypothesis, given that some observations have already been made. The theorem states:

Posterior probability = some × likelihood of × prior probability
of a hypothesis constant hypothesis of the hypothesis

In this equation prior (or ***a priori***) probability means the probability of the hypothesis being true *before* making the observations under consideration. The posterior (or ***a posteriori***) probability is the probability *after* making the observations, and the likelihood of the hypothesis is defined as the probability of making the given observations if the hypothesis under consideration were in fact true. The wrangle about the interpretation of Bayes' theorem continues to the present day. Is 'the probability of an hypothesis being true' a meaningful idea? The great mathematician Laplace assumed that, if nothing were known of the merits of rival hypotheses, then their prior probabilities should be considered equal ('the equipartition of ignorance'). Later it was suggested that Bayes' theorem was not really applicable except in a small proportion of cases in which valid prior probabilities were known. This view is still probably the most common, but there is now a strong school of thought that believes the only sound method of inference is Bayesian. Bayesian methods have also been criticized on the grounds that the assigning of prior probabilities is subjective, that to apply the theorem rigorously implies the need to identify *all* possible hypotheses and to assign a prior probability to each, and that although the theorem is conceptually simple, it is computationally difficult to implement. The Bayesian statistician might counter these objections by stating that all estimation of probabilities is subjective, however it is done, that it is impossible to come to logical conclusions about the truth of hypotheses without considering all the possibilities, and finally that modern computers make complex computations relatively easy.
- The theorem was proposed by the Reverend Thomas Bayes (1701–1761), amateur statistician, in his *Essay towards solving a problem in the doctrine of chances* which was published posthumously in 1763 (*Royal Society of London, Philosophical Transactions*).
- Bayesian interim analysis of randomized clinical trials may occasionally provide a clearer interpretation of the data than standard statistical analysis and assist in the sometimes difficult task of deciding whether a trial should continue.
- Bayesian analysis integrates the summation of our past knowledge (via the prior distribution) with the newly acquired data (through the likelihood function) by Bayes' theorem to arrive at a newer understanding of the studied phenomena (summarized by the posterior distribution) (*JM Brophy, L Joseph*). **See true**

behavioural toxicity (Early Eng. *be-have*; L. *habere*, to have; Gr. *toxikon*, poison)
- *Behaviour*: the aggregate of psychological and physical responses in a particular situation.

- *Behavioural toxicity:* a somewhat unhappy term meaning effects (as judged by orthodox or traditional values) on behaviour of an extent that adversely affects human individuals' mental function or performance in society. In toxicological studies in animals, behavioural tests may detect changes before there is any histopathological evidence of injury. Behavioural tests also provide evidence of defective *integrated* function of physiological systems that cannot be detected by histological or even physiological tests of organs taken separately.

benefit/risk evaluation or ratio
(L. *bene + facere*, to do well; It. *risco*, danger; L. *ratus*, to reckon)
- *Risk* is the probability that something bad will happen, and *benefit* is the probability that something good will happen. Although often not explicit, the concept is fundamental to the use of medicines. Its practical application is often limited by the lack of accurate estimates of the probabilities and *relative magnitude* of benefit and of **risk**.

Berkson's paradox
(Gr. *para,* beyond, beside; *doxa,* opinion)
See **selection bias (in clinical studies)**

Bernoulli random variable
(*Jakob Bernoulli,* 1654–1705, mathematician, Switzerland) (see **random**; **variable**)
- A random variable that is capable of assuming one of two values, e.g. 0 or 1, with fixed probabilities, p and 1 − p, respectively (after **FDA**). For example, blood samples from a number of individuals are tested for the presence of antibody to a particular virus. Each blood sample is a trial, and the outcome is either 1 (*antibody present*) or 0 (*antibody absent*).
See **binomial probability distribution**

Bernoulli trial
(*Jakob Bernoulli,* 1654–1705, mathematician, Switzerland)
- A single replication of an experimental procedure on a defined observational unit with a **Bernoulli random variable** as the outcome (**FDA**).

β-ARK
- β-adrenergic-receptor kinase.
- An enzyme that phosphorylates the occupied form of the β-adrenoceptor preferentially, causing uncoupling of the receptor–**G-protein** complex leading to rapid **desensitization**. It probably also phosphorylates other receptors and rhodopsin.
See **-ergic**

beta-(β-)adrenoceptor antagonists/blockers
- Drugs that **block** competitively the activation of β-adrenoceptors. Used in angina pectoris, cardiac dysrhythmias, hypertension, anxiety, etc.

'beta-blockers'
See **beta-(β-)adrenoceptor antagonists/blockers, adrenoceptor**

betel nut
- The seed of *Areca catechu* (South-East Asia). Contains arecoline, a **cholinomimetic** alkaloid. It is used socially, being chewed mixed with lime and leaves of a climbing pepper plant (*Piper betle*) as '*pan*'. The leaves of *Piper betle* also contain psychoactive substances.

between-patient (subject) trial
- A therapeutic trial or other study in which each subject receives one treatment only, i.e. the controls are other subjects. See **within-patient trial**

bias   (Old Fr. *biasis*, from Gr. *epikarsios*, oblique, or L. *bifax*, looking two ways)
- A latent influence that disturbs an analysis or allocation.
- A mental tendency, particularly when this is irrational.
- A *systematic* deviation from the truth that distorts the results of research. There are four principal categories: **selection bias**, information bias, attention bias, **confounding**; to which may be added, intervention bias, measurement bias, follow-up bias, analysis bias, **reporting bias, recall bias** and interpretation bias.
          See **John Henry effect, Hawthorne effect**, **publication** (*Publication bias*)

bibliography   (Gr. *biblion*, book; *graphos*, writing)
- We recommend all who consult this book to have *at least* (preferably recent editions of):
    - A substantial English language dictionary for reference.
    - A *small English language dictionary* at the bedside for browsing in a manner that will keep you awake or help you go to sleep according to your preference.
    - A *thesaurus* (L. Gr. storehouse): a book containing synonyms (Gr. *sun*, together, with; *onoma*, name). Some people, fearing they will be thought inadequate, are reluctant to admit they use a thesaurus to find a better word to replace one that is not quite right. We have no such scruple and we strongly recommend the use of a thesaurus when in need and for profitable browsing. Single-volume dictionary/thesaurus combinations are available.
- Works worth considering for your personal reference library:
    - Brewer's dictionary of phrase and fable.
    - A medical/scientific dictionary.
    - A dictionary of synonyms and antonyms.
    - A book of *quotations*: choice is wide. The biggest by far (*c.* 65 000 quotations) is *The home book of quotations*, B Stevenson (ed), (Dodd Mead & Co., New York).
    - A dictionary of *etymology* (general dictionaries are adequate for most needs).
    - *Fowler's modern English usage* (Oxford University Press).
    - *The complete plain words, Sir Ernest Gowers*.
    - *The Oxford companion to the English language*, T McArthur (ed).

bicuculline   See **drugs as tools**

billion   (L. *bi*, two; Old Fr. *mille*, thousand)
- Traditionally, a billion is 10^{12} (i.e. a million millions), but "tradition has been overwhelmed by others' usage" and, to avoid confusion there is now a consensus that a billion is 10^9 (i.e. a thousand millions). *Trillion* is best avoided as there is no consensus whether it is 10^{12} or 10^{18} (*Nature* 1992;358:2).

bimodal distribution   (L. *bi*, two; *modus*, measure, manner)
- A distribution (or density function) with two peaks, as opposed to the more common single peak of distributions such as the **normal distribution**, which are described as unimodal. Bimodal distributions commonly arise by superposition of two unimodal distributions (with different **means**). For example, the distribution of the rate of isoniazid acetylation is bimodal as a result of the presence in the population of two distinct genetically-determined subpopulations (slow and fast acetylators), each subpopulation having a unimodal distribution of acetylation rate. Other *(multimodal)* distributions are possible, e.g. *trimodal.*

binary outcome measure   (L. *bini*, two together)
- A measure that can assume only one of two values, e.g. death or survival.

binding domain   See **domain**

binding site   (Old Eng. *bindan*, to tie, fasten, attach)
- That part of any molecule, generally a macromolecule, with which another molecule can form a complex, and that does not necessarily mediate a biological response.   See **acceptor site, receptor**

binomial probability distribution   (L. *bi*, two; *nomen*, name;
                                                         dis, apart; *tribuere*, to give)
- The basis of binomial distribution is a series of *Bernoulli trials* in which there are only two possible (and mutually exclusive) outcomes, e.g. alive or dead, success or failure (*J Bernoulli*, mathematician, 1654–1705, Switzerland).
- The binomial distribution gives the probability, *P(r)*, of observing any specified number, *r*, of 'successes' in a series of *n* independent 'trials' when the outcome of a single 'trial' can be of only two sorts ('success' or 'failure'), and when the probability of obtaining a 'success' at a single trial is constant from trial to trial. In order to calculate *P(r)*, this probability of obtaining success at a single trial must be known and specified. For example, a 'trial' might be administration of a drug to one patient, 'success' being an improvement in the patient's condition, 'failure' being no improvement. Each such observation is sometimes called a **Bernoulli trial**. The binomial distribution would then allow calculation of the probability of observing any specified number of improvements (e.g. *r* = 90 improved out of *n* = 110 patients) given the probability of improvement in a single patient.

bioadhesive polymer   (Gr. *bios*, life; L. *ad*, to; *haerere*, to stick)
- The polymer expands by absorbing water, diffuses into mucin or a tissue surface, and adheres to that surface, often by **hydrogen bonding**. Thus, tissue contact time is increased and absorption of any drug carried by the polymer is enhanced. The polymers may also be used as mucin substitutes, e.g. for a dry mouth or vagina. They also act as moisturizers by promoting the passage of water into surface cells.

bioassay   See **biological assay**

bioavailability   (Gr. *bios*, life; L. *ad*, to; *valere*, (loosely) of value to)
- For pharmaceutical purposes: the amount of drug in a formulation that is released and becomes available for absorption. For oral preparations it is predicted by an *in vitro* dissolution test. Where *in vivo* tests are used, the area under the plasma concentration–time curve **(AUC)** is measured, i.e. the proportion of the dose that enters the systemic circulation. This is the common use. Plainly, the AUC is affected by factors such as intestinal function and **hepatic first-pass metabolism**.
- There is no general agreement on the precise meaning – the term is also loosely used to refer to the fraction of the drug, after absorption, that is 'available' (i.e. is not sequestered, rapidly metabolized, e.g. hepatic first-pass, or rapidly excreted) for action at the treatment site. Since it cannot be quantitatively defined, and is affected by disease, for example, this usage is more likely to engender confusion than clarification.
- The term is also used to mean the proportion of a drug that is absorbed from the gut when presented in solution. This, also, is not particularly useful and is irrelevant if the drug is given for its action in the gut lumen. The term is also difficult to apply to ointments, etc.
- *Absolute bioavailability (f)* is the proportion of a dose contained within a particular **formulation** that enters the body after administration of that formulation (usually oral). It is usually calculated from the $AUC_{0-\infty}$ (see **area under the curve**) after administration of the (oral) formulation and the $AUC_{0-\infty}$ after intravenous administration.   See **bioequivalence, suprabioavailability**

bioburden (microbial)   (Gr. *bios*, life; Old Eng. *byrthen*, load)
- The type and number of microorganisms found in a product before sterilization.

biodegradable polymer   (Gr. *bios*, life; L. *de*, down; Gr. *gradus*, rank;
                                                   Gr. *polumeres*, having many parts)
- Synthetic polymer in which a labile drug can be suspended. This can be inserted under the skin, where the drug is released as the polymer is slowly broken down under the influence of enzymes in body fluids, i.e. a **depot formulation**.

bioequivalence   (Gr. *bios*, life; L. *aequus*, equal; *valere*, to be worth)
- Bioequivalence obtains where the *rate* and *extent* of absorption (**bioavailability)** of two formulations do not differ significantly. The assumption that

bioequivalence equals **therapeutic equivalence** is often, but not invariably, justified. This can be of great significance if a patient needing a **steady state** plasma concentration obtains a supply of medicine from different manufacturing sources. See **substitute or alternative formulation, area under the curve, pharmaceutical equivalence**

bioethics (Gr. *bios*, life; *ethikos*, character, manners)
- To prefix **ethics** with bio- seems hardly necessary; nevertheless the term has gained currency.

biogenic substance (e.g. **biogenic amine**) (Gr. *bios*, life; *gen*, to be produced)
- A substance formed by metabolic processes in living organisms: biogenic amines include **dopamine, adrenaline, noradrenaline, serotonin, histamine**.

bioidentity (Gr. *bios*, life; L. *idem*, the same)
- For a substance whose structure cannot be demonstrated adequately by physiochemical analysis, biological tests are used (see **biological assay**). But they do not provide proof of chemical structure and the use of the term bioidentity test has been powerfully questioned (*S Jeffcoate*, The bioidentity test; illogical, unnecessary, unethical and unscientific? *Pharmaceutical Medicine* 1995;9:191).

biologic product (Gr. *bios*, life, *logy*, subject of study)
- A class of drug product manufactured by biologic process as opposed to *in vitro* chemical process. Biologic products pose special problems (regarding quality and safety) for regulatory bodies.

biological assay/bioassay (Gr. *bios*, life; *logy*, subject of study; L. *exagium*, weighing)
- Measurement of the concentration or potency of biologically active substances by means of the responses of living tissue or cells in comparison with a standard preparation. A technique used when chemical or physical methods do not exist or are impracticable, e.g. when impure substances or mixtures of unknown constitution are measured. It is the only technique by which *biological* or *therapeutic* potencies can be measured. **Therapeutic trials** are a form of bioassay. See **biological standardization**

biological response modifiers (BRM)
- Term introduced by the USA National Cancer Institute (1978) to comprise substances (natural or synthetic) that modify biological responses to tumour cells or immune responses, e.g. **cytokines, immune effectors, interleukins**.

biological standardization (Gr. *bios*, life; *logy*, subject of study; L. *extendere*, to stretch out)
- Determination of the activity of a preparation intended for therapeutic or laboratory use by its effect on living tissues as compared with a national or international standard or reference preparation. It is used where physical and

chemical methods are not available. The International Unit (IU) is defined by the **WHO**.

biomedical research (categories of)
- Categorization is important and highly relevant to the distribution of national funding:
  - *Critical health needs*: improving public health.
  - *Critical technologies*: creating new (better) technologies.
  - *Intellectual capital*: training the next generation of scientists. See **research**

biopharmaceutics   (Gr. *bios*, life; *pharmakeia*, making of drugs)
- The study of the influence of the chemical and physical form and formulation of a drug or medicine on the **pharmacodynamic** and **pharmacokinetic** events consequent on administration.   See **formulation**

biophase   (Gr. *bios*, life; *phasis*, appearance)
- An imprecise term for the locality in which drugs have access to receptors without intervention of diffusional barriers. It has been used with the following meanings:
  - The extracellular environment of the receptor in which the steady state concentration of the drug is determined.
  - A hypothetical 'well-stirred' compartment that contains the receptors, and into which the drug diffuses at a finite rate.   See **well-stirred model**
  - In the previous sense, sometimes identifies with the extracellular space of an isolated tissue, as opposed to the external solution.
  - The 'unstirred' layer adjacent to a surface that contains receptors.
  - A lipid phase that contains receptors (on the assumption that the drug concentration in this phase is important for the effect of the drug).

bioreductive drug   (Gr. *bios*, life; L. *re*, back; *ducere*, to lead)
- A substance that becomes biologically active in the presence of low oxygen tension, e.g. in the centre of solid tumours.

biotechnology   (Gr. *bios*, life; *tekhne*, craft)
- The application of biological processes to manufacture. Strictly interpreted, it includes processes such as fermentation (wine, cheese, antibiotics). No better term (than *biotechnology*) has been introduced to describe such processes.
- The term is particularly applied to the use of **recombinant DNA** technology (**genetic engineering**) to alter cells, especially bacteria, to produce, for example, insulin and **biological response modifiers**.
- Molecular structure may vary with different manufacturing processes, presenting special problems of establishing **bioidentity** and **bioequivalence**.
- Regulatory authorities give special attention to biotechnology products both to protect the public and to encourage development of a strong industry.
    See **transgenic animal bioreactors**

biotransformation   (Gr. *bios*, life; L. *trans*, across; *forma*, shape)

- Chemical modification of a substance within the body.

See **metabolism of drugs**

biphasic   (L. *bi*, two; *phasis*, appearance)
- Term used to describe:
  - A curve that appears, to the observer's eye, to be of a complex shape that could be decomposed into the sum of two curves of simpler shape.
  - A response that consists of the superposition of two separate and different responses.
  - A response to a single stimulus that is composed of two components separated in time.
  - More complex forms are *tri*phasic or *multi*phasic.

Black & Leff model
- An operational **model** that provides a mathematical interpretation of the observed behaviour of a system. The model is controversial, and although it describes **dose–response curves** in a convenient mathematical form and predicts useful **parameters** that can be measured in the laboratory, there is debate over whether these measurable parameters have any physical meaning. The operational model of agonism described by Black & Leff (1983) relates a hypothesis about agonist concentration–effect curves. The model stemmed from the finding that concentration–effect curves are often hyperbolic. From this it can be deduced that the relationship between occupancy and effect must be hyperbolic if the law of **mass action** applies at the agonist–receptor level. This deduction relies upon the fact that if a process comprises several other processes in sequence, each of which can be described by a hyperbolic curve, then the overall process will be described by a **hyperbola**. The model was also extended to account for the more frequently encountered **logistic (equation)** concentration–effect curves. Black & Leff demonstrated that the model could be represented in a three-dimensional graph in which the three axes are receptor occupancy, agonist concentration and effect. The model describes agonism in terms of three **parameters**:
  - An agonist–receptor **dissociation equilibrium constant** (K_A in Black & Leff's terminology – see K_A, K_B, K_d).
  - The total receptor concentration ($[R_0]$).
  - The midpoint location (K_E) of the function defining the **transduction** of the agonist–receptor complex (AR) into effect.
  - The ratio between $[R_0]$ and K_E is defined as the *transducer ratio*, τ, and provides a measure of the **efficacy** of an agonist in a system. The general equation takes the following form:

$$\frac{E}{E_m} = \frac{[R_0][A]}{K_A K_E + ([R_0] + K_E)[A]}$$

where E represents effect (response), E_m, the maximal effect that is possible in the system, and $[A]$ is the agonist concentration. The transducer ratio, τ, is related to the equilibrium dissociation constant for the agonist–receptor interaction (K_A), the total receptor concentration ($[R_0]$) and the midway location parameter for the transduction step (K_E) as follows:

$$\frac{K_A}{1+\tau} = \frac{K_A}{1+[R_0]/K_E}$$

and

$$\frac{\tau}{1+\tau} = \frac{1}{1+K_E/[R_0]}$$

(*JW Black, P Leff; Proceedings of the Royal Society of London B* 1983; B220:141–162.)

blind, blinding   (Old Eng)
                                              See **double-blind, single-blind**

block/blockade/blocker   (Old Fr. *bloc*, obstruction)
– A drug (**antagonist**) is known as a (receptor) blocker when it occupies a **receptor** without activating it, thereby excluding the active **ligand**. Although it is the case that an antagonist can be given in a dose sufficient to prevent (block) normal physiological activation completely, it is not true that a reversible antagonist can completely 'block' an exogenous **agonist**. This is because the effect of the antagonist depends upon the relative concentrations of the agonist and antagonist, and their relative **affinities** for the receptor. The term 'block' has connotations of a static situation. Some would therefore argue that the term **antagonism** is better, except when the effect of the drug is upon physiological transmission. **Nonequilibrium antagonists** can completely block **exogenous** agonists.   See **competitive antagonism**

'blockbuster drug'
– The term derives from aerial warfare with its use of bombs capable of destroying a city block of buildings. The figurative use of the term for a medicine tells us something of the thought processes of the pharmaceutical industry. It refers to a compound that recoups its research and development costs, and much more. Amongst its qualities, listed by the president of a multinational company, are:
  – It is a novel (breakthrough) or **fast-follower** product.
  – It should have regulatory approval (be licensed) in the eight major markets within 5 years of its first licence.
  – It should generate at least 50 per cent of its sales in North America.
  – It should gain and maintain at least 30 per cent of the market share in its class.
  – Its use must be for chronic disease (except anti-infectives and life-saving drugs).
  – It should have adequate [generous] patent protection.
  – Demonstrated *cost–benefit* (see **economics**) advantages should support a high price.
  – It should be easy for patients to use (*Scrip Magazine* 1992).

blood–brain/cerebrospinal fluid barrier
- The blood–brain barrier is the endothelium of the cerebral capillaries. The blood–cerebrospinal fluid (CSF) barrier is the choroid plexus epithelium. Drugs may pass through these differentially, although there are fundamental similarities. Drugs in the CSF may pass into the brain; passive **diffusion** and carrier-mediated processes are involved. See **diffusion (facilitated)**.
- The mechanism in the central nervous system that excludes substances carried in the blood, largely depends on reduced capillary permeability relating to the attachment of tight junction astrocytes to the endothelial basement membrane.

BNF and manufacturers' compendia
- *British National Formulary*. The BNF lists formulations of drugs licensed for prescription in the UK. It is revised twice yearly and is sent free to all doctors practising in the National Health Service. It also contains advice on the choice of medicine, some prescribing information and tables of drug interactions, prescribing in liver disease and renal impairment, as well as an indication of the status of the drug, e.g. **controlled drug**, **prescription-only medicine**, or new product. It is produced independently of the pharmaceutical industry, which produces compendia of its proprietary products, e.g. the Physicians' Desk Reference (USA) and the **ABPI** Compendium of Data Sheets and Summaries of Product Characteristics (UK).

body-count budgeting
- A term in biomedical politics that refers to the allocation of available (government) research funds proportionately according to the numbers suffering from a disease.

'body packing'
- The practice of smuggling illegal drugs in impermeable plastic wrappings, including condoms, inside body cavities (rectum, vagina, stomach). Packs have leaked and have killed the couriers, who are usually poor people risking their lives for payments that are small in relation to the gains of their employers (exploiters).

bolus   (Gr. *bolos*, clod)
- Quantity of food at moment of swallowing.
- Obsolete term for large **pill**.
- Currently used in pharmacology for an injection (intravenous) of a single dose over a short period (e.g. seconds) as distinct from a continuous infusion.

bombesin   See **drugs as tools**

bootstrapping
- With the continual increase in computation power and decrease in its cost, mathematicians and statisticians have devised ways to substitute theoretical analysis of intractable problems by computation. Bootstrapping can be

thought of as an example of this, and there is much theoretical analysis confirming its validity. The technique of bootstrapping was devised by B Efron, and represents an attempt to reconstruct properties of the population, from which samples have been drawn, using the best information available: the existing samples. It is a form of '**Monte Carlo**' simulation where no particular distribution or model is imposed. The samples are re-sampled, randomly with replacement, a large number of times, and the distribution of the resulting parameters approaches their true population distribution. The name comes from the idea of pulling oneself up by the bootstraps (*TiPS*). It requires no assumptions about underlying distributions.

botulinum toxin   See **drugs as tools**

box and whisker plot   See **quantile**

BP
– British Pharmacopoeia.

BPC
– *British Pharmaceutical Codex* (superseded by **PC**, but still seen in references).

bradykinin   (Gr. *bradus*, slow; *kinein*, to move)
– A nonapeptide **autacoid** produced from a plasma protein precursor. Named because it produces slowly developing contractions of smooth muscle preparations *in vitro*.

brainstorming meeting (slang)
– A group of people convened to tackle a problem by speaking freely whatever even remotely relevant thoughts come into their heads with the objective of generating creative ideas. The meeting is unstructured, the status or seniority of participants is ignored and adverse criticism disallowed in order to maximize the free flow of ideas – though prudence suggests that someone should be designated to bring the meeting to order if that should become necessary. Brainstorming originated in business and marketing practice.
                                          See **consensus meeting**

brand equity/loyalty
              (Ger. *brant*, burn, to show ownership; L. *aequus*, fair; *legalis*, legal)
– "Brand equity may be defined as the difference between the value of the brand to the consumer and the value of the product without that branding. Brand equity drives consumer loyalty, and planning for that brand equity is fundamental to planning for profit, the Procter and Gamble executive advised...
– "Brand loyalty is a complex form of consumer behaviour but it can be measured and it can be managed, he maintained, provided the company is able to offer the best performance at a price that represents good value, market the

right range of product offerings, and is prepared consistently to sell the benefits of loyal use directly or indirectly in its advertising" (*Scrip*).

brand name   See **proprietary name**

bridging studies   (Ger. *brucca*, bridge)
– The transition from phase I clinical studies of a **new active substance** to determine safety and tolerance in healthy volunteers and to allow prediction of the likely effective range of dose in phase II efficacy studies in patients becomes complicated where the disease pathology itself alters the dose–response to the drug; for example where there are differences in receptor physiology or pathology, or in neurotransmitters, as in schizophrenia. In such circumstance phase I studies may include patients under particularly close ethical and scientific monitoring. These studies are called *bridging studies* (*NR Cutler, JJ Sramek*).   See **ethics committee, phases of clinical studies**

buccal drug administration   (L. *bucca*, cheek)
– A dose of a drug in solid form is placed between the cheek and the jaw (buccal sulcus) and allowed to dissolve, offering kinetics similar to that of **sublingual drug administration**.

'bundling'   (Old Eng. *byndelle*, binding)
– A marketing practice whereby the manufacturer/supplier of a drug restricts availability, making supply conditional on acceptance by the prescriber/user of a system of distribution and monitoring (of adverse reactions) designated by the manufacturer, e.g. clozapine *re* agranulocytosis. Bundling, with its removal of monitoring discretion from physicians, can greatly increase the cost of treatment. A significant motive that induces manufacturers to 'bundle' is legal **product liability**, but the medical profession objects to this intervention in clinical practice so much that it is unlikely to achieve wide acceptance.

α-bungarotoxin   See **drugs as tools**

bureaucracy/-t   (L. *burra*, red-brown shaggy cloth used for
                                            covering writing tables; Gr. *kratos*, power)
– A system of administration based on organization in divisions (bureaux) and having a hierarchy of authority. Often used pejoratively, meaning administrative requirements characterized by vexatious complexity, detail, caution and delay; the self-protective occupational disease of bureaucrats. However much bureaucracy is derided, it is essential in technically complex societies. Good bureaucrats facilitate the activities that they administer and govern, and know when to seek independent advice, e.g. from scientists. Therefore, they should be honoured and encouraged, not subjected to mindless abuse. If this is done, perhaps we shall get more good bureaucrats.
– "An organization that cannot correct its behaviour by learning from its mistakes" (*M Crozier*).

– *Administratium:* The heaviest element known to science, discovered on All Fools' Day at a UK nuclear research station. It has neither protons nor electrons and the atomic number is zero. However, it does have one neutron, eight deputy neutrons, 64 vice-neutrons and 256 assistant neutrons. Although completely inert it can be detected chemically because it impedes every reaction with which it comes into contact.

See **management and administration**

bush teas
– A West Indian term for a herbal infusion made from wild plants. Sometimes *Crotalaria fulve,* or other leaves containing toxic pyrrolizidine alkaloids, has been included, leading to veno-occlusive disease of the liver.

$(C_1)_{max}$
- The peak plasma concentration reached after a single dose; or $(C_{inf})_{max}$ during constant infusion, of a drug.

CABAL
- A group of ministers of King Charles II (England) (1630–85) named **C**lifford, **A**shley, **B**uckingham, **A**rlington, and **L**auderdale.
- A small group of powerful intriguers, such as occurs in any large institution or department, academic or otherwise.

cachet   (L. *coactare*, to constrain)
- Powdered drug enclosed in a rice-paper shell, becoming soft and easy to swallow when wet. Obsolete.

cacao (cocoa, chocolate)   (Nahuatl. *cacauatl* tree)
- The seed of *Theobroma cacao* contains about 2% theobromine (a xanthine alkaloid allied to caffeine). It is used to make a drink or a solid confection.

caffeine   (Fr. *café*, coffee, from Arabic *kahwa*)
- A xanthine **alkaloid**, the major active psychostimulant ingredient of **tea**, **coffee** and **cola**. Reputedly, all caffeine-containing plants were in use for beverages before recorded history.   See **xanthines and methylxanthines**

caged   (L. *cavea*, stall, coop)
- Chemical structure in which a labile molecule is embedded to render it stable, but which will release the labile molecule when exposed to an appropriate stimulus, e.g. light. Useful for introducing putative **mediators, second messengers**, etc. into cells, and for the rapid application of **agonists.**
                                                                                 See **targeting of drugs**

calcium antagonist   See **calcium-channel blocker**

calcium-channel blocker
- Drug that prevents the passage of Ca^{2+} ions through calcium channels in the cell membrane. Originally referred to as *calcium antagonists*.

cancer cures   (Gr. *karkinos*, crab; L. *cura*, care)
                                                                                          See **laetrile**

CANDA/CAPLA/CARS
- Computer-assisted/new drug/product licence application/regulatory submission. Regulatory terms for applications in which magnetic media largely replace paper.

cannabinoids   (Gr. *kannabis*, hemp)
- Drugs related to the active constituents of **cannabis**, the most abundant of which is Δ^1-tetrahydrocannabinol (also called Δ^9-tetrahydrocannabinol, depending upon which numbering system is used).   See **anandamines**

cannabis (Gr. *kannabis*, hemp)
– Preparations (flowers, leaves, resin) of *Cannabis sativa* used chiefly for social or recreational purposes. There are many regional names – *ganja* (India), *dagga* (Africa), etc. The principal euphoriant components are designated *cannabinols*. Related compounds are called **cannabinoids**.
See **anandamines**

capsaicin See **drugs as tools**

CAPLA See **CANDA/CAPLA/CARS**

capsule (L. *capsula*, a case)
– A gelatin (usually) shell containing a solid or liquid drug.

captive agonist (L. *capere*, to take; G. *agon*, contest, struggle)
– An agonist with a pharmacodynamic action that greatly outlasts its presence in body fluids, presumably because part of the molecule binds in some way to a part of the cell near the receptor from where the **pharmacophore** can interact with the receptor, e.g. salmeterol (*D Jack*).
See **hit-and-run drug, exosite/exoreceptor**

carcinogen/-icity (Gr. *karkinos*, crab; *gen*, produced)
– Carcinogens are substances that produce a significant increase in tumour incidence when administered at any dose level by any route of administration in any species of animal, as compared to concurrent controls. It has been said that if one cannot produce an increase in the incidence of tumours in some species of animal with some dose of a substance by some route, then one is not trying hard enough.
– A *complete* carcinogen acts both as **initiator** and **tumour promoter**.
See **co-carcinogen**

carcinogenesis (Gr. *karkinos*, crab; *gen*, produced)
– The development of cancer, for example by a **carcinogen**.

carcinoid tumour (Gr. *karkinos*, crab; *eidos*, form; L. *tumor*, swelling)
– A tumour of **argentaffin** cells of the gut (usually), which secretes 5-hydroxytryptamine (**serotonin**) and other **autacoids**; clinically characterized by episodes of bronchospasm, diarrhoea and flushing.

cardiac glycoside (Gr. *kardia*, heart; *glukus*, sweet)
– A glycoside having important effects on the heart. A glycoside is a sugar in which a hydroxyl group has been replaced by another group.

cardioprotection (Gr. *kardia*, heart; L. *pro*, in front; *tegere*, to cover)
– An imprecise term that refers to reduction of the **incidence** and/or severity of 'heart attacks', e.g. by beta-adrenoceptor antagonists.

carminative (L. *carminare*, to card wool)
– An agent that assists in expelling gas from the stomach or intestines, e.g. by relaxing the oesophageal sphincter (e.g. peppermint, dill).

carrier (Middle English, one that carries)
- A molecule, often a protein, that circulates in the blood or extracellular fluid and has **binding sites** for other small molecules (**ligands**) which are then carried in the circulation from their site of origin, or injection, to their site of function.
- A specialized molecule within a cell membrane that binds substances insoluble in the cell membrane and transports/carries them across the membrane (facilitated diffusion/*carrier-mediated diffusion*).

See **diffusion (facilitated), transporter protein**

carry-over effect
- A drug effect that substantially outlasts the duration of its administration.
- In therapeutic trials in which each patient may receive more than one treatment (within-patient comparison) the possibility of carry-over effects must be taken into account in the design, e.g. order and duration of treatment periods, periods of no treatment (**wash-out periods**) which may last about ten half-lives of the withdrawn drug. See **hit-and-run drug**

CARS See **CANDA/CAPLA/CARS**

cascade (L. *cadere*, to fall)
- A series of events, the first leading to the second, which leads to the third, and so on, e.g. the stages of blood coagulation. Amplification at each step is implied.

cascade superfusion (L. *cadere*, to fall; *super*, above, over; *fundere*, pour)
- **Superfusion** of several organ preparations in sequence, with the fluid from one flowing immediately over the next in the sequence. A useful technique for identifying unstable mediators.

case-control study
- Patients with the feature of interest (e.g. an adverse drug reaction) are compared with other patients, not having the feature, but selected so as to be comparable, it is intended, in all other ways, in the hope of detecting causal associations. A **control** group is required (but see **risk, floating absolute risk**). It has all the disadvantages of introducing serious bias that occurs with any **retrospective** study. Such studies have been called **trohoc** (**cohort** spelled backwards) studies. A Feinstein (*Journal of Chronic Diseases* 1981; 34:375) has refined the technique by applying to patients the same criteria for admission as would be used in a randomized controlled trial (**cohort study**) and excluding those who did not meet these criteria, and by introducing stratification for severity of disease (modified case-control study).

See **cohort study**

case reports See **anecdotal studies**

'cash-cow' (L. *capsa*, case, money box; Old Eng. *cu*, cow)
- A medicinal product, usually long established, that, without promotion or advertising, continues to yield profits.

cassette dosing   (Old Fr. *casse*, a container)
- Administration of multiple drugs simultaneously (five or more) and tracking their **pharmacokinetics** and/or other properties.

casuistry   (L. *casus*, case)
- A method of reasoning to derive guidance on decision-taking in situations of moral uncertainty. The modern (1980s) casuist approaches a difficult individual case by reasoning from like (but often extreme) cases about which there is little or no disagreement (because the moral arguments are clear), and uses these to approach gradually the difficult or morally clouded case at issue. For example, it is easy to get general assent that patients have the right to make an informed choice whether or not to participate as a subject of research; and it is fairly easy to get agreement that research may sometimes proceed without individuals' consent (otherwise patients with acute severe illnesses and/or impaired consciousness would become therapeutic orphans). Using these poles of opinion, an approach to an intermediate morally clouded issue can be argued with greater clarity.
- Casuistry, in its traditional form, developed in the Middle Ages. It gained a bad reputation from the use of devious moral reasoning to justify the evasion of moral duties.   See **ethics**, **ethics review committee**

catabolize   (Gr. *kata*, down; *ballo*, throw)
- The complement of **anabolize**, i.e. an enzymatically mediated process in which a chemical group (or groups) is (or are) removed from a molecule.

catalysis/catalyst   (Gr. *kata*, down; *lusein*, to loose or release)
- Effect produced by a substance that, without itself undergoing change, aids/causes a chemical change in other substances: the substance is a catalyst.   See **enzyme**

catalytic subunit   (Gr. *kata*, down; *lusein*, to loose or release;
                                                                        L. *sub*, under; *unus*, one)
- That part of a **multimeric** protein which has enzymatic properties.

catch-phrase or word: cliché   (Fr. *cliché*, a stereotype or cast metal
                                        printing plate; Gr. *stereos*, solid; *tupto*, strike)
- A phrase or word that *catches* one's attention.
- A phrase or word, once memorable for its felicity, when tired from overuse becomes a cliché. The user is perceived to be a bore or even ridiculous or illiterate (below).
- Scientists should be ambitious to write and speak well, and it is greatly to their advantage to have a reputation for doing so.
- If you must employ a cliché, recognize that you are doing so and do not allow its familiarity to deceive you into uncritical misuse; for example, where you wish to say that something is important, do not write "the importance of x cannot be underestimated" (a common error), when what you mean is "cannot be overestimated" or "should not be underestimated".

– Fashions in clichés come and go, and, at the time of writing this, it seems that nothing, including the weather, simply stops; it "*grinds* to a halt".

catecholamine (Probably from Malay *kachu*, a resinous plant substance; *amine*, from Gr. *ammonikos*, of Ammon, a town in Libya)
– Ethylamine derivative of catechol (1,3-dihydroxyphenol). Some catecholamines act as **hormones** or **neurotransmitters**, including **adrenaline (epinephrine), noradrenaline (norepinephrine), dopamine**.

cathartic (Gr. *kathairein*, to purge, purify)
See **purgative**

cation (Gr. *kata*, down, positive; *ion*, going)
– Ion bearing a positive charge (i.e. moves towards the cathode).

causation of injury (L. *causa*, cause; *injurius*, unjust)
– When making a claim in law for drug-caused injury, the Court will use the civil law criterion of 'balance of probability' rather than 'beyond reasonable doubt' which is the criterion of criminal law. See **compensation for injury , liability**

cause, causation (L. *causa*, cause)
– That which produces an effect: regular connection between two events.
– Causation of an association, see adverse drug reaction, science/scientific method (in pharmacology).
– If you think, or just have a 'gut feeling', that a run of ten heads in tossing a (properly made) coin will cause it to be more probable that the next toss will be tails you are a victim of the *gamblers' fallacy*. See **causation of injury**

CD
– **Controlled drug.**

CDER
– Center for Drug Evaluation and Research: The regulatory and scientific body of the **FDA** that oversees the development and marketing of all new drugs.

CDO
– Contract Development Organization.

ceiling (of drug effect) (perhaps from Gr. *caelum*, heaven)
– The maximum effect of which a drug is capable. Drugs of the same therapeutic class may have different ceiling effects according to their different modes or sites of action, e.g. **analgesic** (morphine versus **aspirin**), **diuretic** (frusemide versus hydrochlorothiazide).

cell membranes and biological reactions
– Cell membranes are key sites for biological reactions because the limiting probability for two molecules to collide in three dimensions is vanishingly small, but on a two dimensional membrane it approaches near certainty (*M Eigen*).

censored observations   (L. *censere*, to assess; *observare*, to watch)
- An analysis of a study in which the endpoint is time-to-an-event (outcome) done while some patients in the study have not yet attained that outcome, e.g. an analysis of survival done while some patients remain alive. The word censored lacks its usual pejorative sense.

centile/percentile   (L. *centum*, hundred)
- The value below which a given percentage of values of a set of data lie. Its use avoids the disadvantage of including extreme (outlying) values that may distort a picture as a consequence of unknown factors/peculiarities.
                                                    See **outlier, quantile**

cephalosporins
- **Antibiotics** (numerous) obtained from *Cephalosporium* species fungi. Members of the β-lactam group of antibiotics which includes the penicillins.

CFC
- **Chlorofluorocarbon**

chance   (L. *cadere*, to fall)
- Absence of design or discoverable cause, fortuitous possibility of any occurrence. **Randomization** is used to allow chance to operate (e.g. to form groups in a **therapeutic trial**), which is preferable to allowing human **bias**.

channel   See **ion channel**

channel blockade/-er   See **ion channel blocker**

chaos   (Gr. *chaos*, vast chasm, void)
- A state of confusion.
- A technical term for the irregular, unpredictable and apparently random behaviour of a wide variety of deterministic dynamical systems, such as fluctuating biological populations, cardiac dysrhythmias, oscillating electrical circuits (*RV Jensen*).
- Chaotic systems are characterized by extreme sensitivity to tiny perturbations, whereas the reverse is the case in nonchaotic systems. *Chaos theory* is "an attempt to describe the operation of persistently unstable systems" (*B Jones*).

chaperone/-in   (O. Fr. *chape*, hood or cape)
- Molecular chaperones are proteins that enhance the proper conformational folding of newly-produced proteins and also enhance the assembly of proteins into complexes. Some small proteins appear to be able to fold without the help of chaperones, but many proteins need several passes through a chaperone complex to achieve their final conformation. Many chaperones are **heat shock proteins.**
- The origin of the term (coined in 1987 by UK botanist *RJ Ellis* from the social practice of chaperoning young women), is that molecular chaperones prevent illicit liaisons during the assembly of the new protein.

charcoal, activated (*char*, origin obscure; Sanskrit *jval*, to blaze; L. *actum*, a thing done)

- A preparation of charcoal granules that has been heated to drive off adsorbed water and other substances in order to maximize the adsorptive surface available for taking up such other substances as may be wished. It can be used in gas masks, by the oral route in the treatment of poisoning, and in **haemoperfusion**. Coconut shell is a source of medicinal charcoal.

See **adsorption**, **dialysis**

charybdotoxin See **drugs as tools**

chauvinism in publication (*Nicholas Chauvin*, 19th century French soldier noted for mindless aggressive patriotism)

- It has been pointed out that the nationality of a journal is strongly associated with the nationality of the authors whose work it publishes (which is no surprise). In the case of journals that have achieved international recognition (regardless of whether they are titled 'international') this can lead to adverse effects on the careers of scientists working in countries (small and/or less developed and using minority languages) that have no journals with major international impact that will accord them priority. Whether such internationally successful journals (not having 'international' in their titles) have a *duty* to represent research in a geographically 'balanced' fashion is a matter of debate. For example, does the *New England Journal of Medicine* (publication in which carries prestige) have a duty, first to New England (USA), secondly to the USA in general, and thirdly to the worldwide medical scientific community? In fact the Journal formally promotes itself as a journal "that goes beyond nationality and medical specialty" and suggests to potential advertisers that it makes sense for them to put their new product information in the Journal; in 1997 the *British Journal of Clinical Pharmacology* added to its cover "an *international* journal". In the competitive 'rat race' of modern science, the slogan 'publish or perish' seems to have become 'publish in certain journals or perish', e.g. in journals listed in *Current Contents*.

See **impact factor of a journal**

chelate/chelation (Gr. *khele*, claw)

- Inorganic metal complex in which there is a closed ring of atoms caused by attachment of a ligand to a metal atom at two or more points. Chelating agents coordinate to metal atoms at more than one point and render them biologically inert. They are useful in treating poisoning by metals.

chemical antagonism See **antagonism**

chemokine (Gr. *khemeia*, the art of transmutation, alchemy and so chemical; *kinein*, to move)

- A family of chemotactic **cytokines** with molecular masses of 8–10 kDa having amino acid sequence **homologies** of 20–90%. Their principal role is the recruitment and activation of leukocytes in inflammation. See **chemotaxis**

chemoprophylaxis   (Gr. *khemeia*, the art of transmutation, alchemy
                                and so chemical; *pro*, before; *phulaxis*, guarding)
- Prevention of infective disease by drugs.   See **chemotherapy, prophylaxis**

chemotaxis   (Gr. *khemeia*, the art of transmutation, alchemy
                                        and so chemical; *taxis*, arrangement)
- Process by which mobile cells move towards or away from a source of chemicals such as inflammatory mediators.

chemotherapy   (Gr. *khemeia*, the art of transmutation, alchemy
                                        and so chemical; *therapeuein*, to minister to)
- Term proposed by P Ehrlich (1854–1915, bacteriologist, Germany), who defined it as "use of drugs to injure the invading organism without injury to the host". Despite this definition the term has come to be used in relation to cancer because of the similarities between cancer and infections. Its use as synonym for any drug therapy removes a useful distinction and so is objectionable.   **See cytocidal, cytotoxic**

chemotransmitter   (Gr. *khemeia*, the art of transmutation, alchemy
                                    and so chemical; L. *trans*, across; *mittere*, to send)
                                                        See neurotransmitter

Cheng & Prusoff equation
- Equation originally developed for enzymology. It describes the interaction between substrate, S, and **competitive** inhibitor, I.

$$K_i = IC_{50}/(1 + [S]/K_m)$$

where K_i is the **dissociation equilibrium constant** of I; IC_{50} is the concentration of I which produces a 50 per cent inhibition of the enzyme; K_m is the dissociation equilibrium constant of the substrate; and $[S]$ is the concentration of the substrate.
The pharmacological equivalent of this is:

$$K_A = IC_{50}/(1 + [A]/EC_{50})$$

where K_A is the dissociation equilibrium constant for the competitive antagonist; IC_{50} is the concentration of antagonist that produces half-maximal reduction of effect; $[A]$ is the concentration of agonist; and EC_{50} is the midpoint **location parameter** for the concentration–effect curve.
- Another form of the equation is sometimes used in radioligand-binding assays:

$$K_i = IC_{50}/(1 + [L]/K_L)$$

where K_i is the dissociation equilibrium constant of the competing (nonradiolabelled) ligand; IC_{50} is the concentration of competing ligand causing 50 per cent inhibition of specific binding of the radioligand; $[L]$ is the concentration of the radioligand; and K_L is the dissociation equilibrium constant of the radioligand. When $[L]$ is much less than K_L then K_i approximates to the IC_{50}. When

the radioligand occupies a significant fraction of the binding sites, the curve is displaced to the right by a factor of $(1 + [L]/K_L)$.
- The Cheng–Prusoff relationship only applies when the agonist produces a **hyperbolic** concentration–effect curve (or binding curve) and when the antagonism (displacement) is strictly competitive. Unlike the *Schild equation*, use of this modified Cheng & Prusoff equation does not give any indication whether or not the interaction is competitive.

See **ligand–binding assay, Schild equation/plot**

'cherry picking' (Slang: refers to a small fruit of a *Prunus* tree having a short season and considered delectable)
- The selective use in argument or publication of only those results or studies that support the author's preconceived or interested position.

See **data dredging**

child-resistant closures See **packaging and safety**

chimeric receptor (Gr. *chaimera*, she-goat, monster)
- **Receptor** synthesized by **genetic engineering** techniques so that it is composed of protein sequences from two or more types of receptor. Useful in determining the function of different parts of receptor molecules. (In Greek mythology the Chimera was a fire-breathing monster, with a lion's head, a goat's body and a serpent's tail; it was killed by Bellerophon.)

chirality (Gr. *kheir*, hand)
- If a carbon atom in a molecule has four different substituents, the molecule can exist as two **optical isomers** which are mirror images and therefore not superimposable (a pair of human hands is chiral). Such a carbon atom is called a *chiral centre*. Ordinary chemical syntheses usually produce equal amounts of the isomers – a **racemic** mixture. Pharmacological or toxicological activity often resides only, or predominantly, in one isomer; the therapeutically inactive isomer is thus '*isomeric ballast*' (Ariëns). Sometimes pharmacodynamic activity resides in one isomer and toxic activity in the other. If the isomer with the desired activity can be synthesized or separated from an inactive isomer ('resolved'), the drug will be twice as potent, which may matter little. If the other isomer is toxic, such a synthesis or separation will produce a less toxic drug, which matters a lot. Medicines regulatory authorities have turned their attention to chirality.
- *Composite chiral drugs* are mixtures of **stereoisomers**.
- *Homochiral drugs* are single stereoisomers.

See **eudismic-affinity quotient**

chi-square (χ^2) distribution (*chi* (χ) is the 22nd letter of the **Greek alphabet**)
- Chi-square is a **probability density function** that describes the variability from sample to sample of the **variance** calculated from each sample. Most commonly encountered as an approximate statistical test that is used to see whether or not the differences between a set of observed frequencies and the

frequencies that we expected (according to some hypothesis) can plausibly be attributed to **random** sampling errors. For example, it is used to test for association in **contingency tables**, or to test goodness of fit of a theoretical **probability distribution** to observations. This approximate test should now be supplanted by the **Fisher exact test** when $n < 20$ in 2×2 contingency tables.

chi-square (χ^2) test   (*chi* (χ) is the 22nd letter of the **Greek alphabet**)
- A statistical test for the comparison of characteristics of more than two groups. It involves comparison of observed differences and those that may be expected to arise by chance, i.e. **contingency**. It is particularly useful for testing the presence (or absence) of association between characteristics that cannot be expressed quantitatively, e.g. eye colour.

chlorofluorocarbons (CFCs)
- **Aerosol** propellants and refrigerants that have adverse environmental effects (on the ozone layer of the atmosphere). They are replaced in metered dose inhalers by hydrofluoroalkanes which do not have this effect.
See **inhalation of drugs**

cholagogue   (Gr. *khole*, bile; *agogos*, drawing forth)
- Agent that induces bile flow into the intestine. When this is accomplished by stimulating the gallbladder to contract, the more specific term *cholecystagogue* may be used.   See **choleretic**

cholecystagogue   (Gr. *khole*, bile; *kistis*, bladder; *agogos*, drawing forth)
See **cholagogue**

cholera toxin   See **drugs as tools**

choleretic   (Gr. *khole*, bile; *eresis*, removal)
- Agent that stimulates the formation of bile.   See **cholagogue**

cholestasis   (Gr. *khole*, bile, gall; *statikos*, causing to stand)
- An arrest in the flow of bile due to obstruction in small passages (e.g. by oedema and cellular infiltration) or by reduced bile production. Occurs as an allergic drug reaction (e.g. to chlorpromazine), giving rise to cholestatic jaundice.

cholinergic drugs   ([acetyl] Gr. *khole*, bile; *ergon*, work)
- Cholinergic drugs mimic the effects of acetylcholine. (The use of the term *cholinergic* to describe a drug is not desirable on etymological grounds as it implies that the drug works by releasing acetylcholine, e.g. by activating cholinergic nerves. The term **cholinomimetic** is preferred.)
See **-ergic, parasympathomimetic**

cholinergic nerve   ([acetyl] Gr. *khole*, bile; *ergon*, work)
- A nerve that releases acetylcholine as a transmitter.   See **-ergic**

cholinoceptor   See **acetylcholine**

cholinomimetic   ([acetyl] Gr. *khole*, bile; *mimeisthai*, to imitate)
— Drug mimicking the effects of **acetylcholine**.

chromatography   (Gr. *khroma*, colour; *graphein*, to write)
— Technique for the separation of chemicals/**species** by virtue of their differing
   physicochemical properties. For example affinity chromatography, column
   chromatography, paper chromatography, thin-layer chromatography (TLC),
   gas liquid chromatography (GLC), high-pressure (or -performance) liquid
   chromatography (HPLC), high-performance thin-layer chromatography
   (HPTLC).   See **affinity, polar/-ity**

chromodacryorrhoea   (Gr. *khroma*, colour; *dakryon*, tear; *rheo*, flow)
— A flow of tears containing a red pigment from the Harderian gland. Occurs in
   rats overdosed with **cholinomimetic** drugs, especially **anticholinesterases**.

chronic   (Gr. *khronos*, time)
— Long-lasting; the antonym of **acute**.
— The colloquial use of *chronic* to mean severe is widespread and erroneous
   and probably irreversible.

chronobiotic   (Gr. *khronos*, time; *bios*, life)
— Drug having a capacity to modify **circadian** systems.

chronopharmacology   (Gr. *khronos*, time; *pharmakon*, drug; *logy*, study of)
— The study of the action of drugs over periods of time and in relation to biological rhythms.
— The alterations of response to drugs consequent on the passage of time, e.g.
   cyclophosphamide treatment of mouse leukaemia is maximally effective in the
   afternoon and maximally toxic in the morning.
— The prefix *chrono-* is used with many pharmacological terms, e.g. *chrono-
   therapeutics*.   See **circadian, nyctohemeral**

chronotropic   (Gr. *khronos*, time; *tropos*, a turn)
— Affecting rate, e.g. of the heart (positive chronotropism means an increased
   heart rate).

chrysotherapy   (Gr. *khrusos*, gold; *therapeia*, healing)
— Medicinal treatment with gold derivatives, e.g. for rheumatoid arthritis.

-cide/-al   (L. *cidium*, a killing)
— Suffix meaning kill, e.g. bacteri*cidal*.

chunk sample   (*chunk*, etymology uncertain)
                                                         See **convenience sample**

cinchona/cinchonism   (from the Countess of Chinchon, Spain, 17th century)
— The bark of a species of *Cinchona* tree, South America, containing the anti-

malarial alkaloid, quinine. The clinical picture of poisoning is called *cincho-nism*. The Countess of Chinchon, wife of the Spanish Viceroy of Peru, is reputed to have brought the bark to Europe in 1638, but in fact she died before she returned to Spain – "...who took it there, and when, will probably never be settled" (*Encyclopaedia Britannica*).

circa (abbreviation *c.*)   (L. about)
– Particularly used with imprecise numbers, e.g. dates, day (**circadian**).

circadian   (L. *circa*, about; *dies*, day)
– Occurring or recurring *about* once a day (24 hours).   See **nyctohemeral**

cis-/trans- isomerism   (L. *cis-*, on this side of; *trans-*, on the other side of)
– Where two carbon atoms are joined by a double bond, the atoms are not free to rotate as they are when joined by a single bond. Substituents on the two carbons are therefore fixed in their orientation. If two substituents on the two carbons are arranged on opposite sides of the double bond, the structure is *trans*; if on the same side, the structure is *cis*.   See **isomerism**

citation index   See **science citation index**

CL
– **Clearance.**

classical receptor theory   See **receptors**

clathrate   (Gr. *klethra*, lattice bars)
– Compound formed by physical trapping of molecules of one substance in spaces in the crystal lattice of another. No chemical bond is formed between the host compound and the trapped molecule. For example, each water molecule associates (through dipole bonds) with four other water molecules to form an ice lattice. **Hydrophobic** general anaesthetic molecules promote clathrate formation with water associated with neuronal membranes, and these clathrates block ion transport across membranes, stabilizing them.

clavulanic acid
– Clavulanic acid (made by *Streptomyces clavigerus*) inactivates β-lactamases (penicillinases), thus protecting β-lactam antimicrobials from destruction. It is a **suicide (enzyme) inhibitor**.

clearance (CL)   (L. *clarus*, clear)
– The rate of removal of a substance from the blood as it passes through an organ (e.g. liver, kidney) expressed as a *notional volume* of blood plasma that is totally cleared of the substance in unit *time*. If the blood flow through the organ is Q (volume/time), and the concentrations of the substance in the blood entering and leaving the organ are C_{in} (mass/volume) and C_{out} (mass/volume), respectively, then:

$CL = Q(C_{in} - C_{out})/C_{in}$ (units of CL are volume per unit time, usually ml min^{-1}).

– Clearance is the **proportionality constant** for the removal of a substance from the blood by **first-order kinetics.**   See **extraction ratio**

clinical impression   (L. *clinicus*, one on a sick bed, from Gr. *kline*, bed;
L. *im*, in; *premere*, to press)

– The statement by clinicians that patients do better with this or that treatment is due to their having formed an opinion that more patients are helped by the treatment they advocate than by other treatments. The opinion is based on numbers, but having omitted to record exactly how many patients have been treated by different methods and having omitted to ensure that the only variable factor affecting the patient was the treatment in question, only a 'clinical impression', instead of facts, can be stated. This is a pity, for progress is delayed when convinced opinions are offered in place of convincing facts. The former, although not necessarily wrong, are frequently incorrect, despite the great assurance with which they are often advanced. This is not to dismiss the anecdotal clinical survey or the case-report, for they tell what *can* happen, which is useful, although causation remains inconclusive. Also, formal therapeutic trials are frequently carried out because someone has formed an impression which is thought to deserve testing.
See **evidence-based medicine,** *post hoc ergo propter hoc*, **science/
scientific method (in pharmacology), statistics, therapeutic trial**

clinical pharmacology   (L. *clinicus*, one on a sick bed, from Gr. *kline*, bed;
pharmakon, drug; *logy*, study of)

– All aspects of the scientific study of drugs in man.
– It broadly comprises:
  – *Pharmacology* (pharmacodynamics, pharmacokinetics).
  – Therapeutic evaluation.
  – *Control*: rational prescribing, official medicines regulation, social aspects of use and misuse, pharmacoeconomics.   See **pharmacology**

clinical research   (L. *clinicus*, one on a sick bed, from Gr. *kline*, bed;
L. *re*, again; *circare*, to go round in a circle or search)

– Clinical research may be broadly divided into:
  – *Therapeutic*: where the subject may expect/hope to gain personal benefit.
  – *Nontherapeutic*: where the intention is to advance knowledge without any expectation/possibility that the subject, who may be a healthy volunteer or a patient, will gain personal benefit.
See **clinical pharmacology, Declaration of Helsinki, research**

clinical significance or importance   (L. *signum*, a sign; *facere*, to make;
importare, to be of consequence)

– The outcome of a therapeutic trial may show a difference between two treatments that is *statistically significant*. But very small differences can often be measured and **statistical significance** does not necessarily imply that the difference is *clinically important (significant)*, i.e. sufficient to persuade clinicians that it should influence their practice. To avoid misunderstanding it is better to speak of *clinical importance* rather than clinical significance. It is desirable, before a trial begins, for the clinicians to state what level of difference they will regard as worthwhile or important.

clinical trial   (L. *clinicus*, one on a sick bed, from Gr. *kline*, bed;
Old Fr. *trier*, to sort, sift)
- Any systematic study on medicinal products in human subjects, whether in patients or nonpatient volunteers, in order to discover or verify the effects of, and/or identify any adverse reaction to, investigational products, and/or to study their absorption, distribution, metabolism and excretion in order to ascertain the efficacy and safety of the products (*European Community definition*).   See **therapeutic trial**

clinical trials, unreported
- In 1997 over 100 medical journal editors addressed the problem of unpublished **clinical trials.** They agreed that:
  - Many controlled trials (especially those that do not show the sponsor's drug to be superior) are not submitted for publication and that this
  - Reduces the power of **systematic reviews** or **meta-analyses** to detect moderate but clinically important treatment effects (delayed publication of negative results can also **bias** reviews).
  - Trials that do not show promising effects (negative trials) are less likely to be submitted for publication [or be acceptable to editors] which can give rise to misleading conclusions about therapeutic efficacy.
  - Patients may be asked to participate in new studies designed to answer questions that have already been answered.
- The journals sought to remedy this problem by declaring what they called an 'amnesty' (inappropriate word) for authors and invited them to complete an *Unreported trial registration form*, the information to be disseminated on a web site and in other ways. The journal editors have published this offer, for example, *Lancet* 1997;350:756.
                              See **clinical trial, International Committee of Medical**
Journal Editors, therapeutic trial

clioquinol: iodochlorhydroxyquinoline (Entero-Vioform)
- A weak amoebicide that has had widespread popular use for travellers' diarrhoea (generally due to viruses, bacteria or toxins), although there was never much evidence of efficacy. In the late 1960s there was, in Japan, an epidemic of an unusual neurological syndrome of moderately rapid onset, involving the spinal cord, optic nerves and peripheral nerves (hence the name, *subacute myelo-optic-neuropathy or SMON*). The condition was associated with a high consumption of clioquinol and was almost confined to Japan. The drug is not the only causative factor, and hypotheses abound. The pharmaceutical company and the Japanese government joined to compensate the victims. There were many thousands of cases.   See **accidents**

clone   (Gr. *klon*, a young twig or shoot used in plant propagation)
- Cell or cells derived from a single cell by asexual reproduction so that all have

identical genetic constitution. Hence **monoclonal antibody**. The verb 'to clone' means to produce such cells.

- Receptors can be cloned by inserting the gene for that receptor into a suitable cell-line (usually a cell-line which does not normally express the receptor in question, e.g. Chinese hamster ovary). This results in the production of a colony of identical cells, each containing a large number of the receptor under study. See **receptor** (*Cloned receptors*)

co-agonist See **primary agonist**

coated tablet (L. *cotta,* a coat; *tabula*, table)
- Coated Tablets (official name) are tablets covered with one or more layers of mixtures of various substances such as natural or synthetic resins, gums, gelatin, inactive and insoluble fillers, sugars, plasticizers, polyhydric alcohols, waxes, authorized colouring matter and sometimes flavouring agents. The coating may also contain active ingredients. Substances used as coatings are usually applied as a solution or suspension in conditions in which evaporation of the vehicle occurs. When the coating is very thin, the tablets are described as *film-coated* (**BP**).
- The functions of the coating include protection of the tablet, control of disintegration and release of the drug, to eliminate taste and to allow visual identification. See **enteric-coating, tablet**

co-axial bioassay (L. *co, com/cum, con*, with, together, in common, jointly, equally, reciprocally, mutually; *axis*, axle)
- **Bioassay** in which a strip of one type of tissue is set up within the lumen of another type of tissue, e.g. an aortic strip within a trachea (*Fernandez et al.*; *British Journal of Pharmacology* 1989;96:117). Used to detect the release of very labile **mediators**.

co-axial stimulation (L. *co, com/cum, con*, with, together, in common, jointly, equally, reciprocally, mutually; *axis*, axle)
- Field stimulation of an isolated hollow, cylindrical organ *in vitro* (e.g. guinea-pig ileum) by means of two electrodes, one of which is a rod running the length of the lumen, the other a parallel rod in the organ bath outside the lumen. Sometimes loosely called **transmural stimulation**.

coca (Peruvian *cuca*)
- The dried leaves of *Erythroxylon coca* (South America, Indonesia), the natural source of **cocaine**. The drink Coca-Cola, of worldwide popularity, contained cocaine when it was first introduced, but this was eliminated many years ago. It still contains **caffeine** derived from **cola**.

cocaine
- An alkaloid from the South American shrub *Erythroxylon coca* – the first successful local (topical) **anaesthetic** drug. Although still occasionally used for this, it has been superseded by synthetic **congeners** having names ending in -caine.

– A major social drug of abuse. The water-soluble hydrochloride has been largely replaced by '**crack**', the heat-volatile **free base**.

co-carcinogen   (L. *co, com/cum, con*, with, together, in common, jointly, equally, reciprocally, mutually; Gr. *karkinos*, crab; *gen*, to produce)

– An agent which by itself does not induce cancer, but which, when applied to a tissue before, with or after a **carcinogen**, leads to increased or accelerated tumour formation.

(the) Cochrane Collaboration   (established 1993 in memory of *Archie Cochrane*, 1909–1988, epidemiologist, UK.)

– An international network of clinical scientists and others, preparing, maintaining and disseminating **systematic reviews** of (primarily) **randomized controlled (therapeutic) trials**. These are published as the Cochrane Database of Systematic Reviews (a part of the Cochrane Library) on CD-ROM, issued quarterly, also on the Internet (general@cochrane.co.uk). The Cochrane Library also maintains a Cochrane Controlled Trials Register.

See **meta-analysis**

Cochrane plot

– A method for displaying the individual and overall **odds ratios** in a **meta-analysis** or a stratified-design trial. The x-axis is the range of odds ratios. The individual odds ratios (for each **therapeutic trial** or for each *stratum* of a stratified-design trial) (see **stratification**) are plotted one above the other, each represented by a short vertical line drawn across a rectangle, the length of the rectangle on the x-axis representing the confidence interval of each estimate of the odds ratio. The size of the sample used to calculate each value is represented by a solid diamond drawn on the line representing each odds ratio. The overall odds ratio is represented by a line drawn vertically through an unfilled diamond, the horizontal dimension of which latter represents the confidence interval of the overall odds ratio.

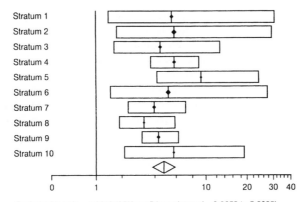

Pooled odds ratio = 4.6816 (95% confidence interval = 3.8659 to 5.6695)

See **Mantel–Haenzsel method**

codon (L. *codex*, book)
- A sequence of three bases (a triplet) in DNA which codes for an amino acid.

coefficient of variation (L. *co, com/cum, con*, with, together, in common, jointly, equally, reciprocally, mutually; *ex-*, before; *facere*, to make, to do; *variare*, to vary)
- The **standard deviation** expressed as a percentage of the **mean**.

coffee (Arabic *kahwa*; Turkish *kahveh*; Dutch *Koffie*)
- A berry (bean) of the plant *Coffea arabica* (or *robusta*), a native of Kaffa, Ethiopia.
- *C. arabica* beans contain 1% caffeine and *C. robusta* 2%; *arabica* is often preferred for taste. Caffeine-free *C. arabica* plants have been developed (1998).
- *Decaffeinated coffee* is prepared by using solvents, methylene chloride, ethyl acetate, water (containing the chemical components of beans except caffeine; the Swiss water process), or supercritical carbon dioxide. The caffeine recovered is often sold to soft-drink manufacturers and to pharmaceutical companies (*SN Katz, Scientific American* 1997;276:124).
See **xanthines and methylxanthines**

cognition enhancer (L. *cognitio*, apprehend; *en*, put in; *altus*, high)
- Agents that enhance attentiveness and the acquisition, storage and retrieval (memory) of information by a variety of mechanisms.
- Drug that increases the ability of the brain to process complex tasks. In the pharmaceutical industry such drugs for therapeutic use against Alzheimer's disease are highly sought after in view of the increasing prevalence of dementia as the population of the planet continues to age. Cognition enhancers are also sought by those wishing to perform better in examinations and similar circumstances. Few drugs have been shown unequivocally and reliably to enhance mental capacity to an important extent; many drugs impair capacity.

cohort/study/analysis (L. *cohors*, company of soldiers; *studere*, to be diligent; Gr. *ana*, up; *luein*, loosen)
- A cohort is a large group of individuals having a shared characteristic.
- A large group of subjects is monitored continuously, **prospectively**. Such studies are more reliable than retrospective **case-control studies**, but are tedious and expensive to perform.
- Strictly, the term cohort in epidemiology is used in relation to a population defined by its birth year or years. It is not properly applied to a group of persons selected by exposure to an environmental factor, e.g. a drug, though this usage is common.
- Cohort studies may be experimental (**therapeutic trials**) or **observational**; a **control** group is required.

cola
- Nuts of the plant *Cola vera*. They contain **caffeine** (about 2%) and are used in cola drinks. See **xanthines and methylxanthines**

cold chain
– Medicinal products required to be stored under refrigerated condition, e.g. vaccines, must be maintained between 2°C and 8°C during transit from manufacturer to user. Carriage may be by means of air, sea, or land transport and vigilance is required to ensure that refrigerated conditions are maintained at all times during such a distribution chain, that is, a *cold chain.*
– Although manufacturers normally deliver their products to some central point such as a regional centre or base hospital, the cold chain may have to be extended over many kilometres, possibly in hot conditions, to outlying clinics or vaccination centres. Special cooling systems, which ensure uninterrupted refrigeration temperature both during storage and transport have been developed (after **PC**).

colloidal solution (sol)/suspension (Gr. *kolla*, glue; *eidos*, form; L. *solutus*, free; *sub*, beneath; *pendere*, to hang)
– Multimolecular particles dispersed in a liquid medium. The particles are too small to be seen by an ordinary light microscope and do not sediment readily as in ordinary suspensions. The suspension may be reversible or nonreversible. Various forms are known as **gels** and **emulsions**. See **aerosol**

combinatorial chemistry (L. *co, com/cum, con*, with, together, in common, jointly, equally, reciprocally, mutually; *bini*, two together; Arabic *khemeia*, the art of transmutation)
– *Combinatorial chemistry* involves the random mixing and matching of large numbers of chemical building blocks (amino acids, nucleotides, simple chemicals) to produce 'libraries' of all possible combinations. This technology can generate **billions** of new compounds that are initially evaluated using an automated *robotic high-throughput screen* that can handle thousands of compounds a day. These screens utilize radio-labelled ligand displacement on single human **receptor** subtypes or enzymes on nucleated (eukaryotic) cells. If the **screen** records a positive response the compound is further investigated using traditional laboratory methods, and the molecule is manipulated to modify **selectivity** and/or **potency**. See **ligand–binding assay**

committee (working party and task force) (L. *co, com/cum, con*, with, together, in common, jointly, equally, reciprocally, mutually; *mittere*, to put)
– A group of people formed to perform a specified service or function. Committees are essential, and anyone working in a substantial institution would be wise to acquire committee skills, if only for self-preservation.
– A committee (or sub-committee) appointed to investigate a problem is called a *working party* or *task force* and is too often used to diffuse responsibility that the originating committee is fearful of taking.
– Committees have an upside insofar as they get things done, but a downside that leads to them being much despised, e.g.:
  – A committee is a group of men [sic] who individually can do nothing, but as a group decide that nothing can be done (*F Allen*, 1894–1956, USA).
  – A committee is a group of the unwilling, chosen from the unfit to do the un-

necessary (*Anon*). But some people are drawn (unhealthily) to seek membership as a source of personal influence and prestige.
- A camel is a horse designed by a committee (*A Issigonis*, 1906–1988, UK, engineer and designer speaking of his dislike of working in teams).
- AB Bergman recommended 'all-out war' on the 'rampant phenomenon' of 'meeting mania' (*New England Journal of Medicine* 1994;330:1622). A few months later a correspondent (*RM Wachter*) reported that the University of California had set up a committee to consider the matter.
- *Commitology*: **EU** jargon (Eurospeak) for "the proliferation of committees with considerable powers and unclear reporting lines and accountability" (*Scrip*, Nov 1, 1994).   See **agenda, upside/downside**

Committee on Safety of Medicines (UK)
- This group of independent advisers was set up under advice to the government from the **Medicines Commission**. It gives advice only (it does not regulate) to the Licensing Authority (in theory the Ministers of Health) via the Medicines Control Agency (which is the arm of government operating the Medicines Act).   See **QUANGO, regulation (official) of medicines**

company observational postmarketing study (COPS)
- A form of **post-marketing surveillance** noted for according promotional values priority over science.

compartment
(L. *co, com/cum, con*, with, together, in common, jointly, equally, reciprocally, mutually; *partiri*, to apportion)
- For pharmacological purposes, a region of the body (blood, extracellular fluid, intracellular fluid, fat, muscle, brain) within which the concentration of a drug is taken to be uniform at all times, although it may be different from the concentration of the drug in other compartments, due to the physicochemical characteristics of the drug. The blood is commonly deemed the 'central' compartment and, with unequal distribution, the kinetics of a drug may be described as in one, two, three, etc. compartments.
                    See **distribution of drugs, efflux coefficient**

compassionate drug use
(L. *co, com/cum, con*, with, together, in common, jointly, equally, reciprocally, mutually; *pati*, suffer)
- Restriction of the supply of medicines to those that are officially licensed is intended to protect the public. But sometimes, in resistant or desperate cases of disease, when licensed medicines are inadequate, the last hope for a patient may lie with a drug that has not passed through the licensing process for one reason or another. National medicines laws ordinarily, in one way or another, permit the supply of an unlicensed medicine in these restricted circumstances, termed (single patient) compassionate use or supply (USA). In the UK the Medicines Act provision for supply of an unlicensed product "for administration to a particular patient" is known as the *named patient exemption*. It is not permissible to exploit this exemption from regulatory requirement in order to conduct research.   See **unlabeled (off label) use**

compatibility (of medicines)   See **incompatibility**

compensation for injury due to participation in research
— Although serious injury caused by participation in **research** is rare, (research) **ethics committees** have long seen it as an important role to ensure that if something goes wrong, research subjects are adequately compensated. There are *four elements* to compensation:
  — The circumstances in which compensation becomes payable and, in particular, whether payment depends on proof of negligence under the ordinary law, or will be made even if there is no-one at fault;
  — The machinery for compensation: litigation in the courts, with its attendant expense and delay, or a speedy, more informal process;
  — The provision of full information on these issues to research subjects so that they may take it into account in deciding whether to participate; (see **consent**).
  — The mundane but important question: if compensation is payable, whatever the basis, will the money actually be available?
                    See **contract, ex gratia payment, liability, negligence**

competition/competitive antagonism/inhibition   (L. *co, com/cum, con,* with, together, in common, jointly, equally, reciprocally, mutually; *petere,* to seek; Gr. *anti,* against; *agon,* contest; L. *inhibere,* to restrain)
— An **antagonist** that inhibits the response to an **agonist** by excluding the agonist from its **receptor** by occupying the same receptor (or sufficiently nearly the same site to result in **steric exclusion** of the agonist, i.e. the receptor can bind only one drug molecule at a time), is said to be acting by competition. The agonist and antagonist compete for the same receptor. This results in a parallel shift of the equilibrium response–log concentration curve for the agonist (see **Schild plot**). The maximal response is not reduced, because increasing the concentration of agonist sufficiently allows the agonist to replace the antagonist on the receptors by binding during the periods for which no antagonist happens to be on them. The term **competitive** is often used to describe antagonism that is **surmountable**. There is no general agreement about whether very slowly reversible (or irreversible) antagonists that compete with the agonist for unoccupied receptors should be called competitive. They clearly satisfy the definition given above, but it may not be practicable to measure responses at equilibrium (which will take a long time to achieve) for such drugs, and if equilibrium is not achieved, the drug may appear to be not competitive. Some would argue that it is better to reserve the term 'competitive' for interactions that fulfil the law of **mass action**, i.e. reactions that come to equilibrium. The term **syntopic**, which implies only that the two drugs act at the same site, avoids this confusion.
— If the agonist and antagonist form only short-lasting combinations with the receptor, so that equilibrium between agonist, antagonist and receptors is reached during the presence of the agonist, the antagonism will be *surmountable* over a wide range of concentrations (*reversible competitive antagonism*). In contrast, some antagonists, when in close enough proximity to their binding

site, may form a stable **covalent bond** with it (*irreversible competitive antagonism*), and the antagonism becomes *insurmountable* when no spare receptors remain (see **receptor** (*Spare receptors*)). More generally, the extent to which the action of a competitive antagonist can be overcome by increasing the concentration of antagonist is determined by the relative concentrations of the two agents, by their association and dissociation rate constants for their binding, and by the duration of the exposure to each. The action of a competitive antagonist can therefore be surmountable under one set of experimental conditions and insurmountable under another (**IUPHAR**, with permission; *Pharmacological Reviews* 1995;47:255–266).

See **block, non-equilibrium antagonists**

complement   (L. *co, com/cum, con*, with, together, in common, jointly, equally, reciprocally, mutually; *plere*, to fill)
– A system of proteins, circulating in blood, that combine with antibody to destroy bacteria and other cells. At present it comprises at least 17 proteins.

See **anaphylatoxin**

complementary medicine/s   (L. *co, com/cum, con*, with, together, in common, jointly, equally, reciprocally, mutually; *plere*, to fill; *medere*, to heal)
– The term is used to embrace traditional medical systems; also cults. The essential feature is that the practices and beliefs are not supported by scientific evidence. Any practice supported by scientific evaluation becomes, by definition, part of scientific medicine. In general, complementary medicine comprises cults or practices occupying niches where conventional scientific medicine has little or nothing to offer, or is not available. The term *alternative* medicine makes a much larger claim than does *complementary* medicine, which is the preferred term.
– For licensing of complementary medicines see **homoeopathy.**

See **cult, regulation (official) of medicines**

complex   (L. *co, com/cum, con*, with, together, in common, jointly, equally, reciprocally, mutually; *plectere*, to braid)
– A compound in which atoms or groups are bound to metal atoms or ions by co-ordinate bonds.
– More generally, an aggregate of two or more molecules. By convention at least one of the reacting **species** is a macromolecule, e.g. drug–receptor complex, antigen–antibody complex.

compliance   (Sp. *complir*, to complete, to do what is fitting)
– Strict *adherence* to a prescribed treatment plan.
– There are two kinds of compliance – *doctor* compliance and *patient* compliance:
  – *Doctor compliance*: the extent to which the behaviour of doctors fulfils their duty not to be ignorant, to adopt **evidence-based** advances, to refrain from inappropriate prescribing, to tell patients what they need to know and to warn, i.e. to recognize the importance of the act of prescribing.

- *Patient compliance*: the extent to which the behaviour of patients coincides with medical advice or instructions; action in accordance with advice. Patient non-compliance with the prescriber's instructions has three major aspects:
  - nonretention of oral instructions, or nonreading of written instructions
  - comprehension of instructions, but failure to carry them out
  - noncomprehension of instructions, so that the patient cannot comply.
- The terms **concordance**, *adherence* (L. *adhere*, to stick to, to follow closely) now often are advocated as seemingly less authoritarian.
- In *research*, where strict **protocols** are necessary for scientific validity, the term *compliance* is entirely appropriate and is applied to both the investigator and the research subject.   See **monitored dosage systems**

compliance (physical)
- A measure of distensibility – the change in volume for unit change in (transmural) pressure. Compliance is the reciprocal of elastance.

composite chiral drugs   See **chirality**

composite event   (L. *co, com/cum, con*, with, together, in common, jointly, equally, reciprocally, mutually; *ponere*, to put; *e(x)*, out; *venire*, come)
- An event that is considered to have occurred if any one of several different outcomes is observed (**FDA**).

compound 48/80   See **drugs as tools**

computer   (L. *co, com/cum, con*, with, together, in common, jointly, equally, reciprocally, mutually; *putare*, to think)
- A device (usually electronic) that processes data or makes calculations according to a set of instructions.
- An *analog* computer uses a continuous input of a variable physical quantity, e.g. voltage, to represent numbers. It is used in monitoring systems. It has no storage capacity.
- A *digital* computer uses a discrete input of data, a set of instructions (program) written in an appropriate programming 'language', e.g. **FORTRAN** (**for**mula **tran**slation), **ALGOL** (**algo**rithmic **o**riented **l**anguage), **BASIC** (**be**ginners' **a**ll-purpose **s**equential **i**nstruction **c**ode). It has huge storage capacity.
- Computers enormously outperform humans for speed, storage capacity and reliability, but their utility is totally dependent on competent programming, hence the aphorism, '**garbage in, garbage out**' (GIGO). Despite the etymology of computer, computers cannot yet think, only calculate.

computer pests
- *Viruses*: "Small but deadly, readily transmitted but with unpredictable latencies, capable of widespread infection and with the ability to replicate but un-

able to live outside a host – computer viruses sound startlingly like the real thing. They originate with a programmer, perhaps one who is bored with standard tasks or hacking (gaining unauthorized access to other computer systems)...The essential component is a set of instructions which, when executed, copies itself onto previously unaffected programs or files. Sometimes after a specified number of replications or on a specific date, the virus executes whatever other instructions have been encoded, e.g. displaying a message, subtly altering data, or destroying files. Even without activation the virus can cause damage by replicating and consuming disk storage space, networking connections, and computer time" (*Lancet*).
– Viruses are similar to, but should not be confused with other computer pests – *bombs* and *Trojan horses*, which cannot replicate, and *worms*, which are self-contained and do not infect other programs (*Lancet*).

concanavalin A   See **drugs as tools**

concentration   (L. *co, com/cum, con*, with, together, in common,
                          jointly, equally, reciprocally, mutually; Gr. *kentron*, sharp point)
– The amount (mass or weight) of dissolved substance in a given volume.
– Amount/volume.
– Use of *level* where *concentration* is intended is undesirable, as being less precise.
– Concentrations (percentage):
  – The term *'per cent'* or the symbol '%' is used with one of four different meanings in the expression of concentrations according to circumstances:
  – Per cent w/w (% w/w) (percentage weight in weight) expresses the number of grams of solute in 100 g of product.
  – Per cent w/v (% w/v) (percentage weight in volume) expresses the number of grams of solute in 100 ml of product.
  – Per cent v/v (% v/v) (percentage volume in volume) expresses the number of millilitres of solute in 100 ml of product.
  – Per cent v/w (% v/w) (percentage volume in weight) expresses the number of millilitres of solute in 100 g of product.
  – The term *percent* used without qualification means, for mixtures of solids and semisolids, percent weight in weight; for solutions or suspensions of solids in liquids, percent weight in volume; for solutions of liquids in liquids, percent volume in volume; and for solutions of gases in liquids, percent weight in volume. For example a 1 percent solution is prepared by dissolving 1 g of a solid or semisolid, or 1 ml of a liquid, in sufficient solvent to make 100 ml of the solution.
– In some areas of clinical practice the expression of concentrations (w/v) as 1 in 1000 or 1 in 10 000 is used because found convenient. But confident calculations of dose, e.g. of adrenaline (epinephrine), by weight from fluid volumes designated by dilution are best and most safely made by people having daily familiarity with this system (**BP**).
Note: 1 in 1000 means 1 gram (1000 mg) of drug in 1000 ml liquid, i.e. 1 mg/ml, or 0.1%; and 1 in 10 000 is 100 micrograms/ml (100 μg/ml), or 0.01%.
                                                    See **displacement values**

concentration–effect curve   See **dose–response curve**

concentration ratio (*r*)
- The term is used to describe the effect of an **antagonist**, being the **ratio** of molar concentrations of a single agonist that cause the same biological effect in the absence and presence of an antagonist. If the two concentration-response curves (in the absence and presence of the antagonist) are separated by the same horizontal distance over the whole range of response level (such curves are often described by the pharmacologist as being *parallel*), then the **equieffective molar concentration ratio** (EMR) is independent of the response level chosen, depending only upon the concentration of the antagonist and its **dissociation equilibrium constant**.
- The term is to be preferred to the traditional, less precise **jargon** term *dose ratio.*

concentration–response data
- It is useful to plot the intensity of response against the **logarithm** of the drug concentration. "This **transformation** is popular because it expands the initial part of the curve, where response is changing markedly with a small change in concentration, and contracts the latter part, where a large change in concentration produces only a slight change in response. It also shows that, between approximately 20 and 80 per cent of maximum, response appears to be proportional to the logarithm of the concentration" (*Rowland & Tozer*, see Acknowledgements).
- The **semilogarithmic transform** is also valuable because concentration data (e.g. **EC$_{50}$**, **potency**, **antagonism**, etc.) are themselves log-normally distributed.   See **heteroscedasticity, logarithmic transformation**

conceptual pharmaceuticals (L. *co, com/cum, con*, with, together, in common, jointly, equally, reciprocally, mutually; *copere*, to take)
- These are the pharmaceutical industry's 'designer products'; marketing motives predominate over considerations of efficacy; sale to the public depends on 'patient appeal' (after *K Helliwell, B Jones*).

concertation   (L. *concertare*, to harmonize)
- **Jargon** ('Eurospeak') for the requirement that member states of the **EC/EU** consult each other on drug regulation (and other topics).

concomitant/concurrent   (L. *co, com/cum, con*, with, together, in common, jointly, equally, reciprocally, mutually; *comitare*, to accompany; *currere*, to run)
- Concomitant, at the same place; concurrent, at the same time (a convenient but not authoritative distinction); used regarding treatment groups in **therapeutic trials**.   See **concomitant event**

concomitant event   (L. *co, com/cum, con*, with, together, in common, jointly, equally, reciprocally, mutually; *comitare*, to accompany; *eventus*, happening)

– **Adverse event** occurring during a clinical trial and which the investigator considers to be unrelated to the study medication.

concordance (L. *co, com/cum, con*, with, together, in common, jointly, equally, reciprocally, mutually; *cor, cordis*, of the heart)

– A term offered as preferable to *compliance,* as implying a co-operation or partnership between prescriber and patient as equals, rather than direction of the patient by the prescriber. See **compliance**

concurrent See **concomitant**

conductance (L. *conductus*, drawn together)

– The inverse of resistance. In *electrical* terminology, conductance is measured as the current flow per unit of potential difference (1 siemen = 1 amp volt^{-1}). In *hydrodynamic* terminology, conductance is measured as the rate of flow per unit of pressure difference. In *thermal* terminology, conductance is measured as the rate of flow of heat per unit of temperature difference.

Note: the definitions given above refer strictly to chord conductances (i.e. the slope of the current–voltage curve between two points). In electrical systems, the relation between current and voltage is often nonlinear, and *slope conductance, dI/dV* (i.e. the slope of the curve relating current to voltage) at a specific voltage is often measured.

– *Ionic conductance*: a measure of the ease with which ions of any one species move across a membrane in response to a potential gradient. In calculating ionic conductances, the potential gradient is taken as $E_m - E_x$ where E_m is the actual potential difference and E_x is the equilibrium potential for the ion in question. Thus the ionic conductance, $G_I = I_I/(E_m - E_x)$, where I_I is the current carried by ions of the relevant species.

conference venues (L. *co, com/cum, con*, with, together, in common, jointly, equally, reciprocally, mutually; *ferre*, bring; *venire*, come)

– Hotels increasingly provide convenient venues for the proliferating conference business. Many pharmacologists find themselves involved in organizing conferences, and MJ Rand gives advice from long experience:

"What is needed in the field of design of conference hotels is an architect who has actually experienced sitting beyond the first twenty or so rows of seats and who is prepared to enlist the aid of an audio-visual specialist with expertise in communication. In the meantime, meetings will be held, and conference hotels offer many advantages, so I suggest the best method for influencing a choice of venue in the future is to reserve the last two rows in the auditorium for the organizers of the conference and for the speakers, who might finally come to understand that slides resembling a page of a telephone directory do not convey a lot of useful information (even from the front row)".

confidence interval and limits (L. *co, com/cum, con*, with, together, in common, jointly, equally, reciprocally, mutually; *fidere*, to trust; *inter*, between; *vallum*, rampart; *limes*, boundary)

- The *confidence interval* (CI) is the range of values with a specified high **probability** (usually 95%) of containing the population or test group value (mean, or other); the CI is usually symmetrical about the value.
- *Confidence limits* (CL) are the boundary or end-point values of the CI.
- CIs reveal the *precision* of an estimate.
- A *wide* CI, and overlapping ranges between groups implies less precision, as does spanning of the zero point (+ and –); it is often the consequence of too-small numbers of subjects.
- A *narrow* CI with no overlapping between groups implies high precision and may only be attainable with large number of subjects.
- *Confidence intervals* are extremely helpful in interpretation, particularly for small studies, as they show the degree of uncertainly related to a result – such as the difference between two means – *whether or not it was statistically significant*. Their use in conjunction with non-significant results may be especially enlightening (*SM Gore*).
- Editors should encourage the reporting of *confidence intervals* for better communication of trial results and so banish for all time the mistake of identifying 'not statistically significant' with 'no difference'(*SM Gore*).
- When an average (mean) value or a proportion is calculated from a sample of a population, the calculation of the limits or interval between which the true population value will lie can be made; e.g. if in a random sample of 100 observations it is found that 18 per cent have the characteristic concerned, it is reasonable to be confident that the proportion in the whole population (from which the sample was drawn) will be between 10 and 26 per cent. If it is desired to be more precise, a larger sample will be required.
- Calculation of CI or CL necessitates the making of certain assumptions, the nature of which depends on the method of calculation used. The most common calculation involves the assumption that the variable in question has a **normal distribution**, although the evidence for this is often flimsy. For example the 95 per cent confidence limits are such that (if the assumptions are correct and there are no systematic errors) if it were possible to repeat the experiment many times under identical conditions (each experiment giving a set of 95 per cent confidence limits, which would differ from one experiment to another), then, in the long run, in 95 experiments out of a 100 the limits would include the true value; in practice, the limits are usually overoptimistic.

See **fiducial inference/limit, power in statistics**

confidentiality (in clinical drug studies)   (L. *co, com/cum, con*, with, together, in common, jointly, equally, reciprocally, mutually; *fidere*, to trust)
- *Confidentiality (regarding trial subjects):* maintenance of the privacy of trial subjects including their personal identity and all personal medical information. If data verification procedures demand inspection of such details, this may only be done by a properly authorized person. Identifiable personal details must always be kept in confidence. The trial subject's consent to the use of records for data verification purposes should be obtained prior to the trials and assurance should be given that confidentiality will be maintained.

- When reporting **adverse events** or any other information to the sponsor and/or the relevant authorities, the investigator should assure that the subject's privacy is not violated (**EC/EU**).
- *Confidentiality (regarding material from* **sponsor***):* maintenance of secrecy of confidential information from the sponsor in connection with the planning, execution, reviewing, auditing or evaluation of a clinical trial (**EC/EU**).

confirmation/replication   (L. *co, com/cum, con*, with, together, in common, jointly, equally, reciprocally, mutually; *firmus*, firm)
- Important experimental/research results commonly need independent confirmation if they are to be generally accepted, particularly so where acceptance means major changes in practice in **science**, medicine or society.
- It is common, in the clinical testing of medicines to hear investigators say: "I am doing a trial to confirm that drug x benefits disease y." This is incorrect thinking, and it promotes biased planning. The objective of research is to find out *whether* a **hypothesis** is true, not to confirm what is wished to be true.
                                        See **bias, truth**

conflict of interest   See **interest, conflict of**

conformer   (L. *co, com/cum, con*, with, together, in common, jointly, equally, reciprocally, mutually; *forma*, mould, shape)
- A term used to describe one particular shape of a flexible molecule. If, for example, only one conformation of a flexible drug molecule is capable of activating the receptor, that conformation can be referred to as the *active conformer*. (*Note*: pronounced with the stress on *con*.)

confounding   (L. *co, com/cum, con*, with, together, in common, jointly, equally, reciprocally, mutually; *fundere*, to mix up)
- The interpretation of observed associations between two variables (to determine causality) may be affected where there is strong association with a third variable, or by hidden or unknown variables or by inseparability of causal factors, i.e. there is confounding. The possibility of confounding has led to sometimes bitter debates on, for example, whether the association between smoking and lung cancer is or is not causal, and whether alcohol consumption (associated with smoking) is a confounding factor.
                                        See **Simpson's paradox**

confrontation meeting   (L. *co, com/cum, con*, with, together, in common, jointly, equally, reciprocally, mutually; *frons*, face, forehead)
- Meeting at which the various parties (protagonists) are invited to support their assertions, explain their differences, and fight them out there and then. Resorted to when all agree that change is necessary but it is prevented by unreconciled differences.   See **consensus meeting**

congener   (L. *co, com/cum, con*, with, together, in common, jointly, equally, reciprocally, mutually; *genus*, race, kind)

- Of the same kind.
- The (non-ethanol) ingredients of alcoholic drinks that contribute to taste, odour and, perhaps, to 'hangover', e.g. other alcohols and aldehydes are loosely described as congeners.
- Chemicals with close structural similarities. A common approach to the search for new drugs is to synthesize a series of closely-related compounds, each with a small **systematic** structural modification. Pharmacological testing of these *congeners*, it is hoped, will lead to an understanding of the structural requirements for the desired activity.　　See **structure-activity relationship**

consensus meeting/conference　　　　(L. *co, com/cum, con*, with, together, in common, jointly, equally, reciprocally, mutually; *sentire*, to feel)
- *Consensus*: agreement of opinion or testimony.
- Where evidence for a course of action or for a hypothesis is equivocal it may be useful to arrange a meeting to determine whether provisional agreement as to the likely truth can or cannot be reached among a group of people who have independently studied the matter. Plainly, selection of the participants is all-important because a desired outcome (e.g. by a pharmaceutical company, by government) can be ensured by biased selection.
　　　　　　See **brainstorming meeting, confrontation meeting, expert**

consent (informed consent) to research　　　(L. *co, com/cum, con*, with, together, in common, jointly, equally, reciprocally, mutually; *sentire*, to feel, perceive)
- Acceptance of something done or planned by another.
- Subjects should know that they are involved in research, although to ensure this can sometimes be difficult or even impossible, e.g. in community projects, mentally handicapped subjects, medical emergencies.
- Potential research subjects are entitled to choose whether or not they will participate in research, and obtaining valid (informed, understanding, voluntary) consent is central to the ethical conduct of clinical investigation. The terms 'valid', 'informed' and 'voluntary' imply that subjects have enough information, in a form that is comprehensible, to enable them to make an autonomous, deliberated (proper) judgement whether or not to participate. The word 'consent' encompasses these requirements, for if they are not met there is no consent. The use of qualifying adjectives is thus strictly unnecessary and may even be confusing. But the term *informed consent* is now standard and may be considered a useful reminder to unthinking doctors and investigators. The obvious impracticability of giving *full* information has led to the saying "there is no such thing as informed consent", a criticism which is most easily rebutted by stressing that it is *adequate* or *sufficient* information that is required. The difficulties of defining adequate information are recognized in the various ways that are used to obtain consent in practice (*Royal College of Physicians of London*).
- *'Informed consent'*: the voluntary confirmation of a subject's willingness to participate in a particular trial, and the documentation thereof. This confirmation should be sought only after information has been given about the trial, in-

cluding an explanation of its objectives, potential benefits and risks and inconveniences, and of the subject's rights and responsibilities in accordance with the current revision of the Declaration of Helsinki (*definition of the European Community*).
- *Where a research subject is incapable of giving personal consent*, the inclusion (in research) may be acceptable if the Research Ethics Committee is in agreement and other precautions are taken (*European Community*).
- The difficulty of determining what is to count as informed consent and what to do about those who are, for one reason or another, deemed incapable of consent cannot be resolved in general terms; it must be left to local ethics committees presented with actual research proposals. *Informed consent* is the name of an ideal rather than an exact and specific condition of research (after *M Warnock*).
- *Concealment and deception of research subjects.* A properly informed subject may give valid consent to *concealment*, e.g. to accept the use of a **placebo**, but to be kept in ignorance (for scientific reasons), of *when* it will be used. But the deliberate withholding of information that might affect a subject's consent (in a way that might displease or embarrass an investigator) is *deception* and is unethical. "If trialists are dishonest with their patients, what right have they to expect honesty in return?" (*S Senn*).   See **contract,**
Declaration of Helsinki, ethics committee, natural justice/rights

CONSORT
- Acronym for consolidated standards of reporting trials.
- The CONSORT statement (1996) comprises a checklist of 21 items that pertain mainly to the methods, results and discussion of a report of a **randomized controlled trial** (RCT) plus a flow diagram providing information about the progress of patients through a (two) **parallel groups design** RCT, "perhaps the type of trial most commonly reported".
- The CONSORT group invites all journal editors and clinical trialists to use the checklist and flow diagram which are published (*Journal of the American Medical Association* 1996;276:637–639) and which will be revised in the light of experience in use.

conspiracy theory (of life)   (L. *co, com/cum, con*, with, together, in common, jointly, equally, reciprocally, mutually; *spirare*, to breathe)
- An individual's belief that if life events in general, but especially events concerning the individual's own promotion, do not proceed satisfactorily, this must be caused by others combining together with malicious intent.
- Where human incompetence, muddle or laziness provide a sufficient explanation for an event, there is no need to have recourse to any other, e.g. conspiracy (*Anon*).

constant   (L. *constare*, to be steadfast)
- A quantity that remains invariable throughout a particular series of experiments or calculations. A mathematical symbol representing the same, often k.
                   See **proportionality constant**

constitutive activity   (L. *co, com/cum, con*, with, together, in common, jointly, equally, reciprocally, mutually; *stituere*, from *statuere*, to set up)
- Basal activity (for example generation of a low level of second messenger) in a **receptor**–effector system (usually a **G-protein**-linked system) in the absence of occupation of the receptors by **agonist** molecules. This depends upon the receptor being able to exist in two forms, an active form that activates the effector system and an inactive form that does not. If the active form can exist in the absence of agonist, then a low level of activation of the effector system occurs.   See **inverse agonist**
- Those properties of a substance that depend upon the arrangement of atoms within the molecule rather than upon their nature or number.

contingency, contingent variables, contingency tables   (L. *co, com/cum, con*, with, together, in common, jointly, equally, reciprocally, mutually; *tangere*, to touch)
- A possible or not very likely event.
- Dependence on chance.
- Degree of association between theoretical and observed frequencies.
- A relationship between **variables** such that each influences the other; dependent variables.
- A table in which, usually two variables, entities or frequencies (2 × 2 contingency tables) are displayed, one in the rows (r) and the other in the columns (c). It allows use of the **chi-square test** to determine whether one entity is related to (contingent on) the other entity, or whether it is independent (i.e. it tests the **null hypothesis**, which is that the variables are *not* dependent).
                      See **Fisher's exact test**

continuation protocols for therapeutic trials
- When a new drug is under trial (to determine whether it will become a medicine) and the **protocol** period of administration is completed, patients who have benefited are sometimes dismayed to find that they can no longer take the drug (whether for reasons of limited supply, regulatory restriction or because they will have to pay). Provision for this situation should, where appropriate, be made at the outset in a *continuation protocol.*

contraceptive   (L. *contra*, against; *concipere*, to take in)
- A drug or device that prevents, by a variety of means, the fertilization of an ovum and/or implantation. The inclusion of drugs that cause early abortion is controversial.

contract   (L. *co, com/cum, con*, with, together, in common, jointly, equally, reciprocally, mutually; *trahere*, to draw)
- Many new drug development studies, especially clinical, are conducted on contracts between companies and investigators and research subjects. To a lawyer a contract is an agreement between two or more persons which is legally enforceable. But for most contracts no formality is necessary, and an oral (including telephone) agreement can be as binding as one embodied in a

formal document. The word is also used by some members of the caring professions, such as social workers, to denote a sincere commitment without the implications of legal enforceability.

– Promises by a pharmaceutical company to compensate research subjects for injury due to participation in a study should be formally recorded. It is recommended that companies should enter into legally binding contracts with each healthy volunteer, but for patients an agreement "favourably to consider" compensation, without legal commitment, may be all that can be obtained. But **EU** guidelines state that research sponsors should provide adequate compensation for trial-related injury and that subjects should be satisfactorily insured.

– Agreements by prospective research subjects to enter into research, including the signature of consent forms, while entitling the researcher to proceed, do not commit the subject to maintain his or her consent in the future. Research ethics committees normally require consent forms to refer to the subject's right to withdraw from the trial at any time without giving reasons, but even without this it is difficult to think that a consent form would ever be treated as a contract to remain in the research. See **compensation for injury, ethics committee/research ethics committee, liability**

contractility   (L. *co, com/cum, con*, with, together, in common, jointly, equally, reciprocally, mutually; *trahere*, to draw)
– The ability of a muscle or other type of cell to contract.
– The velocity of and force of contraction of muscle (e.g. digoxin increases myocardial contractility).
– An imprecise term comprising a mixture of properties. Agents that affect the force of contraction of a muscle, other than those that cause a change in resting length, are said to affect its contractility.

contract research organization (CRO)
– A scientific body (commercial, academic or other) to which a **sponsor** may transfer some of his tasks and obligations. Any such transfer should be defined in writing (*European Community definition*). See **contract**

contragonist   (L. *contra*: against; Gr. *agon*, to struggle)
See **inverse agonist**

contraindicate/-ion   (L. *contra*, against; *in*, in; *dicare*, to proclaim)
– A generally accepted procedure or treatment is contraindicated when there is a special aspect of the patient's condition that predicts hazard or renders an unfavourable outcome certain. It is considered (in prescribing literature) to be a stronger warning than 'precaution' (or special precaution), where the drug may be used with 'special care' e.g. closer than usual monitoring, lower than usual dose.

control   (Old Fr. *contrerolle*, duplicate register, system of checking, from L. *contra*, against; *rota*, a wheel)
– Standard of comparison for checking inferences deduced from experience

(e.g. experimental subject, untreated or treated in a previously accepted way). In therapeutic studies controls may be concurrent or **retrospective**. Generally, but not always, **concomitant/concurrent** (not *historical*) controls are preferred. (Feinstein discussed 12 different types of control in *Clinical Pharmacology and Therapeutics* 1973;14:112. It may be doubted whether he would regard the above definition as sufficient.)

Controlled Substances/Drugs (regulatory term)
– Many countries have legislation designed to minimize social and medical misuse of designated substances by controlling the manufacture, distribution, prescription, and dispensing of such drugs or substances, e.g. opioid analgesics, amphetamines, solvents.   See **opiate/opioid**

controlled-release formulation   See **modified-release formulations**

convenience sample   (L. *co, com/cum, con*, with, together, in common, jointly, equally, reciprocally, mutually; *venire*, to come)
– Where it is impracticable to obtain a random (or a sufficiently large) sample of a population/subjects, e.g. a rare disease, investigators have to rely on recruiting individuals who are conveniently available; also known as a **grab sample** (Old Ger. *grabben*, seize), or a *chunk* (etymol unknown) sample.

convulsant   (L. *co, com/cum, con*, with, together, in common, jointly, equally, reciprocally, mutually; *vellere*, to pull)
– Agent that induces convulsions.

cooperativity   (L. *co, com/cum, con*, with, together, in common, jointly, equally, reciprocally, mutually; *operari*, work)
– A term used to describe the shape of the curve relating the fraction of sites occupied by a **ligand** to the ligand concentration. By extension, the term can be used to describe the shape of the concentration–effect curve for a drug. Cooperativity is commonly found when enzyme or receptor molecules consist of several subunits, each possessing one or more binding sites. The degree of cooperativity can be expressed in terms of the *Hill coefficient, n* (see **Hill equation**). If $n < 1$, the reaction is said to show *negative cooperativity*. If $n > 1$, the reaction is said to show *positive cooperativity*, which is manifest as a sigmoid (S-shaped) rather than a **hyperbolic** binding curve. Binding of a ligand molecule to one site may either enhance (giving rise to positive cooperativity) or reduce (giving rise to negative cooperativity) the **affinity** of the remaining site(s) for ligand molecules. If more than one population of binding sites exists, differing in affinity (but showing no interaction between sites), a spurious appearance of negative cooperativity will result, since for the composite binding curve $n < 1$.   See **allosteric interaction**

COPS
– **Company observational postmarketing study.**

- A product that is **essentially similar** to an already-licensed product; it may be submitted to a regulatory (licensing) body in an **abridged application**, i.e. without full pharmaco-toxicological and clinical documentation.

copyright and moral rights in published works
- Pharmacologists are involved in publishing (see **publication**) in one way or another. Those who publish only in the principal scientific and medical journals need little concern for the subject of this entry. Those who write books and are involved in negotiating publishers' contracts (agreements) are prudent if they understand at least the outlines of these matters.
- *Copyright* constitutes a group of rights relating to literary (and other) creative works, which accord the creator the right to reproduce the work and to authorise others to do so for a (variable) period defined by law.
- Publishers commonly offer to authors contracts that transfer to themselves copyright (as well as the right to publish). This is generally acceptable for journals but is often inappropriate for books. Authors' copyrights cannot be lost accidentally, they must be formally transferred; failure of an author to read carefully a publisher's agreement does not count as an accident. The fact that publishers offer to authors an agreement in printed form means only that that is what the publishers would like to have. It does not mean that the authors are not free to alter it and to negotiate revisions at their discretion; such printed general-purpose agreements often contain inappropriate clauses, e.g. a potential publisher of this book whose draft contract required that the book should be provided with an index, thus showing that as far as he was concerned all books are the same – not a view taken by authors.
- *Moral rights* of authors are the rights of 'integrity and paternity' of the work. They are held by anyone who writes other than for an employer. They protect the author against distortion, mutilation or adaptation of the text and ensure that the author is identified in any uses of the work, including for example, translation and abbreviation. Authors need to assert these rights (which is not the case with copyright, above) and commonly do so in a sentence such as, "[The authors] assert the moral right to be identified as the authors of this work", placed alongside the statement of copyright of the work near the title page.
- The law on these matters is complex and varies between countries. There are books and societies that give to authors explanation, advice and protection.
- Authors should be wary of agreeing to conditions without first ensuring that they understand their full implications. Modern academic/medical publishing is increasingly competitive and increasingly accountant-dominated.
    See **authorship, intellectual property, quotation and permission to quote**

correlation analysis   (L. *co, com/cum, con,* with, together, in common, jointly, equally, reciprocally, mutually; *relatio,* bring back)
- This measures the *strength* of a relationship between two numerical variables; it gives no information on causation.
- *Correlation* is the mutual relationship between variables.
    See **science/scientific method in pharmacology**

correlation coefficient/Pearson correlation coefficient   (L. *co, com/cum, con,* with, together, in common, jointly, equally, reciprocally, mutually; *relatio*, bring back; *efficere*, to accomplish)

- A measure of the degree (strength) of linear association between two continuous **variables** (*K Pearson*, 1857–1936, mathematician and biologist, UK).
- The correlation coefficient gives as a single number an assessment of the extent to which two variables are related (associated), i.e. the extent to which the points on a **scatter diagram** (in which one variable is plotted against the other) are clustered around a curve. If the points fit perfectly (usually on a straight line), the correlation coefficient is +1.0 (if the slope of the line is positive) or −1.0 (if the slope is negative). If the points are scattered at random, the correlation coefficient will be near zero. A positive correlation, e.g. between medical provision and average income in different areas, means that areas with high income are observed usually to have high medical provision, but it does *not*, of course, necessarily imply that imposition of an increase in one variable (e.g. medical provision) will cause a rise in the other (e.g. income).   See **regression analysis**

correlations between variables   (L. *co, com/cum, con,* with, together, in common, jointly, equally, reciprocally, mutually; *relatio*, bring back)

- To seek correlations that we have postulated *in advance* is a useful activity. But if correlations are sought *after* the collection of multiple variables (i.e. *post hoc*), it is likely that something unexpected or unusual (and therefore 'interesting') will be found. This is called 'going on a fishing expedition' or **data dredging**. Such correlations are commonly not replicated in subsequent studies. It is salutary, at the end of an ordinary day, to consider the many extremely rare events that have occurred, e.g. passing other individuals in the street who are completely unknown to us, and how insignificant in every sense these events are. It has been pointed out that the occurrence of improbable events/correlations is extremely probable.   See **correlation coefficient**

cosmeceutical   (Gr. *kosmetikos*, adorn; *pharmakeia*, making of drugs)
- A blend word of *cosmetic* and *pharmaceutical*. It applies to preparations that have both **cosmetic** and medicinal use, e.g. skin camouflage and masking preparations, oestrogen-containing creams. Cosmeceuticals pose problems for the official regulation of medicines.

cosmetic   (Gr. *kosmetikos*, adorn)
- Any substance intended for placing in contact with any parts of the body exclusively to clean, protect or perfume them, change their appearance, or control body odours (*Scrip*). The definition has importance to official medicines regulators.   See **cosmeceutical**

COSTART
- Coding Symbols for a Thesaurus of Adverse Reaction Terms. This thesaurus (Gr. *treasure*) is a dictionary/encyclopaedia devised to bring coherence into

what would otherwise be incoherence – the vocabulary of **adverse drug reactions** reported from many different sources. It is maintained by the Center for Drugs and Biologics of **FDA**.

See **ADROIT, adverse drug reactions (international terminology)**

cost–benefit analysis   See **economics**

cotransmitter   (L. *co, com/cum, con*, with, together, in common, jointly, equally, reciprocally, mutually; *trans*, across; *mittere*, to send)
– A **neurotransmitter** stored in the same neuron as, and released together with, the 'main' neurotransmitter; for example parasympathetic nerves supplying the salivary glands release both **acetylcholine**, which stimulates salivation, and *vasoactive intestinal peptide* (VIP), which causes vasodilatation.

cough mixture defence
– The response ("I took a cough mixture and did not know what it contained") made by an athlete in whose drug-test sample (generally urine) an illicit, for sport, drug has been found.   See **hip flask defence**

counterfeit drugs   (L. *contra*, against; *facere*, to make)
– Fraudulent medicines make up as much as 6 per cent of pharmaceutical sales worldwide.
– The trade may involve false labelling of legally manufactured products, in order to play one national market against another; also low-quality manufacture of correct ingredients; wrong ingredients, including added ingredients (e.g. corticosteroids added to herbal medicine for arthritis); no active ingredient; false packaging.
– The trail from raw material to appearance on a **pharmacy** shelf may involve as many as four countries, with the final stages (importer, wholesaler) quite innocent, so well has the process been obscured.

counterfeit incorporation mechanism   (L. *contra*, against; *facere*, to make)
– This occurs where a structural **analogue** of a physiological substance is incorporated into the normal cell chemistry and alters its function, e.g. purine analogues in cancer chemotherapy, methyldopa in arterial hypertension.
See **antimetabolite, false transmitter**

counter-irritant   (L. *contra*, against; *irritare*, to provoke)
– A substance (e.g. methyl salicylate, turpentine) that stimulates sensory nerve endings in intact skin, the aim being to relieve pain in tissues/organs supplied by the same nerve root. The mechanism is uncertain, but local vasodilatation and release of **autacoids** and **endorphins** in the nervous system may be important.

covalent bond   (L. *co, com/cum, con*, with, together, in common, jointly, equally, reciprocally, mutually; *valentia*, strength; Old Norse *band*, a fetter)
– A bond formed between two atoms by the mutual sharing of electrons in their

outer orbits. Double or triple bonds are formed when two or three electrons are shared. The energy of a covalent bond is generally high compared to other types of atomic interactions, so the bond will usually be broken only during the course of a chemical reaction in which the atoms are able to form new covalent bonds. Some drugs (e.g. **alkylating agents**) act by forming covalent bonds with target molecules in the body.

covariance   (L. *co, com/cum, con*, with, together, in common, jointly, equally, reciprocally, mutually; *variare*, to diversify)
- A measure of the extent to which two variables are correlated. Uncorrelated events have zero covariance.   See **correlation analysis**

covariate   (L. *co, com/cum, con*, with, together, in common, jointly, equally, reciprocally, mutually; *variare*, to vary)
- In determining the effect of a treatment on a certain characteristic, other characteristics may also be measured. These are *covariates*; they may or may not be altered by the treatment.

COX
- **Cyclooxygenase.**

Cox proportional hazards/regression model
- A statistical device to test associations between variables (*DR Cox*).
- A rank test of maximal local power for detecting dependence of prognosis on a continuous variable (*R Peto*).
- The model allows independent variables (**covariates**) in a **regression** equation to be taken into account. It assumes relative **risk** between each independent variable adjusted for the effect of all the other variables. It is an alternative to the **logrank test**. Its multiple regression approach allows for variable periods of follow-up and so for correction for confounders (see **confounding**).   See **variables and analysis of variables**

CPMP
- Committee on proprietary medicinal products. Part of the **EU** drug regulatory machinery.

CRA
- Clinical research associate.

'crack'   (Onomatopoeic from the sound made by the heated crystals)
- The free alkaloid **base** form of **cocaine**. When heated to create **aerosol** and vapour for inhalation, the crystals ('rocks') make a cracking sound. At one time illegally used cocaine was taken only in the form of the hydrochloride salt (a white powder), usually by nasal insufflation or intravenous injection. Recently, the free base (nonsalt) form of cocaine has become more popular as the effects are about as rapid and intense as those of intravenous injection. Use by inhalation (or preparation of the free base from the hydrochloride by

heating with bicarbonate followed by solvent extraction) is known as 'free-basing'.

craving (drug)   (Old Eng. *crafian*)
- Drug craving is the desire for previously experienced effects of a psycho-active substance. This desire can become compelling and can increase in the presence of both internal and external cues, particularly with substance availability. It is characterized by an increased likelihood of drug-seeking behaviour and, in humans, of drug-related thoughts (*United Nations International Drug Control Program – World Health Organization – UNIDCP–WHO*).
- In Italy, for two months in 1992, cigarette supplies were interrupted by an industrial dispute. Once supplies were exhausted, people smoked whatever they could get, including even cigarettes made from aromatic herbs and sold to help people stop smoking tobacco. It is recorded that some people snatched lighted cigarettes from the lips of others in the street.
- *Anti-craving compounds* are sought using biological **models** involving conditioned drug reinforcement, withdrawal, tolerance and sensitization processes, and so on.   See **dependence**

CRC
- Child-resistant closure (of a medicine container).

cream   (Etym. uncertain: Gr. *khrisma*, anything smeared on;
                                                  L. *cramum*, the top of the milk)
                                                            See **ointment**

CRO
- **Contract research organization.**
- Clinical research officer.

cross-over (clinical) trial   (L. *crux*, cross; Old Norse *yfir*, over;
                                                  Old Fr. *trier*, to sort, sift)
- A design of clinical trial in which each subject or group of subjects receives each treatment in turn. This is obviously suitable only for chronic diseases or for clinical pharmacological studies in stable or healthy subjects.
                          See **carry-over effect, parallel groups,
                          single-patient trial ($n = 1$), within-patient trial**

cross-sectional study
- A study on a representative sample of a population or sub-population recruited at one point in time.   See **longitudinal study**

cross-talk
- The phenomenon that can occur if two types of **receptor** exist on a cell surface and either share a single **effector coupler** or are each coupled to more than one effector coupler, one or more of which they share. Binding of a **ligand** (**agonist** or **antagonist**) to one receptor type may alter responses of

the other receptor type to another ligand, or may cause a response via one receptor that could be mistaken for having been initiated through the other receptor.
- A situation in which two pathways are mutually dependent upon each other so that the function of one pathway is constantly modified or **modulated** by a constituent or constituents of the second pathway which is itself subject to modification or modulation by a constituent or constituents of the first pathway, e.g. the inter-relation between nitric oxide and Ca^{2+} in cell homeostasis.

cross-tolerance   (L. *crux*, cross; *tolere*, to bear up; Old Norse *thola*, to endure)
- **Tolerance** that extends to drugs of a similar structural group or pharmacological action (e.g. opioid analgesics).   See **analgesic, opiate/opioid**

cryopreservation   (Gr. *kryos*, frost; L. *pre*, pre-; *servare*, keep, protect)
- Technique for the preservation of living cells, tissues, organs or even whole bodies at low (subfreezing) temperature.
- Some commercial companies offer to store, for a fee, the bodies or severed heads of recently dead people in liquid nitrogen until a cure for the disease that killed the person becomes available, or until it becomes possible to transfer the personality from a frozen brain to another, living body.

CSM
- **Committee on Safety of Medicines (UK).**

CTC
- Clinical trial certificate (UK).   See **regulation (official) of medicines**

CTX
- Clinical trial exemption (certificate) (UK).
                                   See **regulation (official) of medicines**

cult   (L. *cultus*, worship)
- Devotion to a person, idea or activity.
- A practice that follows a dogma, tenet or principle based on the theories or beliefs of its promulgator to the exclusion of demonstrable scientific experience (*American Medical Association*).
              See **homoeopathy, science/scientific method (in pharmacology)**

culture, drug   (L. *cultus*, worship)
- From time to time it is asserted that drug use can be the basis for a 'culture' (or subculture). The phrase 'drug culture' implies that drugs can provide the spiritual, emotional and intellectual experiences and development that are the basis of a way of life that can reasonably be described as a culture, i.e. the total range of activities and traditions. It is inherently unlikely that chemicals could be central to a constructive culture, and no support for the claim, other than mere assertion, has been produced. That like-minded people seeking mental experiences and practising drug-taking may gather into closely knit

groups (social and/or religious) for mutual support and relaxation, is to be expected, but that is hardly a culture, unless the definition (Japan, 1950s) of culture as 'socially transmitted adjustable behaviour' is used. Even when drug-using subgroups are accepted as representing a culture (or subculture), it may be doubted if drugs are sufficiently central to their ideology to justify using 'drug' in the title, i.e. drug use is secondary, associated, and not a primary phenomenon. The use of drugs for *religious purposes* may be considered an allied practice.

- In the 1960s there appeared in the USA "a messiah, martyr and high priest of the **psychedelic**" who had experienced 'illumination' after eating Mexican 'sacred mushrooms' (**magic mushrooms**). His deep religious experiences over the next 5 hours led him to ask such profound questions as "Why?" and "So what?" He called on the people of America to "turn on [with the aid of drugs], tune in, and drop out" (see *T Leary, The politics of ecstasy*, 1970). Hallucinogens of vegetable origin (including fungi and cacti) have been widely used for centuries in religious and social rituals, but have been largely replaced by synthetic drugs, e.g. **lysergic acid diethylamide (LSD, lysergide)**.

cumulation (L. *cumulus*, a heap)
- Formed by successive additions, e.g. of data, of drug doses.
See **accumulation**

curare (from *Carib*, the name of the aboriginal inhabitants of northern South America)
- The first identified voluntary neuromuscular blocking drug, used as an arrow poison in South America and obtained from plants (*Strychnos* and *Chondrodendron*). It acts by **competition*** with acetylcholine. The principal **alkaloid** is named *tubocurarine* because the Amazonian Indians stored their plant extracts in bamboo tubes (tube curare). Some tribes stored their extracts in gourds or calabashes (calabash curare).
(*Although the interaction between acetylcholine and tubocurarine, in organ-bath studies and *in vivo*, appears to be one of **competition**, in reality tubocurarine is an **ion channel blocker**.)

curriculum vitae (CV) (L. *currere*, to run; *vitalis*, life)
- A summary or outline (not too little, not too much) of an individual's education and professional or working life. A well prepared CV is of the utmost assistance when applying for jobs. A CV is also known as a *resume* in American (business) English.

cusum
- **Cu**mulative **sum** (cusum) techniques are among the simplest statistical techniques known. They are used to determine trends in clinical and laboratory data. First a reference value (e.g. the approximate **means** of initial data points) or an established reference point (e.g. normal body temperature) is taken. This reference value is then subtracted from each of the data points in succession, and any remainder is added algebraically to the previous sum

(hence 'cusum') and graphed. Cusums were developed for industrial process control.

cybernetics   (Gr. *kubernetes*, steersman)
– General term for control theory.   See **feedback**

cyclic-AMP; cAMP   (Gr. *kuklos*, circle, ring)
– Cyclic adenosine 3′,5′-monophosphate. A substance found in many cells, produced from **ATP** (adenosine 5′-triphosphate) by the membrane-bound enzyme, adenylyl cyclase. cAMP serves as an intracellular **second messenger**, by which many drugs and hormones produce their intracellular effects. cAMP usually acts by regulating the activity of a protein kinase that phosphorylates other enzymes, mediating a variety of physiological responses (e.g. glycogenolysis, changes in **contractility**).   See **first messenger**

cyclic-GMP; cGMP
– Cyclic guanosine monophosphate is a **second messenger**. See **cyclic-AMP**

cycling (of receptors)   See **receptor** *(Endocytosis)*

cyclooxygenase (COX)
– The **enzyme** responsible for generating the prostaglandins and thromboxanes from **arachidonic acid**. It represents the major site of action of the **nonsteroidal anti-inflammatory drugs**, e.g. **aspirin**.

cycloplegia   (Gr. *kuklos*, circle, ring; *plege*, stroke, and so, paralysis)
– Paralysis of the ocular ciliary muscle and therefore of ocular accommodation, e.g. by **parasympatholytic** drugs such as atropine.

CYP   See **cytochrome P450**

cyto-   (Gr. *kutos*, vessel, cell)
– Prefix meaning pertaining to a cell, e.g. **cytocidal**.

cytochalasin   See **drugs as tools**

cytochrome P450   (Gr. *kutos*, vessel, cell; *chromos*, colour; *450*, optical absorption peak at 450 nm)
– A mixed-function oxidase enzyme system present in the rough endoplasmic reticulum of (liver) cells and in the **microsomal fraction**, comprising close to 100 **isoenzymes** (isozymes). It is important in phase I drug metabolism. The activity of the enzyme complex depends upon oxidoreduction of iron which is present in the form of haem. Cytochrome P450 is inducible, e.g. by phenobarbitone.
– The designation *450* derives from the finding that when poisoned with carbon monoxide, this family of cytochromes absorb light at a wavelength of 450 nm.
– The abbreviation CYP is now widely used for cytochrome P450.

– The hepatic cytochromes comprise a number of closely related **superfamilies** of enzymes.   See **enzyme induction, metabolism of drugs, phases of drug metabolism**

cytocidal   (Gr. *kutos*, vessel, cell; L. *caedere*, to kill)
– Killing living cells.

cytokines   (Gr. *kutos*, vessel, cell; *kinein*, to move)
– Polypeptides belonging to a **supergene family** of inflammatory mediators. They are currently grouped into six classes:
    – The interferons.
    – The interleukins.
    – Tumour necrosis factor.
    – Human growth factors.
    – Chemokines.
    – Miscellaneous growth factors.
– The cytokines act by recruiting and activating specific cells of the immune system.   See **biological response modifiers**

cytopempis   (Gr. *kutos,* cell; *pempis*, send through)
                    See **transcytosis**

cytoprotection   (Gr. *kutos*, vessel, cell; L. *pro*, for; *tegere*, cover)
– A term introduced for the effect of **prostaglandins** in the protection of the stomach from chemical injury (due to ethanol, acid or alkali). The mechanisms are unknown and the term has lapsed into confusion due to misuse and excessive use.

cytostatic   (Gr. *kutos*, cell, vessel; *stasis*, standing)
– Agent that inhibits multiplication of living cells.

cytotoxic   (Gr. *kutos*, cell, vessel; *toxicon*, poison)
– Killing or injuring living cells, e.g. anticancer drugs, antibiotics.
                    See **chemotherapy**

cytotoxic drug, handling precautions
– Many cytotoxic drugs pose a potential risk to staff who handle them, e.g. by inhalation, skin contact, ingestion. Safety precautions include specially designated handling areas, use of laminar flow cabinets, protective clothing, special labelling and packaging and disposal procedures.

DALY
- Disability-adjusted life year.   See **quality of life**

4-DAMP
- 4-Diphenylacetoxy-*N*-methylpiperidine methiodide; an antagonist at **muscarinic acetylcholine receptors**; it has selectivity for the M_3 subtype.

data   (L. *dare*, to give, and so *data*, things given)
- Facts or information, especially as a basis for inference.
- The word is the plural of *datum*. The common misuse of the word data as singular (e.g. '*this* data *is* important') is uneducated but has been adopted by the computing and allied disciplines, which means that it is likely to become standard (**Fowler**, 1996). Similar misuse occurs with the word medium/media, and, more esoterically, agendum/**agenda**.   See **laws (various)** (*Leahy's law*)

data dredging/torturing   (Old Scandin. *dreg*, to bring up, clear out)
- The *unplanned* (in advance) analysis of sub-groups.
- Data that do not at first give an interesting or desired result are regrouped (**stratified**) and analyzed and re-analyzed in different ways until a 'significant' difference is obtained in favour of the investigators' ideas (or financial or academic interest), and this result alone is reported. *Data torturing* is a variant.
- However, it is claimed that there do exist statistical techniques that render appropriate ***post hoc*** comparisons to be as acceptable (in relation to error) as ***a priori*** (pre-planned) comparisons (*R Persaud; Lancet* 1993;342:373).
                  See **correlation coefficient, correlation between variables**

data sheet (for a medicine)   (L. *dare*, to give, and so *data*, things given;
                                              Old Eng. *skeat*, cloth)
- Manufacturer's written information about a medicine for prescribers. Its claims must be compatible with any official regulatory license. The term is giving place to **summary of product characteristics**.   See **patient package insert**

data transformation
- Many biomedical variables are positively **skewed**, with some very high values, and they may require mathematical transformation to render the data appropriate for analysis. In such circumstances the **logarithmic transformation** is often applicable, although occasionally other **transformations** (such as square root or reciprocal) may be more suitable (*British Medical Journal*).
      See **heteroscedasticity**

DDD
- **Defined daily dose.**   See **drug consumption studies**

DDX
- Doctor/dentist exemption (from need to hold a **CTC**) (regulatory term).
                          See **regulation (official) of medicines**

decile, centile, percentile   (Gr. *deka*, ten; L. *centrum*, hundred; *per*, by, for each)
– Division of a set of values into tenths, hundredths or a given percentage.

See **quantiles**

Declaration of Helsinki and Nuremberg Code   (L. *declarare*, to make clear)
– *The Declaration of Helsinki*: The code of ethics of the World Medical Association adopted by the World Medical Assembly (Helsinki, 1964) for guidance of clinical investigators. It is revised from time to time. The South Africa Revision was published in 1996 – *it includes the following statements*:
  – The purpose of biomedical research involving human subjects must be to improve diagnostic, therapeutic and prophylactic procedures and the understanding of the aetiology and pathogenesis of disease.
  – In current medical practice most diagnostic, therapeutic or prophylactic procedures involve hazards. This applies especially to biomedical research.
  – Medical progress is based on research which ultimately must rest in part on experimentation involving human subjects...the design and performance of each experimental procedure involving human subjects should be clearly formulated in an experimental protocol which should be transmitted for consideration, comment and guidance to a specially appointed committee independent of the investigator and the sponsor [see **ethics committee**]...Biomedical research involving human subjects cannot legitimately be carried out unless the importance of the objective is in proportion to the inherent risk to the subject...each potential subject must be adequately informed of the aims, methods, anticipated benefits and potential hazards of the study and the discomfort it may entail. He or she should be informed that he or she is at liberty to abstain from participation in the study and that he or she is free to withdraw his or her consent to participation at any time. The physician should then obtain the subject's freely given informed consent, preferably in writing. (For full text see *Journal of the American Medical Association* 1997;277:925–926: further revision in progress.)
  – In 1991 a European Community Directive stated that "All **clinical trials** [in the development of medicinal products] shall be carried out in accordance with the ethical principles laid down in the current revision of the Declaration of Helsinki". Governments in **EU** countries are under an obligation to incorporate EU directives into national law (for medicinal products).
– "*The Nuremberg Code* is the most important document in the history of the ethics of medical research." It provides the basis for all subsequent codes of ethical research practice including the Declaration of Helsinki, codes of the World Health Organization and the United Nations (Civil and Political Rights). The Code is an outcome of the trial, following the 1939–1945 War, of certain doctors charged with atrocious experimentation on human subjects. "The judges articulated a sophisticated set of 10 principles" (after *E Shuster*, Fifty years later: the significance of the Nuremberg Code. *New England Journal of Medicine* 1997;337:1436–1440). *The Code follows*:
  1. The voluntary consent of the human subject is absolutely essential. This means that the person involved should have legal capacity to give consent; should be so situated as to be able to exercise free power of

choice, without the intervention of any element of force, fraud, deceit, duress, overreaching, or other ulterior form of constraint or coercion; and should have sufficient knowledge and comprehension of the elements of the subject matter involved as to enable him to make an understanding and enlightened decision. This latter element requires that before the acceptance of an affirmative decision by the experimental subject there should be made known to him the nature, duration, and purpose of the experiment; the method and means by which it is to be conducted; all inconveniences and hazards reasonably to be expected; and the effects upon his health or person which may possibly come from his participation in the experiment. The duty and responsibility for ascertaining the quality of the consent rests upon each individual who initiates, directs or engages in the experiment. It is a personal duty and responsibility which may not be delegated to another with impunity.

2. The experiment should be such as to yield fruitful results for the good of society, unprocurable by other methods or means of study, and not random or unnecessary in nature.

3. The experiment should be so designed and based on the results of animal experimentation and a knowledge of the natural history of the disease or other problem under study that the anticipated results will justify the performance of the experiment.

4. The experiment should be so conducted as to avoid all unnecessary physical and mental suffering and injury.

5. No experiment should be conducted where there is an *a priori* reason to believe that death or disabling injury will occur; except, perhaps, in those experiments where the experimental physicians also serve as subjects.

6. The degree of risk to be taken should never exceed that determined by the humanitarian importance of the problem to be solved by the experiment.

7. Proper preparation should be made and adequate facilities provided to protect the experimental subject against even remote possibilities of injury, disability, or death.

8. The experiment should be conducted only by scientifically qualified persons. The highest degree of skill and care should be required through all stages of the experiment of those who conduct or engage in the experiment.

9. During the course of the experiment the human subject should be at liberty to bring the experiment to an end if he has reached the physical or mental state where continuation of the experiment seems to him to be impossible.

10. During the course of the experiment the scientist in charge must be prepared to terminate the experiment at any stage, if he has probable cause to believe, in the exercise of the good faith, superior skill, and careful judgement required of him, that a continuation of the experiment is likely to result in injury, disability, or death to the experimental subject. See **clinical research, consent**

decongestant   (L. *de*, remove; *con-gero*, bring together)
- An agent that reduces congestion or swelling, ordinarily by vasoconstriction, as with 'nasal decongestant'.

deduction   (L. *de*, from; *ducere*, to lead)
- Inference by reasoning from generals to particulars.
- *A priori*: a phrase describing reasoning from causes to effects, i.e. deductive reasoning.
- Arguing from assumed **axioms** and not from experience.
- "The scientific method is not deductive in character" (*PB Medawar*).

See **induction, logic**

defective drug/product   (L. *deficere*, to fall short; *deficiens*, lacking)
See **product liability**

defensins   (L. *defendere*, to ward off)
- Peptides synthesized and stored in neutrophils and which have antimicrobial activity.

define   (L. *definire*, to set bounds to)
- To make clear.
- To mark out limits.
- To set forth the essence of.
- To declare the exact meaning or scope of.
- "Though defining be thought the proper way to make known the proper signification, yet there are some words that will not be defined" (*J Locke*, 1632–1704, philosopher, England).

defined daily dose (DDD)   (L. *definere*, to set bounds to)
- An estimate of the average maintenance dose of a drug for its principal indication. The term is used in studies of drug consumption or utilization.

See **drug consumption studies, drug utilization**

definition   (L. *definire*, to set bounds to)
- Statement of the precise nature of a thing or the meaning of a word, or the form of words in which this is done.   **See meaning**

degrees of freedom
- The number of degrees of freedom is the number of choices that can be made in fixing the values of expected frequencies (*Erricker*).
- The size of degrees of freedom reflects the number of observations that are free to vary after certain restrictions (inherent in the organization of the data) have been placed on the data (*Mould*).
- The number of independent comparisons that can be made amongst a set of observations.
- The concept of degrees of freedom is one of the more elusive statistical ideas (*Altman*).

Delaney clause
- A clause (sponsored by Senator Delaney) of the Food Additive Amendment (1958) to the USA Federal Food, Drug and Cosmetic Act (1938) that prohibits the addition to *food stuffs*, of *any substance* that has been shown, *at any dose*, to produce cancer in *any* experimental animal. It has been said that if you cannot produce a cancer in some animal with a substance at a high enough dose, by some route, then you're not trying hard enough. Strict application made illegal many pesticides now regarded as safe (in the context of their use) which enter foods in previously undetectable amounts. The clause has been replaced (1996) by one that allows substances in foods provided that there is "reasonable certainty of no harm".
- For *drugs*, regulatory agencies examine the benefit/risk ratio in relation to the proposed therapeutic use. **See carcinogen, proposition 65**

delayed hypersensitivity reaction
- A local inflammatory skin reaction occurring 12–24 hours after intracutaneous application of a drug or **antigen**. The reaction is mediated by sensitized T lymphocytes rather than by circulating antibodies. **See hypersensitivity**

delayed-release formulation **See modified-release formulations**

delivery systems of drugs
- Modes of selectively delivering drugs (or other therapeutic agents) to sites where they are wanted (**targeting**), and for sustaining desired concentrations of drugs. The simplest forms are tablets, fluids for injection, fluids or solids for inhalation, ointments, suppositories. More complex forms include **antibodies, liposomes, modified-release drug delivery systems, gene therapy**.

demography (Gr. *demos*, the populace; *graphein*, to write)
- Science of population statistics illustrating the pattern or conditions of life in the community, e.g. births, deaths, diseases, social habits, drug use or abuse.

demulcent (L. *demulcere*, to caress soothingly)
- An agent, such as an oil or mucilage, that coats dried mucosal surfaces and relieves irritation (e.g. in throat **lozenges**).

dendrogram (Gr. *dendron*, tree; *gramma*, something written)
- An organizational diagram showing the relationship of things as though they were branches on a tree, e.g. evolutionary charts. It is also used in the branch of **statistics** known as **multivariable analysis**.

dendrotoxin **See drugs as tools**

denervation supersensitivity **See supersensitivity**

dependence (drug) (L. *de*, from; *pendere*, to hang)
- Drug dependence is a state arising from repeated, periodic or continuous

administration of a drug, resulting in harm to the individual and sometimes to society. One or more of the following phenomena occur: emotional dependence, physical dependence, tolerance.

- The compulsive use of a drug that has psychoactivity and that may be associated with tolerance and physical dependence (i.e. may be associated with withdrawal symptoms after cessation of drug use) (US Surgeon General's Report on Nicotine Addiction, 1988).
- A state in which symptoms occurring after withdrawal of a drug are most easily alleviated by further doses of the drug.
  See **craving, discontinuation syndrome, tolerance, withdrawal syndrome**

depilatory   (L. *de*, down, from, reverse; *pilus*, hair)
- Agent that removes skin hair.

depolarization   (L. *de*, down, from, reverse; *polos*, end of an axis)
- To reduce or abolish a state of polarization. Excitable cells function mainly because they are able to maintain an electrical charge separation, i.e. they are polarized, with the inside of the cell more negative than the outside. During activation (e.g. during propagation of an action potential) the inside of the cell becomes less negative, so that the size of the potential difference between the inside and outside of the cell becomes less. This is depolarization, even though the actual potential difference appears to 'move upwards' when represented graphically or on an oscilloscope screen.

depolarization/-ing block   (L. *de*, from, down, reverse; *polos*, end of an axis; Old Fr. *bloc*, interruption, obstruction)
- A mechanism of neuromuscular block that occurs when the muscle endplate is held in a depolarized state by the continued presence of an agonist, and the voltage-sensitive sodium channels (in the membrane of the muscle fibre adjacent to the endplate) become inactivated so that they can no longer open to propagate an action potential in the muscle fibre in response to endplate depolarization.   See **inactivation, ion channel**

depot formulation   (L. *depositus*, to put down; *forma*, a shape, model)
- A drug in a slowly absorbed form (e.g. dissolved in oil or as a suspension of an insoluble salt), usually for intramuscular injection, which allows decreased frequency of administration (e.g. antipsychotic drugs such as fluphenazine oenanthate in sesame seed oil, given once every 2–6 weeks; iodized oil for the treatment of endemic goitre, given once every 5 years).
                    See **modified-release formulations, implant**

depression, amine hypothesis of   (L. *de*, down; *premere*, to press; Gr. *hupothesis*, foundation)
- **Hypothesis** that mental depression involves deficiencies of **noradrenergic, dopaminergic** or **serotonergic** mechanisms of the central nervous system.

descriptor   (L. *de*, off, from; *scribere*, to write)
- A term used in **molecular design**. Starting with a molecule with the desired

properties, the first step is to characterize the molecule in terms of a set of *descriptors*. Descriptors can be such properties as the boiling point or the octanol/water partition coefficient. In modern, computer-aided approaches, descriptors can be purely mathematical expressions. A popular modern descriptor is the *topological index*, based upon the skeletal structure of the molecule. This index is a single number that is characteristic of the molecule; it can be used to search chemical structure databases for similar structures (i.e. substances with similar descriptors and, hopefully, with similar pharmacological properties). See **topology**

desensitization (L. *de*, down; *sentire*, to feel)
− *In pharmacology*:
  − A change (e.g. in receptors) that results in the given effect occurring only at a higher concentration, i.e. the system becomes less **sensitive** to the drug. By convention desensitization usually refers to changes occurring on a timescale of seconds or minutes. A slow decrease of responsiveness is often referred to as **tolerance,** and a fast as **tachyphylaxis**. However, desensitization is not the same as tolerance and tachyphylaxis, which may be due to a variety of mechanisms.
  − A decreased **responsiveness** to a drug when it is administered repeatedly or continuously. This use is less valuable than the preceding one as it reduces the precision of the term. This phenomenon is more properly described as tachyphylaxis.
  − It is probably best to avoid using the term desensitization unless there is evidence that the concentration (dose)−response curve is shifted to the right on the concentration (dose) axis. Evidence of a decreased response to a given concentration (dose) is not sufficient evidence of desensitization.
  − The **IUPHAR** committee on receptor nomenclature and drug classification recommends that the term *desensitization* be reserved for phenomena that involve the **receptor** rather than other elements in the stimulus-response chain.
− *In immunology*: the abolition of an allergic response by repeated small doses of **antigen**. See **fade, hyposensitization**

'designer' drug (L. *de*, down; *signare*, to mark)
− This unhappily chosen term is applied to drugs of abuse specially made for the illegal drug market, i.e. for nonmedical, recreational purposes. It also includes agents legitimately synthesized for research but which are found to have recreational use only, e.g. some derivatives of fentanyl (an opioid) and tenamfetamine (**MDA**).
− Designer drugs are invented by chemists working in illegal laboratories. Originally they were designed and synthesized to avoid US drug laws which prohibited specifically named drugs and structures. Because they were novel compounds, designer drugs were not specifically proscribed and so it was legal to make and possess them. This loophole has now been closed. The structures are novel but an intention to produce similar effects to those of the

commonly abused drugs, e.g. amphetamine-like, heroin-like, hallucinogenic, is prohibited.

detergent   (L. *de*, off; *tegere*, to wipe)
- A substance that increases the spreading or wetting properties of a liquid by lowering the surface tension (**surfactant**): a cleansing agent. Detergents are classed as anionic, cationic and non-ionic.

development risk   See **product liability**

dialysis/haemodialysis/peritoneal d.   (Gr. *dia*, through; *lusis*, set free)
- Separation of substances in a liquid by differences in their capacities to pass through a membrane into another liquid. Dialysis is commonly used in biochemistry as a means of removing low molecular weight components from solutions of proteins. In medicine, haemodialysis (passing blood through a system of semipermeable plastic tubes bathed in a suitable electrolyte solution) is used to remove toxic waste products from the blood of patients with renal failure, or, in cases of poisoning, to remove the drug or poison responsible. Peritoneal dialysis can be used as an alternative to haemodialysis, electrolyte solution being perfused continuously through the peritoneal cavity (the peritoneum is a semipermeable membrane).   See **haemoperfusion**

dialysability   (Gr. *dia*, through; *lusis*, set free)
- The ability of a substance to pass through a semipermeable membrane.
- In clinical practice the terms *dialysable* and *nondialysable* are used to describe whether or not a drug or other substance is removed from the body in a *clinically significant* amount during a standard 3–4 hour period of dialysis treatment (*Rowland & Tozer*, see Acknowledgements).

diaphoresis   (Gr. *dia*, through; *phorein*, to carry)
- Sweating: a drug having **muscarinic** effects on sweat glands is said to be diaphoretic.

diastereoisomer   (Gr. *dia*, through; *stereos*, solid; *isos*, equal; *meros*, shape)
- Optically active isomers that are *not* mirror images, e.g. glucose.
                                            See **chirality**, **optical isomerism**

dichotomy/-ous: polychotomy/-ous   (Gr. *dicha*, in two; *tomia,* cutting)
- Division into two parts (*di*) or many parts (*poly*). A general term also used for classifying or stratifying data. The parts may be equal or unequal.

dictionary   (L. *dictio*, word)
- "A book containing the words of any language in alphabetical order, with explanations of their meaning; a lexicon; a vocabulary; a word book" (*Samuel Johnson,* 1755).
- "A malevolent literary device for cramping the growth of language" (*A Bierce*; satirist, USA, 1842–1914: *The Devil's dictionary*).
                                            See the **preface** to this book, **bibliography**

diffusion (L. *diffusus*, to spread abroad, from; *dis*, away; *fundere*, to pour)
- Bulk movement of a substance resulting from random thermal agitation of individual molecules. The direction of the bulk movement is necessarily such as to reduce the electrochemical gradient of the substance between different regions. The process is sometimes tautologically referred to as passive diffusion, although, strictly, there is no other kind; but see **diffusion (facilitated)**.

diffusion (facilitated) (L. *dis*, away; *fundere*, to pour; *facilis*, easy)
- Transfer of a substance across a cell membrane by a process involving association of its molecules with carrier (transporter) molecules within the membrane, and translocation of the complex in such a way that dissociation can occur on the other side of the membrane. As with any diffusion process, the net movement is always down the electrochemical gradient, and no source of energy is required (in contrast to active transport). In contrast to passive diffusion, facilitated diffusion shows the characteristics of saturability (in that increasing the ligand concentration beyond a certain point fails to increase the rate of transfer, because the carrier molecules are fully occupied), and of competitive inhibition by other substances that have an affinity for the carrier.
See **transport (active)**, **transporter proteins**

diffusion hypoxia (L. *dis*, away; *fundere*, to pour; Gr. *hypo*, below; *oxy*, acidic)
- On cessation of inhalation of a relatively insoluble anaesthetic gas, the flow of gas out of the blood into the alveoli can, for a few minutes, be sufficient to dilute significantly the available oxygen. The process is probably clinically important only with nitrous oxide. See **second gas effect**

digestant (L. *di(s)*, apart; *gerere*, carry)
- A drug that may promote digestion in the gut by replacing deficiencies in, for example, bile or pancreatic enzymes; a loose term.

digital (L. *digitus*, finger or toe, hence any number from 0–9)
See **analogue**

dilution (L. *diluere*, to wash away)
- The process by which a solution is made less concentrated, i.e. the addition of solvent to a solution.
- The reciprocal of **concentration**.
- Its units are volume per unit mass (e.g. L g^{-1}).

dipole:electric dipole (L. *di*, two; *polos*, end of an axis; Gr. *elektron*, amber, since this substance develops an electrostatic charge when rubbed)
- A molecule in which positive and negative charges are separated.

directly observed treatment (or therapy) (DOT)
- This involves health workers watching each patient take the prescribed medicine, and evaluating their progress. It is used to ensure **compliance** where

this is vital, and particularly where the health or safety of other persons is at stake, e.g. oral therapy of tuberculosis, in which DOTS (directly observed treatment, short course) has made a major therapeutic contribution.

'dirty' drug   (Old Norse *drit*, faeces; *drug*, disputed origin)
– A drug with low **selectivity** so that it acts on several/many receptors. Properties other than the main or desired property are sometimes known as **parallel pharmacology**. The term '*dirty drug*' has pejorative implications. Dirty drugs are more euphoniously known as **promiscuous drugs** or as having a 'rich' pharmacology.   See **adverse drug reactions, side-effects**

discontinuation syndrome   (L. *dis*, apart, reversal of previous state; *continuare*, join together; see **syndrome**)
– Any clinical change associated with discontinuation of a drug treatment, e.g. after a course of a benzodiazepine. Changes may be classed as:
  – *Recurrence or resurgence* of the condition for which the drug was originally given.
  – *Rebound*, in which the original condition is transiently more intense.
  – *Withdrawal*, in which symptoms implying physical **dependence** occur, e.g. increased autonomic activity.
All three may occur in any one patient.   See **withdrawal syndrome**

discontinuous variable   (L. *dis*, apart, reversal of previous state; *continuare*, join together; *variare*, to diversify)
                    See **continuous variable, quantum/quantal response**

discretionary fund   (L. *discretio*, separation, discernment; Old Fr. *fonz*, foundation)
– A fund provided for use at the discretion of a named individual in order to meet minor, unexpected or urgent needs. It is (normally) audited in the usual way. A respectable form of **slush fund**.

disinfectant   (L. *dis*, apart, reversal of previous state; *inficere*, to dip into, stain)
– An agent that kills all medically important microorganisms, but usually not spores. Many disinfectants are toxic to human tissues, e.g. phenol.
– Allied terms (self-explanatory) include *fungicide, sporicide, biocide*, etc. (L. *cidium*, kill).   See **antiseptic, sterilization**

disintegration/dissolution   (L. *dis*, apart, reversal of previous state; *integrare*, to make whole; *solvere*, to loosen)
– *Disintegration*: in pharmacy, the fragmentation of a solid **tablet**, after being swallowed or immersed, into its component particles. "It is a paradox of tablet manufacture that considerable ingenuity is used to make individual particles form a coherent structure and further ingenuity is then often required to ensure the breakdown of that structure into its individual components after ingestion" (**PC**), by incorporating disintegrants, e.g. starch, alginic acid, cellulose.

- *Dissolution*: the process of dissolving.
- Pharmacopoeias may require a disintegration or dissolution test on drug formulations as some *in vitro* prediction of **bioavailability** and **pharmaceutical equivalence.**

dispensing   (L. *dis*, apart; *pendere*, weigh)
- The provision of a medicine to a patient in accordance with a **prescription**.

dispersible tablet   (L. *dis*, apart; *spergere*, to scatter)
- Dispersible **tablets** should **disintegrate** within 3 minutes after being placed in water.   See **soluble tablet**

dispersing agent   See **emulsion**

dispersion   (L. *dis*, apart; *spergere*, to scatter)
- The degree to which the values of a frequency distribution are *scattered* around a central point, which is usually the (arithmetic) **mean** or **median**.
                              See **dispersible tablet, scatter diagram, standard deviation**

displacement values of dissolved powders for injection
- When the recommended volume of water is added to a powdered drug, the volume of solution withdrawn from the ampoule may be (by displacement of diluent) larger by a significant degree than the volume of added water. Where the dose required is the full amount (of the powder) this does not matter. But where the dose is to be a fraction of the full amount, then account of this expansion (where it is not negligible) needs to be taken to ensure the accuracy of the dose. Many manufacturers provide the necessary information in their **summary of product characteristics**.   See **concentration**

disposition (of drugs)   (L. *dis*, apart, reversal of previous state; *ponere*, to place)
- A term covering **pharmacokinetics** after absorption has taken place, i.e. **distribution** in the various tissue compartments of the body, **elimination** and **metabolism**.

dissociation constant   See **dissociation equilibrium constant**

dissociation equilibrium constant (K)   (L. *dissociare*, to separate from;
                      aequus, equal; *libra*, a balance; *con*, together; *stare*, to stand)
- **IUPHAR** recommends the use of the word order *dissociation equilibrium constant* rather than the older *equilibrium dissociation constant*.
- The dissociation (equilibrium) constant of a reversible association/dissociation reaction relates, at equilibrium, the concentrations of the reacting substances. For a drug A interacting reversibly with receptors R:

$$A + R \underset{k_{-1}}{\overset{k_1}{\rightleftharpoons}} AR$$

At equilibrium the rates of association and dissociation are equal, hence:

$$k_1[A](1-y) = k_{-1}y$$

Rearrange:

$$\frac{k_{-1}}{k_1} = K_A = \frac{[A](1-y)}{y}$$

K_A is the dissociation equilibrium constant of A, where y is the fraction of receptors occupied by A (the fraction of free receptors is therefore $1 - y$), and $[A]$ is the molar concentration of A. K_A is thus the concentration of ligand at which half the receptors are occupied (i.e. when $y = 1 - y = 0.5$).

– When the treatment involves two ligands, the respective dissociation equilibrium constants are K_A for **ligand** A and K_B for ligand B. In some texts the term K_d has been used to represent the dissociation equilibrium constant for an **agonist**, with K_d' representing the dissociation equilibrium constant for the **antagonist**. The term K_A has also been used to mean the association equilibrium (affinity) constant. This is a constant source of confusion.

See **affinity, ionization constant, K_A, K_B, K_d, pK$_a$**

dissociative anaesthesia   (L. *dis*, apart; *sociare*, to join together)
– Profound analgesia with light sleep, such as that produced by ketamine.

See **anaesthesia, neuroleptanalgesia, 'special K'**

dissolution   See **disintegration/dissolution**

distomer   (L. *dis*, apart; Gr. *meros*, part, share)
See **eudismic-affinity quotient**

distribution   (L. *dis*, apart; *tribuere*, to give)
See **normal distribution curve, skewed,
probability distribution, distribution of drugs**

distribution-free tests
– Distribution-free, or nonparametric, tests are those that do not require that a certain **distribution** of observed values be assumed. They are particularly useful for small numbers of observations (which are inherently unlikely to be distributed in any particular way).

See **parametric and nonparametric statistics/tests**

distribution of drugs   (L. *dis*, apart; *tribuere,* to assign)
– Except where it acts directly at the site of application/administration, a drug enters the water phase of the blood plasma, is carried (in free and protein-bound forms) throughout the body and is distributed in the interstitial tissues and cells according to blood flow, its molecular physiochemical properties and passive and active transport mechanisms.   See **compartment, diffusion**

distribution rate constant
– The rate at which a drug would leave a tissue if the arterial concentration

were suddenly to drop to zero (expressed as a fraction of any drug remaining in the tissues).   See **elimination rate constant**

distribution volume   See **volume of distribution**

diuretic   (Gr. *dia*, through; *ouron*, urine)
– Substance that increases the rate of production of urine (diuresis). More usefully (therapeutics), a substance that increases the rate of sodium excretion.   See **aquaretic**, **forced alkaline diuresis**, **natriuretic**

DMPP   See **drugs as tools** *(Dimethyl-phenylpiperazinium)*

domain   (L. *dominus*, lord, master)
– Sequence of peptide chains in protein macromolecules that can be identified as serving a special function, or as having distinctive physical properties. For example, in many **slow receptors** seven parts of the peptide chain have sequences of amino acids that favour the formation of **lipophilic** α-helices. These regions are arranged across the lipid membrane and are described as 'seven membrane-spanning domains'.
– The naming hierarchy of e-mail addresses on the Internet involves several domains, the first of which is the name of the computer (often an individual's name), followed by a domain which describes the location of the computer (e.g., a University department), followed by one or more domains which describe the organization providing the service.

DOPA
– Dihydroxyphenylalanine, the precursor of the neurotransmitters **dopamine**, **noradrenaline** (norepinephrine) and **adrenaline** (epinephrine).
– As a medicine it is used as *levodopa* in the management of parkinsonism.

dopamine
– 3,4-Dihydroxyphenylethylamine (or 3-hydroxytyramine) – the amine produced when **DOPA** is decarboxylated. It is the precursor of **noradrenaline** (norepinephrine) and **adrenaline** (epinephrine), and a neurotransmitter in its own right.

dosage form   See **formulation**

dose   (Gr. *dosis*, giving, gift, and so portion of medicine)
– Amount of drug administered.
– *Loading or priming dose*: a single dose sufficient to raise rapidly the amount of drug in the body to therapeutic concentration.
– *Maintenance dose*: a dose smaller than the loading dose, which maintains tissue/blood concentrations in the therapeutic range, i.e. balances input with output (elimination) (**steady state**).
– *Maximum tolerated dose* is used when the ideal therapeutic effect cannot be achieved because of the occurrence of unwanted effects (anticancer drugs,

some antimicrobials). The usual way of finding this is to increase the dose until unwanted effects begin to appear and then to reduce it slightly; or to monitor the plasma concentration.

– *Minimum tolerated dose.* This concept is not so common as the above, but it applies to long term adrenocortical steroid therapy against inflammatory or immunological conditions, e.g. in asthma and rheumatoid arthritis, when the dose that provides full symptomatic relief may be so high that serious adverse effects are inevitable if it is continued indefinitely. The patient must be persuaded to accept incomplete relief on the grounds of safety. This can be difficult to achieve.   See **individual effective dose, concentration, minimum effective dose, therapeutic window**

dose-dependent kinetics
        See **Michaelis–Menten kinetics, saturation kinetics, zero-order kinetics**

dose-dependent/related response   See **graded response**

dose dumping   (see **dose**; Norw. *dumpa*, fall suddenly)
– Dose dumping occurs where a **sustained-release** formulation behaves as an **immediate-release** formulation.

dose ratio   See **concentration ratio**

dose–response curve/relation
– A graph showing the relationship between the administered dose of a drug and the response produced in living tissue.
– A graph showing the relationship between the dose given to a whole animal and the biological effect of the drug. (**In vitro** the term 'concentration' should replace 'dose', but this is often overlooked in pharmacologists' vernacular speech.) It is often plotted as response (ordinate) against logarithm of concentration (abscissa). For continuously variable responses, the lower end of the curve must be **sigmoid**, plotted in this way.
– For a **hyperbolic** dose/concentration–response curve, the **semilogarithmic transformation**, so beloved of pharmacologists, produces a sigmoid curve, which is approximately linear between 20 and 80 per cent of the maximum range, and is symmetrical about the EC_{50}/ED_{50}.
– Responses may be **graded** (0–maximum) or *quantal* (present or absent).
                 See **quantum/quantal response, reciprocal plot**

DOT, DOTS
– **Directly observed treatment,** and DOT short term.

double-blind technique/study   (L. *duplus*, two-fold; Gr. *tekhne*, art)
– An experimental procedure, often used in therapeutic trials or other studies on human subjects, in which neither subject nor observers (nor associated staff) know what is being given, whether inert **dummy** (**placebo**), active new drug or active standard drug, the intention being that the hopes, fears and precon-

ceived ideas of all parties will not cause **bias**. The technique is philosophically and practically sound and can be perfectly ethical, although the contrary has been argued. The consent of the subject to use of a placebo at some (although unspecified) time, should normally be obtained. The technique is used where it is believed that subjective influences may determine the results (e.g. in analgesic trials), but it is unnecessary where measures are truly objective (leukaemia). The term is obviously unsuitable in studies of eye diseases, and 'double-masked' is used in this situation.

See **bias, double dummy, single-blind study, triple-blind study**

double dummy　　　　　　　　　(Old Eng., Ger., Scand. *dummy*, dumb, mute)
− A technique used in **double-blind** trials where two treatments are being compared, when the two treatments have noticeably different dosage forms, e.g. one as capsules, the other as injections. In double dummy trials, patients receive both dosage forms, but only one contains the active drug, the other is a **dummy (placebo)**. Also used to control variations in the number of active doses per day and the number of dose units per dose.

double effect, principle of　　　　　　　　　　　　See **euthanasia**

down-regulation (of receptors)　　　　　　　　(O. Eng. *dun*; L. *regula*, rule)
− When a system is exposed to an agonist in high concentrations for a period of time (days) there is often an adaptive reduction in the number of **receptors** (*down-regulation*). The size of the maximal response may then change (see **receptor reserve**) although the **affinity** of the drug for the remaining receptors is unchanged. Down-regulation is a common mechanism underlying the **withdrawal syndrome**.

Draize test
− A test for **topical** mucosal toxicity, named after JH Draize, scientist of the **FDA** (USA). It is still in use on the rabbit eye, although originally (1944) the penis was also included. It continues to be ethically controversial, especially for testing cosmetics.

drinking toasts　　　　(O. Eng. *drinean*; L. *torrere, torsta*, to scorch or parch;
　　　　　　　　　　　　　　hence the term *toast* from the 17th century practice
　　　　　　　　　　　　　　　　　of adding spiced toast to alcoholic drinks)
− Pharmacology is international, and so are pharmacologists. Exclamatory drinking toasts are commonly made between social takers of (alcoholic) beverages (curiously they are not usually employed with caffeine-containing drinks). Biological and medical scientists travel the world professionally. The following may help to smooth social aspects of their visits to other lands:
　− Amharic (Ethiopia): *letenachin* (to our health).
　− Arabic: *fi sehetak* (to your health); *haniaa* (for your pleasure, health and comfort); used *after* taking coffee or other non-alcoholic drink.
　− Chinese: *gan-bei* (dry up the cups).
　− Danish: *skol* (health).

- Dutch: *proost* (may it prove beneficial).
- English: *good health*; *here's health*; *cheers*; (*here's mud in your eye*); (*bottoms up*) (refers to bottom of the drinking vessel); (*down the hatch*) (the choice of phrase varies with the formality of the occasion: the phrases in brackets are especially informal).
- Finnish: *skool* (health); *kippis* (here is to your health) (informal).
- French: *santé* (health); *à votre* (to you) or *à votre santé*.
- Gaelic: *sláinte* (good health).
- German: *prosit* or *prost* (may it prove beneficial).
- Greek: *eis ygeian* (to [our] health), *stin ygeia sou* (to your health); *'yia mas!* (to our health, after a few drinks have already been consumed); *aspro pato* (empty glasses).
- Hebrew: *l'hayim* (to life).
- Icelandic: *skál* (health).
- International: *chin-chin* (Chinese: please have some drink/food) (originally used by upper classes in old China).
- Inuit (Eskimo): *chimo* (greetings).
- Italian: *salute* (health); Italians commonly use *cin-cin* (see above).
- Japanese: *kanpai* (dry up the cups).
- Norwegian: *skål* (health).
- Polish: *na zdrowie* (to your health).
- Portuguese: *sáude* (health).
- Russian: *vashe zdarovje* (your health) or *na zdarovje* (to health).
- Spanish: *salud* (health).
- Swedish: *skal* (health).

drop-out   (Old Eng. *dropa*, fall by force of gravity; *ut*, out)
- A patient enrolled in a clinical trial who is either unwilling or unable to return to the study clinic for regular [trial or post-trial] follow-up visits (**FDA**).

drug   (Late Middle Eng., disputed origin)
- A drug is a substance that changes a biological system by interacting with it.
- A drug is an active ingredient of a medicine (**medicinal product**).
- A substance other than a nutrient or essential dietary constituent which, when administered to an animal, produces a specific biological effect.
- For regulatory purposes (**FDA**): a substance other than a food intended to affect the structure or any function of the body.
- (*USA Food Drug & Cosmetic Act*), (1) a substance recognized by an official pharmacopoeia or formulary; (2) a substance intended for use in the diagnosis, cure, mitigation, treatment or prevention of disease; (3) a substance other than food intended to affect the structure or function of the body; (4) a substance intended for use as a component of a medicine but not a device or a component part, or accessory of a device. Biologic products are included within this definition and are generally covered by the same laws and regulations, but differences exist regarding their manufacturing processes (chemical process vs biological process) (**FDA**).
- In social usage the word is especially applied to substances of addiction or abuse.

- "An ingredient used in physick: any thing without worth or value: any thing for which no purchaser can be found" (*S Johnson; Dictionary* 1775).
- A drug may or may not be a medicine.
- A medicine may or may not contain a drug.
- A substance which when injected into a guinea-pig produces a research paper.   See **'dirty' drug, drug or medicine, medicine, medicinal product**

drug accidents   (L. *ac, ad*, before; *cidere*, to fall)
                              See **accident, clioquinol, practolol, stilbestrol, thalidomide**

drug bulletins   (L. *bulla*, a seal and hence sealed document)
- Drug bulletins provide prescribers and pharmacists with concise critically evaluated comparative information about drugs and therapeutics, especially new drugs. They are produced independently of industry and contain no advertising. Many bulletins are also independent of **government**. The first bulletin, *The Medical Letter* (USA, 1959), was soon followed by *Drug and Therapeutics Bulletin* and *Prescribers' Journal* (UK, 1962). The International Society of Drug Bulletins (ISDB, BP 459, 75227–Paris, Cedex 11, France) was founded in 1986 and now has above 50 members in all continents, including regional, national and international bulletins. It aims to encourage the further development of independent drug bulletins, to promote the exchange of good quality information on drugs and therapeutics, and to facilitate international cooperation in this field (*A Herxheimer*).

drug candidate   (L. *candere*, to be white (robed) as were
                                                 Roman candidates for office)
- Substance that is deemed worthy of laboratory exploration as a potential medicine.

drug consumption studies   (L. *con*, together; *sumere*, to take up)
- Measures of drug use in the community, often calculated from the incidence of a disease and the known total amount of drug used in the community. These allow an approximate calculation of the doses used, e.g. DDD (**defined daily dose**). They can reveal prescribing preferences in disease, as well as inadequate use of drugs.

drug culture   See **culture, drug**

drug explosion   (L. *ex*, out; *plaudere*, to clap)
- A term used to refer to the enormous increase, over the past 45 years, in the number of drugs used in modern medicine (one of the factors behind the growth of **clinical pharmacology** as a separate discipline).

drug holiday   (Old Eng. *halidaeg*, holy day)
- The deliberate interruption of long-term therapy with the objective of restoring responsiveness (which has been lost) or of reducing toxicity.

drug lag   (Distortion of Old Eng. *latost, last* in childrens' game)
- A delay in the introduction of useful new medicines (between countries).

Caused by differing official regulatory and patent procedures. It may occur as a result of mere procrastination, of adherence to fixed and inflexible regulatory requirements, or of shortage of competent staff. The explosion of **biotechnology**, in particular, presents official regulatory bodies with the need to recruit large numbers of skilled (and therefore costly) staff, e.g. the **FDA** (USA) in 1992 promised to recruit 600 additional scientists and other professionals to cope with the review of the safety and **efficacy** of increasing numbers of **new active substances**.

drug master file (DMF) (regulatory term)
– A DMF is a set of documents submitted voluntarily to an official regulatory authority by the manufacturer of an active ingredient, excipient, or container component (or by his agent). The information is submitted on a commercially confidential basis and access to it is authorised by the person or company originally supplying the information. It also permits the supply of commercially confidential information on chemical synthesis and quality control direct from a *chemical* manufacturer to a regulatory authority, bypassing the pharmaceutical company that is using the chemical in its product. The objective is to maintain confidentiality for the chemical company.

drug or medicine   (L. *mederi*, to heal)
– Terminology is vital for communication. Suggestions have been made that the popular (mis)use of the word **drug** has become so prevalent that pharmacological science (basic and clinical) and medical practice should now use the word drug exclusively to mean substances of abuse, and that the word **medicine** should be used for beneficial substances. Though well-intentioned, such a change of usage would have major unintended consequences. Chemicals are not *either* substances of abuse *or* beneficial, and to force them into such a classification would mean that the word medicine would have to be used for legions of substances used in scientific pharmacology (basic and clinical) that fall into neither category. Indeed, some substances would have to be called drugs in one context and medicines in another; and to term 'medicines' substances newly made in drug development (enormous numbers) before they have even been tested in man would be bizarre (though it has been proposed). In general it is undesirable that scientific terminology should follow popular (demotic) usage and fashion, or that terms used in clinical drug development should depart from their meanings in the supporting sciences. The undoubted problems presented by popular misuse of language are small compared with the (unintended) consequences for science of changing long-standing usage. Changes of language, though well-intended, can have adverse effects, just as do new drugs/medicines.   See **drugs as tools**

drug policy (official)   (L. *politus*, polished)
– "A means of ensuring that the community, within limits set by its resources, benefits from the best in drug therapy which current knowledge can devise" (*MNG Dukes*). Elements include **drug utilization** studies and drug *information*, *education* and **research**.

drug product (regulatory term)
- A finished dosage form (tablet, capsule, solution) that contains a **drug substance**, generally in association with one or more other ingredients (such as disintegrants, colouring agents, or preservatives) (**FDA**).

drug regulation/control, official   See **regulation (official) of medicines**

drug safety
- "No woman should be kept on *The Pill* (see **pill**) for 20 years until, in fact, a sufficient number have been kept on the Pill for 20 years" (*AS Parkes*, pathologist, UK). This statement pinpoints the inescapable dilemmas regarding the *safe development* and *long-term use* of medicines.

drugs as tools   (OE. *tol*, tool)
- Many, if not most, drugs lack sufficient **selectivity** for it to be claimed that any effect they produce provides evidence of a **specific** mechanism. But some are sufficiently selective to be useful as tools to elucidate biological processes. The following list is confined (with some exceptions) to agents that are not used in therapeutics. It is by no means exhaustive:
  - *Aequorin*: a protein obtained from a luminescent jellyfish (*Aequorea forskalea*), which emits light in the presence of free calcium ions. Used as a detector of free calcium within cells.
  - *Alloxan*: causes necrosis of pancreatic insulin-secreting β-islet cells.
  - *Antipyrine (phenazone)*: this is used to measure drug metabolizing capacity. It is readily absorbed from the gut, distributed throughout the body water, is less than 10 per cent protein bound, and is 95 per cent metabolized, mainly by the liver mixed-function enzyme system.
  - *Apamin*: a polypeptide component of bee venom; it blocks small conductance Ca^{2+}-activated K^+ channels in peripheral tissues.
  - *Batrachotoxin*: steroidal alkaloid in the skin of a frog (*Phyllobates aurotaenia*): it irreversibly depolarizes membranes by opening sodium channels.
  - *Bicuculline*: γ-aminobutyric acid (GABA) antagonist.
  - *Bombesin*: a tetradecapeptide extracted from the skin of some European frogs, which stimulates secretion of gastric acids in mammals by releasing gastrin.
  - *Botulinum toxin*: a protein toxin produced by the organism *Clostridium botulinum*. It prevents the release of acetylcholine from nerve endings. (It is now sometimes used to treat human blepharospasm, torticollis and anal fissure).
  - *α-Bungarotoxin*: a protein constituent of the venom of certain elapid (fixed poison-fang) snakes (especially *Bungarus multicinctus*), which combines almost irreversibly with **acetylcholine** receptors at the skeletal neuromuscular junction. Used as a marker for acetylcholine receptors.
  - *Capsaicin*: the active principle of the pepper plant (*Capsicum* spp.), which selectively destroys certain sensory neurons when administered to developing animals, and depletes mature sensory nerves of **substance P**.

- *Charybdotoxin*: toxin of an Israeli scorpion, *Leiurus quinquestriatus*. It is a selective blocker of Ca^{2+}-activated K^+ channels.
- *Cholera (Vibrio cholerae) toxin*: an enzyme that catalyses the **ADP-**ribosylation of the α-subunit of stimulatory **G-protein** (G_s) thereby locking **adenylyl cyclase** in its active state, resulting in the continuous formation of **cyclic-AMP**.
- *Compound 48/80*: synthetic histamine releaser; a basic polymer of *p*-methoxyphenethylamine.
- *Concanavalin A*: a plant lectin that binds to the carbohydrate moiety of membrane glycoproteins, causing a variety of cellular changes (e.g. lymphocyte activation).
- *Cytochalasin*: substances isolated from moulds which inhibit cell cleavage without preventing division of the cell nucleus. They act by disorganizing microfilaments and thus inhibiting cell motility.
- *Dendrotoxin*: toxin (polypeptide) from the **venom** of the green mamba snake (*Dendroaspis angusticeps*). It selectively blocks the delayed rectifier type of voltage-sensitive K^+ channel.
- *Dimethyl-phenylpiperazinium (DMPP)*: an autonomic ganglion stimulant (**nicotinic acetylcholine receptor** agonist).
- *Freund's adjuvant*: a mixture of mineral oil and dead tubercle bacilli which stimulates and prolongs antibody production following the injection of a range of antigens.
- *Hemicholinium*: a synthetic substance containing two choline **moieties** which blocks choline uptake by cells and thus inhibits **acetylcholine** synthesis.
- *Hexamethonium (C-6)*: autonomic ganglion-blocking agent (neuronal-type **nicotinic acetylcholine receptor** antagonist).
- *6-Hydroxydopamine*: a compound that is taken up selectively by dopaminergic and noradrenergic neurons and then destroys them, probably by conversion to a reactive product.
- *Joro spider toxin*: toxin from the venom of a Japanese spider (*Nepila clavata*) which blocks **glutamate** receptors.
- *Kainate/kainic acid*: an amino acid structurally related to **glutamic acid**, one of the excitatory **amino acids**. Kainic acid is extracted from a Japanese seaweed, *Digenea simplex*. Three main types of CNS receptors for excitatory amino acids have been characterized on the basis of their sensitivity to the selective agonists **NMDA**, **AMPA** and **kainate**. (AMPA-sensitive receptors were originally classified by their sensitivity to quisqualate.)
- *Lanthanides*: a group of rare metallic elements, including lanthanum itself, with atomic numbers from 57 to 71, some of which have been shown to block calcium channels of cell membranes.
- *Levamisole*: an **immunostimulant** (and **anthelmintic**).
- *Luciferin/luciferase*: an enzyme system derived from firefly tails that emits light in the presence of **ATP** and thereby provides a sensitive assay method for ATP.
- *Methonium compounds*: Bisquaternary ammonium compounds in which

two nitrogens, each with three methyl substituents, are linked by a polymethylene chain. When, for example, there are six carbon atoms in the chain, the drug is *hexa*methonium (see above).

- *Metirosine (α-methyl-L-tyrosine)*: an inhibitor of tyrosine hydroxylase, preventing the conversion of tyrosine to **DOPA** and thereby depleting transmitter stores of noradrenergic and dopaminergic neurons and chromaffin cells, including **phaeochromocytoma** cells.
- *MPTP*: see main text.
- *Muramyl dipeptide*: an **immunostimulant** derived from *Bordetella pertussis*.
- *Murexide*: a calcium detector (obtained from the gastropod *Murex*) which can be used in biological tissue. It changes its absorption spectrum in the presence of Ca^{2+}.
- *Phorbol esters*: highly irritant, tumour-promoting compounds from certain plants that activate protein kinase C directly, thus bypassing the **second messenger** system which normally stimulates protein kinase C.
- *Proadifen: (SKF–525A)*: inhibits **microsome** drug metabolism.
- *Reserpine*: an alkaloid produced by *Rauwolfia* spp., which depletes noradrenaline stores, probably by preventing its uptake by vesicles.
- *Sarafotoxin*: occurs in the venom of the Israeli burrowing asp (a snake), *Atractaspis engaddensis*. It has a high **homology** with the **endothelins**.
- *Saralasin*: **partial agonist** of angiotensin II.
- *Saxitoxin*: a toxin produced by certain molluscs which blocks the sodium channels of excitable membranes, thus preventing action-potential propagation. Similar in its action to tetrodotoxin (below).
- **SKF–525A**: see Proadifen (above).
- *Streptozotocin*: causes necrosis of pancreatic insulin-secreting β-islet cells.
- *Suramin*: **ATP** (adenosine 5′-triphosphate) antagonist (at P2-**purinoceptors**).
- *Tetraethylammonium (TEA)*: an organic cation with a variety of pharmacological effects, the principal ones being to block the potassium channels of excitable membranes (so that smooth muscle cells, for example, develop action potentials). It is an antagonist at **nicotinic acetylcholine receptors** in autonomic ganglia.
- *Tetrodotoxin*: a toxin produced by the puffer fish (*Tetraodontidae*) and certain amphibia (*Salamandridae*), which selectively blocks the sodium channel associated with action potentials. Used to distinguish between neurally and non-neurally mediated events. Similar in action to saxitoxin (above).
- *Tyramine*: indirectly acting sympathomimetic amine, i.e. acts by releasing stored noradrenaline. It is formed naturally in foods by bacterial decarboxylation of tyrosine.
- *Xylocholine (TM-10)*: noradrenergic-neuron-blocking agent.
- *Yohimbine*: a natural alkaloid from a tropical African tree (*Pausinylstalia yohimbe*) which is a partially selective antagonist at $α_2$-adrenoceptors. Its reputation as an **aphrodisiac** may rest on this action.

drug screening (Old Fr. *escren*, to examine for presence of something)
– Detection of those compounds having a desired effect, by applying a single test or set of biological tests. Screens can be *blind*, in which it is hoped to detect any kind of pharmacological activity, or *specific*, in which a barrage of tests is used to discover whether newly synthesized chemicals have the intended pharmacology. The former is a relatively primitive method of discovering potentially useful drugs. The latter highly sophisticated.
See **combinatorial chemistry, screen/-ing**

drug substance (regulatory term)
– An active ingredient in a drug product that is intended to furnish pharmacological activity or other direct effect in the diagnosis, cure, mitigation, treatment or prevention of disease or to affect the [body] structure (**FDA**).
See **medicine**

drug utilization or consumption (L. *utilis*, useful; *con, cum*, together; *sumere*, take up)
– The marketing, distribution, prescription and use of drugs in a society, with special emphasis on the resulting medical, social and economic consequences (*PKM Lunde*, clinical pharmacologist, Norway).
See **drug consumption studies, DURG**

DTC
– Direct to consumer (advertising). DTC refers to the advertising of prescription-only medicines (PoM) directly to the public. This is a controversial matter with doctors (prescribers), and is illegal in some countries.

dual block (L. *duo*, two; Middle Eng. *blok*)
See **neuromuscular-blocking agent**

dualist See **partial agonist**

dummy (Old Eng., Ger., Scandin. *dummy*, dumb, mute)
– A pharmacologically inert formulation used as a control in the scientific evaluation of drugs. See **double dummy, placebo**

DUMP
– Disposal of unwanted medicines and poisons. An initiative to recover from the public unwanted medicines as a contribution to domestic safety. So large are the amounts sometimes recovered that they have presented problems of waste disposal and cost. There has been an instance (Scotland) where an intended campaign was abandoned for these reasons (*Pharmaceutical Journal*).

DURG
– Drug utilization research group. A system for assessing drug use in the community, including outcomes; introduced by the World Health Organization in

1972 (WHO-DURG). Its use has expanded to individual countries and groups of countries, e.g. UK-DURG, European-DURG.

See **drug consumption studies**

duty/duty of care (L. *debere*, to owe)
– A duty is that which is owed to another. It may be moral or legal, and the test of the latter is that a court of law would recognize it.
– *Duty of care* in relation to professional practice means that clinicians, pharmacologists and drug developers are required by law to take reasonable care to avoid acts and omissions which can reasonably be foreseen as likely to injure persons who are so closely and directly affected that they ought reasonably to have them in contemplation as being affected when their acts or omissions are called in question (after *Lord Atkin*, judge, UK). Where injury occurs as a result of breach of this duty there is liability in law to compensate.

See **liability, negligence**

dynorphins (Gr. *dunamikos*, powerful; *-orphine*, part of the word morphine)
– One family of endogenous opioid peptides. The dynorphins are of intermediate size; dynorphin-A, for example, has 17 amino acid residues. The terminal five amino acids are the same as in leu-enkephalin. Dynorphins are as widely distributed as the **enkephalins** but their concentrations are lower, although they are as effective at opioid receptors. See **endorphins, opiate/opioid**

dys- (Gr. *dus*, diseased, abnormal, faulty)
– A prefix meaning abnormal or disturbed function, e.g. **dysrhythmia, dysphoria**.

dyscrasia/dyscrazia (Gr. *dus*, diseased, abnormal, faulty; *krasis*, a mixing)
– Obsolete term for disease.
– Use is now ordinarily confined to the blood (blood dyscrazia), meaning abnormalities of the cellular elements (**agranulocytosis, thrombocytopenia**, etc.). Drugs are an important cause of blood dyscrazias.

dyskinesia (Gr. *dus*, diseased, abnormal, faulty; *kinesis*, motion)
– Abnormal movements, e.g. **tardive dyskinesia**.

dysphoria (Gr. *dus*, diseased, abnormal, faulty; *pherein*, to bear)
– A feeling of discomfort, lack of sense of wellbeing. See **euphoria**

dysrhythmia (cardiac) (Gr. *dus*, diseased, abnormal, faulty; *rhuthmos*, rhythm, flow)
– Any variation from normal cardiac rhythm (and gross changes in rate).

dystonia (Gr. *dus*, diseased, abnormal, faulty; *tonos*, tension)
– Disorder of muscle tone (increased or decreased).
– As an adverse reaction to drugs acting on the cerebral basal ganglia (e.g. phenothiazine **neuroleptics**), a hypertonic state sometimes mimicking tetanus.

EC
– European Community: for some, but not for all, purposes the EC was re-placed by the European Union (EU) in 1993. It has an official medicines regulatory body, the **EMEA**.

EC$_{50}$/ED$_{50}$
– Effective concentration/dose in 50 per cent of subjects/tissues.
– The concentration of a drug that produces a specified all-or-nothing response in 50 per cent of subjects, **median** effective concentration.
– The concentration (molar) of a drug producing 50 per cent of the maximal possible effect of that agonist in a tissue that gives graded responses. The effect of the agonist may be to stimulate the system or to inhibit it. Other per-centage response levels can be specified (EC$_{20}$, EC$_{70}$, etc.).
– Under some circumstances it may be neither possible nor wise to determine the maximal effect of the drug. This is often the case in laboratory animals and in clinical investigations. Under these circumstances it may be preferable to define a dose or concentration of drug that causes a given change in the variable under investigation, e.g., a 20% increase in cardiac output or a 10 mm Hg fall in diastolic blood pressure. Hence the term would be expressed ED$_{20\%}$ or ED$_{10\ mm\ Hg}$ etc.
– The term is developed from that first proposed by J Trevan for expressing the toxicity of drugs – LD50; note that in Trevan's notation there was no subscript, although the subscripted form is now preferred (**LD$_{50}$**).

eclectic   (Gr. *ek*, out of; *legein*, to gather)
– Selecting what seems best from a variety of ideas, doctrines, hypotheses, methods.

ecological fallacy   (Gr. *oikos,* house, and so, environment; L. *fallax*, deceitful)
– The type of error that occurs when the existence of a group association is used to imply the existence of a relationship that does not exist at the individ-ual level (**FDA**).

ecology   (Gr. *oikos*, house and hence environment; *logia*, subject of study)
– Study of the interrelationships between living organisms and the environment. For example, antimicrobial drugs have ecological effects, e.g. in hospitals, in travellers' diarrhoea.

economics   (Gr. *oikos*, house; *nomos*, a law)
– The science of distribution of wealth/resources.
– The "Dismal Science" (*Thomas Carlyle*, 1795–1881, Scottish philosopher and historian); so-named because economics "maintained that the distribution of the profits of industry depended on natural laws, with which morality had nothing to do. Carlyle insisted that morality was everywhere, through the whole range of human action" (*JA Froude*, biographer and friend of Carlyle).
– Six economic concepts have particular importance to users and developers of drugs:

1. *Costing* provides an estimate of burdens in monetary terms. Alone, it gives little that is useful in determining the priorities of competing demands.
2. *Cost-minimization*: production of a given output (or outcome) at minimum cost.
3. *Cost-benefit* identifies and values costs and outcomes in monetary terms.
4. *Cost-effectiveness* takes a simple outcome measure particular to a therapeutic area and appraises the costs of alternative ways of achieving it.
5. *Cost-utility* is an extension of cost-effectiveness analysis to take account of the quality of life; it gives the cost of producing a given change in outcome, e.g. **quality of life year (QALY)** (after *A Maynard*, health economist, UK).
6. *Opportunity-cost* is the value of the resources foregone (for other purposes) by employing a particular treatment option, i.e. 'If we do this, then there will be no resources to do that'. Opportunity costs are inescapable.

– "Modern medicine born of research saves lives but does not always save money, if for no other reason than that the patient cured of one disease will live to get another" (*BJ Culliton*). See **utility**

'ecstasy' (Gr. *ek*, out of; *histanai*, to place)
– Popular or 'street' name for 3,4-methylenedioxymethamphetamine (*MDMA*), a synthetic amphetamine derivative, patented in 1914 as an appetite suppressant, but without a place in modern therapeutics. Recently it has become a popular recreational drug, particularly at 'raves'. Often referred to as 'E' by users.

ectopic (Gr. *ektopos*, out of position)
– Not in its right or normal position.

ED$_{50}$ See **EC$_{50}$/ED$_{50}$**

EDR
– **Equieffective dose ratio.** See **equieffective molar concentration ratio**

EDRF
– **Endothelium-derived relaxing factor.**

education (L. *e*, from; *ducere*, to lead)
– Pharmacologists are much engaged in education.
– "Education is what survives when what has been learned has been forgotten" (*BF Skinner*, 1904–1990, psychologist, USA).
– "Human history becomes more and more a race between education and catastrophy" (*HG Wells*, 1866–1946, novelist and social philosopher, UK).
– [Education is] "not the filling of a pail but the lighting of a fire" (*WB Yeats*, 1865–1939, poet, Ireland).
– "To be *trained* is to have arrived; to be *educated* is to continue to travel" (*K Calman*).
– "An education in *science* consists of two distinct components – a body of knowledge and understanding sufficient to allow a person with imagination to

stand, as Newton said he had done, on the shoulders of earlier giants, and an appreciation of what it is to confront problems in the real world whose solutions are unknown" (*Nature*).

effectiveness (regulatory term)   (L. *efficax*, efficient, from *efficere,* to achieve)
– The extent to which a treatment produces a beneficial effect when implemented under the usual conditions of clinical care for a particular group of patients (**FDA**).   See **efficacious, efficacy**

effector coupler   (L. *efficere*, to achieve; *copulare*, to join together)
– Molecule that links cell-surface receptors to intracellular responding systems (effectors), e.g., **G-proteins**. Effector couplers transmit to the responding system the information passed to them as a result of the interaction of a **ligand** with the **receptor**, usually by undergoing a conformational change that alters the binding characteristics of the molecule, for example by increasing the **affinity** of the coupler for the effector compared with its affinity for the receptor.

effervescent   (L. *ex*, out; *fervere*, to boil)
– The formation and escape of (small) bubbles in a liquid by reduction of pressure (fizzy drinks) or by chemical action (some medicines).
– *Effervescent Tablets* (official term) are uncoated tablets generally containing acidic substances and either carbonates or bicarbonates which react rapidly in the presence of water to release carbon dioxide. They are intended to be dissolved or dispersed in water before administration (**BP**).

efficacious   (L. *efficax*, efficient, from *efficere*, to achieve)
– Having **efficacy**. *Efficacious* almost invariably means having *therapeutic* efficacy.

efficacy   (L. *efficax*, efficient, from *efficere*, to achieve)
– *General sense*: the capacity to produce the desired result/effect.
– *Therapeutic efficacy*: the capacity (relative to other drugs) of a treatment to produce a desired effect; the ceiling or maximum of such an effect, e.g. morphine has greater therapeutic efficacy than paracetamol in that it relieves pain beyond the reach of paracetamol.
– A relative concept referring to the ability of a drug to elicit a beneficial clinical effect. This may be measured or evaluated using objective or subjective **parameters**, and in terms ranging from global impressions, to highly precise measurements (**FDA**).   See **effectiveness, outcomes research**
– *Pharmacological efficacy*: a particular measure of the ability of an **agonist** or **partial agonist** to elicit a response from the tissue. RP Stephenson (*British Journal of Pharmacology* 1956;11:379–393) proposed that response (*R*) is some function (*f*) (undefined) of **stimulus**, *S*:

$$R = f(S)$$

and that the stimulus is proportional to the fraction of receptors occupied (*p*):

$$S = ep$$

where *e*, the *efficacy*, is the **proportionality constant**. Consequently, two agonists with the same **affinity** for a particular population of receptors may produce different responses because they differ in efficacy.

Stephenson also suggested the convention that if a **partial agonist** occupied all the receptors, and still only produced half the maximal response of a **full agonist** of the same class, it had an efficacy of 1.0. A full agonist would therefore have an efficacy greater than 1.0 and a **competitive antagonist** would have an efficacy of zero. Thus in terms of early 'classical' ideas about **receptor** action, efficacy is a measure of the ability of drugs to activate, as distinct from occupy, receptors.

- A related measure of the maximum action that an agonist can cause is its **intrinsic activity**. This was originally defined (*EJ Ariens*, pharmacologist, the Netherlands) in terms of the size of the signal to the tissue resulting from occupation of the receptors. However, Ariens had assumed that all full agonists have the same intrinsic activity, which he defined as 1.0. Intrinsic activity is now often used simply to indicate the magnitude of the maximum response to a partial agonist as a fraction of that to a full agonist of the same class – (maximal response to partial agonist) ÷ (maximal response to full agonist).

See **maximal agonist effect (α)**

Efficacy and *intrinsic activity* are not synonymous – all full agonists have the same intrinsic activity (1.0 by definition) but may differ in their efficacy – values from zero to a large positive number are possible. (One agonist may need to occupy fewer receptors than another in order to elicit a given response – see also *Spare receptors*, under **receptors**).

- It was subsequently realized that the stimulus depends not only upon the characteristics of the drug, but also upon the characteristics of the tissue, particularly the number of receptors and the coupling mechanism between receptor and response. This led to the introduction (*RW Furchgott*, pharmacologist, USA) of the term **intrinsic efficacy** (not to be confused with **intrinsic activity**), which is solely a drug-dependent property, related to efficacy as follows:

$$\varepsilon = e/[R_t]$$

where ε is the intrinsic efficacy, *e* is Stephenson's efficacy, and $[R_t]$ is the receptor density. Intrinsic efficacy is the stimulus produced by an agonist per receptor molecule.

- Thus a drug may be a full agonist in one tissue and a partial agonist in another. Even in the same tissue, the efficacy and the intrinsic activity of a given agonist may vary, depending on the responses that are measured (e.g. **depolarization** v. **conductance** increase, produced by acetylcholine; increase in heart rate v. rise in cyclic-AMP, elicited by a β-adrenoceptor agonist).

- In the *two-state* model of drug–receptor action (see under **receptor**), efficacy is defined as the ratio of the affinity of the agonist for the 'resting' receptor v. its affinity for the 'activated' forms of the receptor.

efflux   (L. *ex*, out of; *fluere*, to flow)

- Movement of an entity out of a specified compartment or across a specified barrier.

efflux coefficient   (L. *ex*, out of; *fluere*, to flow; *co, com/cum, con*, with,
together, in common, jointly, equally, reciprocally,
mutually; *efficere*, to accomplish)
- One of the constants that can be used to describe a **first-order** efflux from a
compartment. It is the *percentage* of a substance that leaves the compartment in unit time ($\% \ min^{-1}$). It is 100 times the **efflux rate constant**.

efflux rate constant
- The **rate constant** that applies to the **first-order** efflux of a substance from a
compartment. It is the fraction of a substance that leaves the compartment in
unit time (min^{-1}).

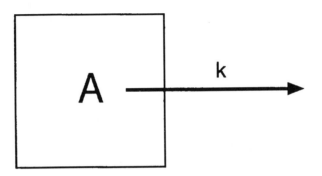

If [*A*] is the concentration of substance A within the compartment, then the
rate of efflux = *k*[*A*], where *k* is the efflux rate constant. At any time, (*t*), the
concentration in the compartment, ([*A*]$_t$), can be obtained from the exponential equation:

$$[A]_t = [A]_0 e^{-kt}$$

where *e* is the base of natural logarithms (see **exponential curve/equation/
function**).

EFPIA
- European Federation of Pharmaceutical Industries Associations.

EGF
- Epidermal growth factor; one of the **cytokines**.

eicosanoids   (Gr. *eikosa*, twenty; *eidos*, form)
- A family of twenty-carbon essential fatty acids, formed principally from
arachidonic acid. They play a major role in physiology and disease throughout the body, and comprise principally the **prostaglandins, thromboxanes**
and **leukotrienes**.

electrophoresis   (Gr. *electron*, amber; *phorein*, to carry)
- An electric current passed through a solution causes electrically charged sol-

ute particles to migrate towards the oppositely charged electrode. Proteins and other molecules can be separated on the basis of charge and size. A gel or other support medium, e.g. cellulose acetate, is added to reduce diffusion and mixing of the separated materials.

electroporation   See **iontophoresis, transdermal**

electuary   (Gr. *e*, out; *leikhein*, to lick)
- An obsolete form of medicine made with honey or syrup for licking rather than swallowing. If the preparation was made too thin it fermented; if too thick, it solidified. In either case it rotted the teeth.

elimination   (L. *e*, out; *limen*, threshold)
- Removal of a drug from the body, unchanged or via biotransformation, e.g. via the kidneys, lungs. The term is generally preferred for *excretion*.
                                                             See **half-life**

elimination rate constant   (L. *e*, out; *limen*, threshold)
- The elimination rate constant (k) is the *fractional rate of drug removal* or *fractional* **turnover** *rate*:

$$k = (\text{rate of elimination}) \div (\text{amount in body})$$

(After *Rowland & Tozer*, see Acknowledgements.)

elixir   (Arabic *al iksir*, the elixir; probably from
                                              Gr. *xerion*, powder for drying wounds)
- *Modern*: clear, pleasantly flavoured liquid preparation of a medicine. The vehicle frequently contains a high proportion of alcohol, sugar, glycerol or propylene glycol.
- *Ancient*: anything that purports to be a sovereign remedy, e.g. 'elixir of life'.

embryotoxicity   (Gr. *embruon*, from *bruein*, to swell; *toxicon*, arrow poison)
- The property of causing damage to the embryo during the period of organogenesis, i.e. the first 12 weeks of gestation (human).
                                                       See **fetotoxic, teratogenesis**

E$_{max}$
- The maximal effect that an **agonist** can produce. The system in which the effect has been measured should be described, as E_{max} can vary depending upon the system (e.g., according to **receptor** density or type of coupling) (after **IUPHAR**, *Pharmacological Reviews* 1995;47:255–266).

EMEA
- European Medicines Evaluation Agency: the agency for harmonizing the licensing of medicines in the European Union.

emetic   (Gr. *emein*, to vomit)
- An agent that causes vomiting. **Ipecacuanha** has use as a liquid emetic mix-

ture in cases of poisoning by mouth, especially in children, provided that the patient is conscious.

emollient (L. *mollis*, soft)
— A thing that softens or soothes, chiefly applied to the skin, which it also hydrates.

empirical/-ism (Gr. *en*, in; *peiria*, experience)
— Based on, or acting on, observation or experiment, not on theory; deriving knowledge from experience alone; without knowledge of principles.
— "Empiricism is not the negation of science, as certain physicians seem to think; it is only its first stage" (*Claude Bernard*, 1813–1878, French physiologist and author of *An introduction to the study of experimental medicine*, 1865, available in translations, highly recommended reading; a seminal book and still relevant today).
— In chemistry: formula showing constituents of a compound in their proportions but not their configuration.

EMR
— **Equieffective molar concentration ratio.**

emulsion/emulsifying agents (L. *e*, out; *mulgere*, to milk)
— *Emulsion*: a colloidal dispersion of one liquid in another.
— *Emulsifying agents*: substances that enhance the dispersion of globules to form an emulsion and/or prevent coalescence after dispersion (e.g. soaps, cetrimide, macrogol).

enantiomer/-morphism (Gr. *enantios*, opposite; *meristikos*, symmetrical; *morphos*, shape)
See **optical isomerism**

encode (L. *en*, in; *codex*, wooden tablets making a book)
— The assigning of **bases** in DNA in such a way that they represent the amino acid sequence of a given protein or polypeptide.

endocrine (Gr. *endo*, within; *krinein*, separate)
— Glands that secrete directly into the bloodstream, i.e. ductless glands, and hence anything pertaining to **hormones**. See **APUD, exocrine**

endocytosis (Gr. *endo*, within; *kutos*, vessel, cell)
— The process by which a cell engulfs a quantity of a material (*endocytosis*): of liquid (*pinocytosis*); of solid (*phagocytosis*). See **exocytosis**

endogenous (Gr. *endo*, within; *gen*, production)
— Produced within an organism.

endorphins (Gr. *endo*, within; *-orphine*, part of the word morphine)
— Naturally occurring polypeptide **ligands** for opioid **receptors**: larger than **enkephalins**. See **dynorphins, exorphins, opiate/opioid**

endothelins   (Gr. *endo*, within; *thele*, nipple)
- A family of vasoconstrictor isopeptides (21 amino acids), similar in sequence to the sarafotoxins produced by a snake, the burrowing asp (*Atractaspis engaddensis*). Endothelin-1 (ET-1) is made by the vascular endothelium and is the most potent vasoconstrictor known, but it also releases potent vasodilators, e.g. prostacyclin and **EDRF**. ET–2 and ET–3 have been identified, but their origin is unknown. There are at least two types of endothelin receptor, tentatively designated ET_A and ET_B.

endothelium-derived relaxing factor (EDRF)
- A term, introduced by RF Furchgott (pharmacologist, USA), for the substance – released from vascular endothelium in response to various stimuli (e.g. **muscarinic** agonists) – which is responsible for the relaxation of adjacent smooth muscle in the blood vessel. Now known to be **nitric oxide** produced from arginine by a specific enzyme system.

enema   (Gr. *enienai*, to send in)
- Liquid introduced into the rectum (by gravity from a reservoir or by syringe) to evacuate the bowel, medicate or diagnose (e.g. barium sulphate for radiology).
- The rectal route also has psychological implications for some people who may come to like it for itself. This can apply both to those who receive and those who administer enemas as, for instance, the exploits of a masked intruder who made late night enema attacks on female University students (particularly) and became known as the "Illinois enema bandit" (1964–1975). After his arrest a list of intended victims was found; it included the President of the USA.

enkephalins   (Gr. *enkephalos*, brain)
- Substances (pentapeptides) found in the central nervous system that are specific for what (in ignorance) had to be called morphine or opioid **receptors**, because it was not then known (although always suspected) that there was an **endogenous ligand** for these receptors. They are smaller than **endorphins**.   See **opiate/opioid**

enteral drug administration   (Gr. *enteron*, intestine)
- Drug administration via the alimentary tract, i.e. by swallowing or by the rectum.   See **parenteral drug administration**

enteric-coating   (Gr. *enteron*, intestine)
- **Tablets**, etc. coated with a substance resistant to gastric acid secretion (e.g. varnish, as in enteric-coated **aspirin**), so that the coating is dissolved and drug release is delayed until after the tablets enter the small intestine; also known as *gastroresistant* tablets.   See **modified-release formulations**

enterohepatic cycle/biliary recirculation   (Gr. *enteron*, intestine; *hepar*, liver)
- Excretion of a substance via the bile into the small intestine, followed by re-

absorption into the hepatic portal vein. This recycling can increase the persistence of a drug in the body. In some cases the drug is conjugated (e.g. with glucuronide) by the hepatocytes, and the conjugate is secreted into the intestine, where it is hydrolysed back to the active drug. Excretion in the bile is dependent on molecular weight (size) and charge.

enthalpy   (Gr. *enthalpein*, to warm in)
– The heat content of a system.
– One of the basic properties of energy and matter described in the science of thermodynamics.
   – Enthalpy (*H*) is one of the thermodynamic 'functions of state'.
   – The change in enthalpy (ΔH) is defined as the quantity of heat absorbed by a closed, isothermal system when, at constant pressure, it undergoes a change of state without performing any work (except that associated with any change in volume).
   – If heat is released into the surroundings, the system undergoes a loss of enthalpy (ΔH is negative) and the reaction is said to be *exothermic*. If the system absorbs heat (ΔH is positive), the reaction is *endothermic*.
                                                          See **entropy**

enthalpy/entropy-stabilized interactions   (Gr. *enthalpein*, to warm in; *entropeia*, turning towards)
– *Enthalpy-stabilized interactions* between **ligands** and **receptors** are usually characterized by the formation of new bonds, e.g. hydrogen bonds and **van der Waals' bonds**.
– In *entropy-stabilized interactions*, new **hydrophobic** interactions occur and ordered water molecules are displaced. Most ligand–receptor interactions are entropy-stabilized at first; then one or more enthalpy-stabilized steps often follow.   See **enthalpy, entropy**

entheogen   (Gr. *en*, in; *theos*, god; *gen*, to be produced)
– Drugs that open the way to supposedly divine inspiration. Not to be confused with **hallucinogens**, which merely cause the perception of non-existent phenomena and which are not used (useful) in the search for eternal truths. Most drugs claimed to be entheogens are hallucinogens; hallucinogens are not necessarily entheogens.

entity   (L. *entitas*, being)
– That which exists or has a being.

entropy   (Gr. *en*, in; *tropos*, a turn)
– A measure of the disorder of a system.
– A measure of the distribution of total energy of a system amongst its constituent atoms.
– In an isothermal thermodynamic system undergoing reversible change, the change of entropy is the energy absorbed divided by the thermodynamic temperature. It is measured in joules per kelvin ($J\ K^{-1}$).

- In statistical mechanics, entropy is a measure of the degree of order, or disorder, of a system, e.g. when water freezes there is a more ordered arrangement of atoms in the ice crystals.
- The application of the concept of entropy to the universe leads to a prediction that there will eventually be no energy available for use – 'entropy death' – (assuming that the universe is a closed system, which may well be untrue). Such a state, if it occurs, need not trouble anyone who reads this.

See **enthalpy, enthalpy/entropy-stabilized interactions, equilibrium**

entropy-stabilized interaction

See **enthalpy/enthalpy-stabilized interactions, entropy**

environmental impact assessment of the manufacture and use of medicines (Old Fr. *environ*, surroundings)
- So great is the scale of chemical manufacturing in the pharmaceutical industry that it poses problems of environmental pollution and general laws in this area are applied to its activities. For example the **EU** requires that applications to the **EMEA** for marketing authorisation for new active substances should be accompanied by an Environmental Risk Assessment (ERA) and an estimate of Predicted Environmental Concentration (PEC) of the drug in clinical use. The industry is subject to Integrated Pollution Control (IPC) and meets its obligations by using Best Available Techniques Not Entailing Excessive Costs (BATNEEC) and so on and on.
- As regulations proliferate, so do **abbreviations** and **acronyms.**
- Packaging also presents a waste problem that is subject to official regulation.
- Abandoned illicit drug factories (in California, USA) are reported (1997) to pose serious problems of leftover toxic chemicals disposal.

enzyme (Gr. *en*, in; *zume*, leaven, yeast; the term 'enzyme' was coined in 1881)
- A protein **catalyst**.
- "Many enzymes have flexible loops, floppy tails, mobile lids or bivalve-like hinged **domains**, which appear to close down over the substrate(s)" (*Knowles*).
- A variety of enzymes have crucial roles in signal transduction subsequent to drug–receptor binding (e.g. adenylyl and guanylyl cyclase, and various protein kinases).
- Enzymes are important targets for drugs (e.g. **aspirin**, benserazide, captopril).

enzyme induction/inhibition (Gr. *en*, on; *zume*, leaven, yeast; L. *in*, in; *ducere*, to lead; *habere*, to have)
- *Induction*: an increase in (hepatic) **microsome** activity, usually by increased enzyme synthesis, caused by a drug or other substance that acts as a substrate. Usually, inducing agents increase the amount of many different microsomal enzymes of hepatic drug metabolism, including oxidases and various conjugation enzymes. This results in increased metabolism of the causative drug (*autoinduction*) or of other drugs and physiological substances.

— *Inhibition*: a decrease in the rate of, or abolition of, an enzymatic reaction, usually by chemical inactivation of the enzyme (which may be reversible or irreversible).   See **cytochrome P450**

EPAR
— European Public Assessment Report, a substantial document made publicly available to 'interested parties' after a product receives **EU** marketing approval.

epinephrine   (Gr. *epi*, upon; *nephros*, kidney)
— The USA name for **adrenaline** (because *Adrenalin* was registered as a proprietary trade mark in the USA); epinephrine is now the recommended **INN** in medicine.

epiphenomenon   (Gr. *epi*, upon, in addition; *phainomai*, appear)
— An event occurring during the course of a disease or experiment that is casual or not necessarily related to it, i.e. is irrelevant or secondary.

epistemology   (Gr. *episteme*, knowledge)
— The theory of knowledge; the study of its validity and methods.
— "What do we really know or what do we think we know, when we think we know something 'scientifically'?" (*J Ziman*, physicist, UK).
                              See **heuristic**, **knowledge**, **science in pharmacology**

epitope   (Gr. *epi*, upon; *topos*, place)
— Antigenic determinant. Those structures on the antigen that cause the activation of B or T cells, i.e. the regions of the antigen molecule that interact with the **receptor** on these cells and with which the specific antibody produced by these cells combines to inactivate the antigen.

epitopic suppression   (Gr. *epi*, upon; *topos*, place;
                                                         L. *sub*, under; *premere*, to press)
— When the host has been pre-immunized against a **carrier** protein to which an **epitope** binds, selective, epitope-specific suppression of antibody production occurs.

equieffective molar concentration ratio (EMR)
— The ratio of the molar concentrations of test and reference substances that produce the same biological effect (whether activation or inhibition) (**IUPHAR**, with permission; *Pharmacological Reviews* 1995;47:255–266).
— When it is not possible to use concentration, as in experiments in man or laboratory animals, the term *equieffective dose ratio* (EDR) is preferred.

equilibrium   (L. *aequus*, equal; *libra*, balance)
— A state of balance; zero **entropy** production.

equilibrium (dissociation) constant   (L. *aequus*, equal; *libra*, balance;
                                                         constans, standing firm)
                  See **association equilibrium constant**, **dissociation equilibrium constant**

equilibrium potential (L. *aequus*, equal; *libra*, balance; *potentia*, power)
- The equilibrium potential for an ion across a biological membrane. The potential difference across the membrane at which there is no net passive flux of the ion. Provided that the movement of the ion across the membrane is independent of the fluxes of other ionic species, the equilibrium potential, E, is given by the **Nernst equation**:

$$E_1 = \frac{R \cdot T}{z \cdot F} \cdot \ln\left(\frac{[I]_1}{[I]_2}\right)$$

where R, T and F are the universal gas constant, the absolute temperature and Faraday's constant, respectively; z is the valency of the ion, I; and $[I]_1$ and $[I]_2$ are the concentrations (strictly speaking, the activities) of I on the two sides of the membrane. For *positively charged* ions the equilibrium potential is given by:

$$E_1 = \frac{R \cdot T}{z \cdot F} \cdot \ln\left(\frac{[I]_o}{[I]_i}\right)$$

For *negatively charged* ions the equation is:

$$E_1 = \frac{R \cdot T}{z \cdot F} \cdot \ln\left(\frac{[I]_i}{[I]_o}\right)$$

where $[I]_o$ and $[I]_i$ are the concentrations of the ion outside and inside the cell, respectively.

equipoise (L. *aequus*, equal; *pensum*, weight)
- The concept that, the **null hypothesis** being true, there is potential equality of benefit and of risk to subjects entering a randomized **therapeutic trial**. This has been seen by some as justifying entering patients into such trials without seeking their (informed) **consent**. It is likely that genuine equipoise does not occur as often as many investigators would wish.
- The concept of equipoise may be applied to the general concept of a particular therapeutic trial, or, perhaps better, applied to each individual patient entering a trial. See **uncertainty principle**

equivalence trial (or superiority trial) (L. *aequalis*, equal; *valere*, to be worth)
- A trial that has the declared objective of demonstrating therapeutic equivalence with existing licensed therapy in order to gain a licence to market. For this purpose proof of superiority is not required.
  See **need clause, therapeutic trial**

-ergic (Gr. *ergon*, work)
- Originally a suffix used to classify nerves in terms of their transmitter, as in noradrenergic nerve, cholinergic nerve, i.e. nerves that release noradrenaline or (acetyl)choline. Now that many nerves are known to contain and to release more than one transmitter, this use of the term is less useful. However, it is

still appropriate for classifying transmission in terms of the chemical involved. The suffix should not be used for **receptors**, e.g. 'adrenergic receptor', since it is unnecessary and can create confusion. The terms **adrenoceptor, acetylcholine** receptor are preferred (also **dopamine** receptor, not dopaminergic receptor). The term adrenergic agent is 'horrible' and ambiguous as it implies that the drug acts by releasing adrenaline. The terms adrenoceptor agonist or antagonist are superior (after *U Trendelenburg*).

ergot (Old Fr. *argot*, cock's spur, because of the appearance of the curved mycelial body)
- Ergot is a fungus that infects grasses, especially rye. It contains many **alkaloids** based on ergoline, which bears a structural resemblance to the biogenic amines **noradrenaline, dopamine** and **serotonin** (5-HT). The alkaloids have both **agonist** and **antagonist** actions, giving rise to extraordinarily complex and important biological effects.

Erice Declaration (The)
- The International Conference on Developing Effective Communications in Pharmacovigilance (Erice, Italy, 1997) issued The Erice Declaration on Communicating Drug Safety Information, published in the **IUPHAR** Newsletter, No. 49, December 1997.

error (L. *errare*, to wander or travel in quest of)
- Mistake: involuntary deviation from truth or accuracy.
- Types of statistical error:
  - *Type I (α) error:* treating a difference as significant when there is, in reality, no difference; false positive finding.
  - *Type II (β) error:* treating a difference as insignificant when in reality there is a difference; false negative finding.
  - *Type III (γ) error:* error in the *direction* of a difference, i.e. to conclude that A is better than B when, in fact, the *reverse* is true.
  - [*Type zero error* has been proposed – the important danger of not studying an association when it actually exists (*KB Michels, BA Rosner*, 1996)].
  - *Systematic error:* error that is consistent in direction and/or amount.

See **bias**

error peptides
- Synthetic peptides (for medicinal use) contain impurities that are variants of the synthesized peptide, e.g. truncated forms, blocked forms and variants of the molecular conformation (but not of the primary structure). These variants are called error peptides.

escalation in drug misuse (L. *e(x)*, out, from; *scala*, a ladder)
- The idea that an individual taking soft-use drugs is especially liable to proceed by successive stages to hard-use drugs. Pharmacologically, it is a doubtful concept. Where escalation occurs it is probably due to social/environmental factors. See **hard drug/soft drug**

escape clause (rescue treatment) in clinical trials (L. *ex*, out; *cappa*, cloak)
- An ethical device providing that where an experimental treatment fails, this is quickly detected and a known effective treatment substituted, e.g. in trials of new analgesics, antihypertensives. **See rescue treatment**

essential drugs(L. *essentia*, the being of something vitally important, fundamental)
- The World Health Organization (WHO) Division of Drug Management and Policies has a programme on the Use of Essential Drugs, as follows:
  - "The concept of essential drugs has been endorsed unanimously by the World Health Assembly. It is intended to be flexible and adaptable to many different situations; exactly which drugs are regarded as essential remains a national responsibility."
  - "There are convincing justifications for WHO to propose 'model' or 'guiding' lists of essential drugs as a contribution to solving the problems of Member States whose health needs far exceed their resources and who may find it difficult to initiate such an endeavour on their own."
  - "Such 'guiding' or 'model' lists should be understood as a tentative identification of a 'common core' of basic needs which has universal relevance and applicability. In certain situations, there is a need to make available additional drugs essential for rare diseases."
  - "Exclusion does not imply rejection."
  - "Many drugs included are an *example of a therapeutic group* and another member of the group could serve as an alternative."
  - The Sixth Model List (*Technical Report* 850; 1995) comprises about 300 items, including some nondrugs, e.g. intravenous electrolyte solutions and condoms. The list is updated at intervals of 2–3 years.

essentially similar (regulatory term) (L. *essentia*, a quality, a being; *similis*, like)
- For licensing purposes, a drug is *essentially similar* to another where it has "the same **qualitative** and **quantitative** composition in terms of active principles *and* the pharmaceutical form is the same *and,* where necessary, appropriate bioavailability studies have been carried out" **(EU)**. The product is not required to be entirely identical regarding minor impurities.
- A variant of the above is "**medicinal product** *of essential similarity*", which is a product made by more than one manufacturer for the same therapeutic use, interchangeable with, and with comparable **bioavailability** to, a medicinal product which has been authorized in the [European] Community for 6–10 years and which is marketed in the Member State concerned **(EU)**.

establishment (L. *stabilire*, to make firm)
- A group or class of people having similar values and posts of influence within society, or sections of it, (civil service, universities, professions, etc.) who formally, but perhaps more importantly, informally, influence policies, generally in a conservative direction. Their control of new appointments in their own fields perpetuates their influence. **See QUANGO**

estimate; point, interval estimate   (L. *punctum*, point; *aestimare*, fix price of)
- *Estimate*: a value or range of values calculated from sample observations that are used to approximate a corresponding population value or parameter (**FDA**).
- *Point estimate*: a single value calculated from sample observations, which is used as an estimate of the population parameter (FDA).
- *Interval estimate*: two numerical values between which the parameter/characteristic is likely to occur.   See **confidence interval**

ethics/-al   (Gr. *ethikos*, custom)
- *Ethics* comprises the moral values of human conduct and the rules and principles that govern it. It is concerned with intentions and motives and with the obligations or duties that people have to their fellows (neighbours). Morals (ethics) are sanctioned, if at all, by social pressure, except when they are so fundamental that society chooses to make them enforceable by law. Thus ethics provides standards that the legal system is devised to promote. Ethics and law have a common concern with justice.
- The use of the term *ethical* for proprietary drugs advertised only to the medical profession (and to describe the companies that market them) implies that the marketing companies can be counted on to put the public good before commercial considerations. Such misuse of language is of a degree that justifies terming it unethical.   See **Declaration of Helsinki and Nuremberg code, duty, interest (conflict of), right**

ethics committee: research ethics committee (REC)
- "An independent body, constituted by medical professionals and nonmedical members, whose responsibility is to verify that the safety, integrity and human rights of the subjects participating in a particular investigation are protected, thereby providing public reassurance. Ethics committees should be constituted and operate so that the suitability of the investigators, facilities, protocols, the eligibility of trial subject groups, and the adequacy of confidentiality safeguards may be objectively and impartially reviewed independently of the investigator, sponsor and relevant authorities. The legal status, constitution and requirements pertaining to ethics committees, review boards or similar institutions may differ among countries. A list of members of the ethics committee, and their positions, and a description of the committee's working procedures, including response times, should be publicly available" (**EC** definition).
- RECs ordinarily serve local districts. To avoid the wasteful need for multiple applications some countries have established special multicentre research ethics committees (MREC).
- The official term Institutional Review Board (IRB) is used in the USA; also the unofficial NRB (non-institutional review board). Generally it is desirable that a committee title should give a hint of its function.
- The title 'Ethics Committee' is also used for a committee that advises on the ethical issues arising in routine medical practice.

- In some countries there are research ethics committees for animals.
See **consent, Declaration of Helsinki, risk**

ethnopharmacology   (Gr. *ethnos*, nation; *pharmakon*, drug, medicine; *logy*, study)
- The identification and investigation of indigenous drugs or traditional medicines; allied to *ethnobotany.*
- The scientific study of plants used by a cultural group for medicinal purposes.
- Also used as synonymous with **pharmacoanthropology**.

ethopharmacology   (Gr. *ethos*, character; *pharmakon*, drug, medicine; *logy*, study)
- Study of the effect of drugs on social behaviour or interaction, in *animals* (e.g. response of a resident group of mice to an intruder; aggression, defence, flight) or in *man* (e.g. effect of drugs on personal and social behaviour in schizophrenia).

EU
- European Union: see **EC**.

eudismic affinity quotient   (Gr. *eu*, well, easily, pleasant; *dus*, bad, ill)
- Where a **ligand** exists as a pair of **enantiomers** the ratio of the **affinity** for the **receptors** of the more potent enantiomer (*eu*tomer) to that of the less potent enantiomer (*dis*tomer) is the *eudismic ratio*, and the logarithm of this ratio is the *eudismic index*. The slope of the line correlating the eudismic index with the affinity of the eutomer (for a series of enantiomers) is the eudismic affinity quotient. This definition clearly supposes that affinities can be measured accurately. The proportion of the concentrations of eutomer and distomer is the *eudismic proportion*.
- In the absence of affinity measurements a similar definition has been used, but with **potency** substituted for affinity.

eudismic ratio/index/proportion   See **eudismic affinity quotient**

euphemism   (Gr. *eu*, good; *pheme*, speech)
- The substitution of a word or phrase that is emotionally neutral for another with high emotional content. It is a device to escape embarrassment or confrontation with unpleasant reality. For example:
  - *In research on animals*: vocalize *for* scream; sacrifice *for* kill
  - *In employment*: let go *for* dismiss.

euphoria   (Gr. *eu*, well, easily, pleasant; *pherein*, to bear)
- A feeling of wellbeing, commonly exaggerated and not necessarily well founded. The opposite of **dysphoria**.

Eur. P
- European Pharmacopoeia.

eutectic   (Gr. *eu*, well, easily, pleasant; *tektos*, melt)
- A mixture of two substances in such proportions that both components of the mixture change state (melt, boil, etc.) evenly throughout at a specific temperature. For a solid it constitutes what has been called a 'solid solution', e.g. some mixtures of local anaesthetics for use on unbroken skin.

euthanasia   (Gr. *eu*, well, easily, pleasant; *thanatos,* death)
- The original meaning of a quiet, peaceful, painless death such as is the objective of all who care for the dying has in modern times been changed to mean a (single) medical act done *deliberately* to end life and at the patient's request. This is properly known as *voluntary* euthanasia and it may be *active* (generally using drugs) or *passive* (withholding treatments that may only add to or prolong suffering). Where life is deliberately ended in a patient who is unable to communicate rationally this is *involuntary* euthanasia *except* where this is done in accordance with a valid *advance directive (living will)*. (*Physician)-assisted suicide* is a variant of voluntary euthanasia. It implies a single or short term series of acts directly intended to end life quickly (see **judicial execution**); it includes providing drugs for self-administration.
- Where adequate relief of pain and suffering may also hasten death it is morally (and legally) permissible to give this relief *provided* the *intention* of the doctor is to relieve and not to kill. This is know as the *principle of double effect*. In individual cases its validity presents difficulties.
- *Terminal sedation* involves the production of a 'sleep-like state' (term used by the American Medical Association, 1997) or unconsciousness in that minority of patients who, in the last days or weeks of life cannot otherwise be relieved of severe pain. Drugs used include opiates, benzodiazepines, barbiturates, neuroleptics and combinations of these.   See **palliative care**

eutomer   See **eudismic–affinity quotient**

evacuant   (L. *e(x)*, from; *vacuus*, empty)
See **purgative**

evaluable patient   (L. *e*, out; *valere*, to be worth; *pati,* suffer)
- A patient in a trial who is regarded by investigators in the trial as having satisfied certain conditions and, as a result, is retained for analysis purposes **(FDA)**. A group of such patients is sometimes called a *valid patient group*.
See **intention to treat, observed case**

event   (L. *e*, out; *venire;*. come)
- An occurrence, incident, or experience, especially one of some significance **(FDA)**.   See **adverse event**

evidence-based medicine   (L. *ex*, out; *videre*, to see)
- "Evidence-based medicine, whose philosophical origins extend back to mid-19th century Paris and earlier, remains a hot topic for clinicians, public health practitioners, purchasers, planners and the public.

- "Evidence-based medicine is the conscientious, explicit and judicious use of current best evidence in making decisions about the care of individual patients. The practice of evidence-based medicine means integrating individual clinical expertise with the best available external clinical evidence from systematic research. By individual clinical expertise we mean the proficiency and judgment that individual clinicians acquire through clinical experience and clinical practice...By best available external clinical evidence we mean clinically relevant research, often from the basic sciences of medicine, but especially from patient-centered clinical research into the accuracy and precision of diagnostic tests (including the clinical examination), the power of prognostic markers, and the efficacy and safety of therapeutic, rehabilitative, and preventive regimens" (*DL Sackett et al.*; *British Medical Journal* 1996;312:71). Advocates of evidence-based medicine are sometimes reluctant to face the question of costs; "The policy and professional conflict between the individual–patient ethic and population–health goals waxes and wanes and is often fought as a political battle" (*A Maynard*).
- The evidential value of *properly conducted* different kinds of drug study (in descending order) is:
  1. **Meta-analysis**/systematic review.
  2. Randomized controlled **therapeutic trial**.
  3. **Cohort study**.
  4. **Case-control study**.
  5. **Cross-sectional study**.
  6. Case report (**anecdotal study**).
  (After *GH Guyatt et al.*; Users' guides to the medical literature. IX. A method for grading health care recommendations. *Journal of the American Medical Association*, 1995;274:1800–1804.)

examinations   (L. *examinare*, to weigh)
- "Examinations are formidable, even to the best prepared, for the greatest fool may ask more than the wisest man can answer" (*CC Colton*, 1780–1832).
- "In an examination those who do not wish to know ask questions of those who cannot tell" (*WA Raleigh*, 1861–1922).

exception proves the rule   See **proof/prove**

excipient   (L. *excipiens*, from *excipere,* to take out)
- Any material, other than the therapeutically active substance(s) present in a pharmaceutical **formulation**. *Functions of excipients* include adjustment of bulk; physical coherence of particles with the active drug/s; assistance with flow of powder and prevention of sticking to manufacturing machinery; to control disintegration of the tablet; to provide a protective coating; to eliminate taste; to control release of the drug/s; colouring (for visual identification).

excitatory amino acids   See **amino acids, glutamate, kainate**

excretion   (L. *ex*, out; *cernere*, to shift)
                                                    See **elimination**

exemplary (L. *ex*, out of; *emere*, to take)
- Fit to be imitated.
- Serves as a warning.

***ex gratia* payment** (L. *ex*, out of; *gratia*, favour)
- A payment that is voluntarily made without an admission that it is legally due.

exocrine (Gr. *ex*, out of; *krinein*, separate)
- Glands that release their secretions outwardly through a duct (e.g. pancreas, sweat glands, lachrymal glands), hence the term is used to describe things pertaining to this type of gland. See **endocrine**

exocytosis (Gr. *ex*, out of; *kutos*, vessel, cell)
- The process whereby the envelope of secretory granules or vesicles fuses with the cell membrane so that their contents are released from the cell. See **endocytosis**

exogenous (Gr. *ex*, out of; *gen*, production)
- Originating outside an organism.

exon
- The sequence of bases on DNA (**codon**) that **encodes** a specific amino acid. Non-coding sequences are called *introns*.

exoreceptor See **exosite/exoreceptor**

exosite/exoreceptor   (L. *ex*, out; *situs*, local position; *re*, again; *capere*, to take)
- Postulated *additional* **binding site** for a **ligand**, either on the **receptor** itself, or in its immediate vicinity. The ligand (or part of the ligand with affinity for the receptor or active part of the receptor) is free to transfer between the active receptor site and the exosite, but not free to diffuse away. The exosite is not normally involved in agonist **recognition** by the receptor and it does not mediate a biological response; it may act as a store and contribute to prolonged action, e.g. salmeterol and analogues. See **captive agonist**

exorphins (Gr. *ex*, out of; *-orphine*, part of the word morphine)
- Opioid substances (including peptides and alkaloids) formed outside the body (**exogenously**); e.g. morphine, an alkaloid, and the products of digestion of many dietary proteins, including casein and gluten, and other peptides from the digestion of meat. See **endorphins, opiate/opioid**

expectorant (L. *ex*, out of; *pectus*, breast, chest)
- An agent that promotes coughing up and out. Expectorants reduce the viscosity and/or increase the volume and water content of bronchial secretion. Sticky secretions, which may block smaller bronchi, thereby become easily eliminated by ciliary action and cough, at least that is the theory. The clinical efficacy of these agents is dubious.

experiment   (L. *experimentum*, proof, trial, from *experiri*, to test)
- Procedure adopted for testing a **hypothesis**.
- To find out by trial.
- An experiment is a hypothesis-testing or estimation procedure in which the investigator creates a situation according to a plan.
- An experiment is a research situation created according to the wishes of an investigator, as opposed to simply observing what occurs without interference (observation).
- The word is also (inappropriately) used to include the demonstration of a known fact, as in student practical classes, where the student alone (perhaps) is unknowing.   See **science in pharmacology**

expert   (L. *experiri*, to test)
- People whose knowledge, experience or skill causes them to be regarded as authorities, to have intellectual ascendancy over the opinions of others and to be entitled to be believed.
- As experts are increasingly seen to be fallible where their failures cannot be concealed and to be working for particular interests in society, [public] trust is disappearing (*New Scientist*).
- "No lesson seems to be so deeply inculcated by the experience of life as that you should never trust experts...they all require to have their strong wine diluted by a very large admixture of common sense" (*Lord Salisbury*, 1830–1903, Prime Minister, UK).
- The occupational disease of experts is arrogance – intellectual and technocratic.
- "One who knows more and more about less and less" (*NM Butler*, 1862–1947, President of Columbia University, USA).
- *Experto crede* (or *credite*) (L.): Believe one who has experience in the matter (*Virgil*, Roman poet, 70–19 BCE).
- A President of France (*G Pompidou*) stated that there are three roads to ruin (for a man): women, gambling and taking the advice of experts. Women, he designated the most pleasant, gambling the quickest, but the last as the surest.
- The common observation that experts disagree is due to the fact that as individuals they have all the faults of human beings, including vanity, as well as that their advice is sought on matters of particular difficulty.

Expert Reports (to a regulatory authority)   (L. *ex*, out; *perire*, try;
                                                              re, back; *portare*, to bring)
- For a marketing application three Expert Reports are ordinarily required, (1) pharmaceutical (2) pharmaco-toxicological, (3) clinical. They are submitted by the applicant and their function is to provide a summary and critical overview to assist regulatory decision-making on the enormous volumes of data nowadays supplied. The experts may be from within the development company or recruited from outside. Their qualifications to be regarded as experts must be stated.   See **expert**

expiry date
(L. *expirare*, to breathe one's last)
See **shelf-life**

exponential curve/equation/function (L. *exponere*, to set out; *fungio*, to perform)
- One of the class of functions that approaches an **asymptote** at an ever-decreasing rate.
- Exponential processes occur when the rate of change of a quantity at a given moment is directly proportional to its size at that moment; i.e. the exponential function $y = e^{-kt}$ is a solution of the equation $-dy/dt = ky$.
- More generally, an exponential function is any function that is linearly related to e^{-kt}, where $e = 1 + 1/1! + 1/2! + 1/3! + ... = 2.71828$ and t is the independent variable (commonly time). (*Note*: e is the base of natural logarithms.) This function decreases with t at a rate measured by k, which is known as the **rate constant** (if t is time). The reciprocal of k has the same units as t and is known as the **time constant**, if t represents time; or **length constant**, if t represents distance. In the former case, for example, the time constant is the time taken for the function to fall to a fraction $1/e$ ($= 36.788$ per cent) of its initial value at $t = 0$.
- The *half-time* is the time taken to fall to 50 per cent of the initial value, and is $0.693/k$. It is a characteristic of the exponential process that the time constant (and *half-time*) are independent of where the initial value is taken (*Note*: 0.693 is the natural log of 2).
- Examples of exponential processes include the growth of microorganisms by binary division (positive exponential growth) and the declining plasma concentration of many drugs, e.g. gentamicin (eliminated unchanged via the kidney) after a single intravenous dose (a negative exponential process).
See **half-life/half-time**

exponential distribution
(L. *exponere*, to set out, expound; *dis*, asunder, reversal of previous state; *tribuere*, to give)
- The **probability distribution** of random lengths of time (or distance). For example, the life-time of a drug–receptor complex, or of an open **ion channel**, is an exponentially distributed random variable. The exponential **probability density function** has the same shape as a decaying **exponential curve** (the mean of the distribution being the **time constant** of the curve). It is therefore a very **skewed** distribution.

exponential kinetics
(L. *exponere*, to set out; Gr. *kinein*, to move)
- The rate of a process is proportional to the amount of the substance present (law of **mass action**).
- A constant *fraction* of a drug is eliminated in unit time whatever the dose/concentration.
- The concept is fundamental to the determination of dose schedules of most drugs. See **first-order (exponential) kinetics, half-life/half-time, zero-order**

expression (gene)
(L. *ex*, out of; *pressare*, to press, squeeze)
- The production of a protein from a particular gene.

extended-release formulation   See **modified-release formulations**

extraction ratio   (L. *ex*, out of; *trahere*, to drag; *ratio*. from *reri*, to think)
– The rate of extraction of a drug by an organ (liver, kidney) relative to the rate of entry. By definition it varies from 0 to 1.   See **clearance, ratio**

extrapolation   (L. *extra*, outside; *polire*, to smooth, polish)
– To estimate from known numbers to others that lie outside the range of those known numbers.

extrapyramidal reactions/side-effects/syndrome   (L. *extra*, outside; the pyramidal part of the central nervous system)
– Disorders of movement due to drugs altering the function of cerebral basal ganglia (the corpus striatum) and associated structures (the substantia nigra, etc.), particularly associated with drugs that block (i.e. are antagonists at) dopamine receptors (e.g. **neuroleptics**).   See **tardive dyskinesia**

extrinsic   (L. *ex*, out of; *secus*, beside)
– Lying outside; originating from without.

ex vivo   (L. *ex*, outside; *vivus*, alive))
– The practice of modifying cells in culture and then returning them to the host.
– Techniques in which part of an experimental procedure is carried out on an intact animal, after which the experiment is completed on cells, tissues or organs removed from the animal, i.e. *in vitro*.

fact (L. *facere*, to do)
- A thing known to be **true**, i.e. verifiable.
- A thing that has really occurred.
- An event known actually to have happened.
- *In law*: in legal controversy, facts are matters determined by admission or by evidence; as distinct from matters of law, which are determined by authority and by argument.

factitious (L. *facere*, to do)
- Artificial rather than natural; fake, sham; used of deliberately induced disease (e.g. factitious dermatitis, factitious hypoglycaemia) – a form of **malingering**.
- Drugs so misused include warfarin, digitalis, atropine (to induce unilateral mydriasis so as to imply serious brain disease), thyroxine, laxatives, antidiabetics.

factor (L. *facere*, to do)
- A fact or influence that contributes to a result/outcome.
- An independent **variable** that influences another variable.
- A number by which another number is multiplied, e.g. the effect is increased by a *factor* of two.
- A number that divides into another number, giving a whole number answer.

factorial design (L. *facere*, to do; *designare*, to mark out)
- The investigation of effects and interaction of effects, and interactions of two or more treatments and/or doses, by assigning patients to all treatment combinations (including a **placebo**). In a study in which two drugs (A and B) were tested at two doses, patients would be allocated thus:
  - high A + high B
  - high A + low B
  - low A + high B
  - low A + low B.

facultative (L. *facultas*, capability)
- Able to live under more than one set of environmental conditions.
- Able to use or develop an alternative metabolic pathway.

fade (L. *fatuus*, silly + *vapidus*, vapid; hence, to dull)
- In the continued presence of an agonist, the response declines. This fade may be due to exhaustion of the responding elements, e.g. because of depletion of an essential substance, or due to **desensitization** or **down-regulation** of receptors. Not to be confused with **tachyphylaxis** or **tolerance**, in which there is a reduction in the size of *discrete* responses to *repeated* doses.

failure: why things go wrong (L. *fallere*, deceive)
- Decision-traps in complex situations include: acting with insufficient reflection, short-sightedness in calculating consequences, becoming enamoured of our own predictions in the teeth of contradictory data, over-involvement with self-

generated projects, excessive focus on small corners of a problem, neglect of early signals of impending catastrophe, and so on (*M Piattelli-Palmarini*).

false transmitter   (L. *fallere*, to deceive; *trans*, across; *mittere*, to send)
– A **counterfeit incorporation mechanism** whereby a drug replaces, by **competition**, a normal metabolite/substrate in the enzymatic synthesis of a neurotransmitter (e.g. methyldopa induces the formation of methylnoradrenaline instead of **noradrenaline**). A false transmitter may be less effective (by way of lesser **efficacy** or **potency**) than the true transmitter. Similarly, its pharmacological profile may differ from that of the true transmitter.

fast-follower drug
– A drug that, during the period of success or market dominance of a novel (breakthrough) drug, takes a major slice of the market from, or even excludes, the initial drug (e.g. chlorothiazide – hydrochlorothiazide; cimetidine – ranitidine: the second of each pair is a fast-follower).

fast receptors (ionotropic receptors)
– **Receptors** that comprise both the **recognition site** and **ionophore (ion channel)** in one molecule. Agonist binding to the recognition site causes a rapid change in conformation, which leads to a change in permeability of the channel to a particular ion species, and therefore a rapid response. In **slow receptors** the response is mediated through a second or third molecule, which catalyses the production of an intracellular **second messenger**.

FDA
– **Food and drug administration** (USA).   See **CDER**

FDCA
– Federal Food Drug and Cosmetic Act (1938) (USA). The pioneer legislation that first introduced *premarketing* regulatory control of new drugs. It followed a major drug accident in the USA in which about 107 people died after taking a liquid formulation of sulphanilamide dissolved in ethylene glycol (antifreeze) for bacterial infection. The rest of the world introduced similar legislation following the thalidomide disaster (1960–1961).

feedback   (Old Eng. *fedan*, feed; *baec*, back)
– The control of performance by the consequences of the act performed.
– *Negative feedback*: the rise in concentration of a hormone in response to pituitary secretion of the appropriate trophic hormone suppresses production of the trophic hormone (e.g. hydrocortisone and adrenocorticotrophic hormone); also neurotransmitters acting via *presynaptic receptors* (**autoreceptors**) to modulate their own release.
– *Positive feedback*: at a party guests raise their voices to make themselves heard, thus adding to the prevailing din so that everyone must shout louder and louder to be heard at all. Positive feedback is a fundamentally unstable and, in extreme cases, a self-destructive process, i.e. guests leave the party;

it occurs in autoimmune disease and ovulation in women (*PB Medawar*, 1915–1987, zoologist/immunologist, UK).   See **cybernetics**

fees   (Middle Eng.)
- Amounts paid for services rendered. A fee is sometimes (deliberately) confused with an *honorarium* (L. *honorarius*, honour), which is a reward given for a service for which payment is not formally required or is inappropriate. An honorarium is sometimes used as a device to blur the implications of receiving money where this may raise ethical issues, e.g. for recruiting patients for a clinical trial.

fetotoxic (USA and UK) **or foetotoxic** (UK) (UK spelling of fetus has the distinction of being wrong for the past 400 years, **Fowler**; see *Leahy's law* in **Laws (various).)**
(L. *fetus*, offspring, brood;
Gr. *toxicon*, arrow poison, widened to mean any poison)
- Toxicity at any stage of pregnancy, or toxicity after 12 weeks' gestation (human).   See **embryotoxicity, teratogenesis, teratothanasia**

fiducial inference/limit   (L. *fiducia*, trust)
- A system of inference originated by RA Fisher. In most (but not all) cases of practical importance, fiducial limits are identical with **confidence limits**. The logical basis of the method is controversial, and most people now prefer the confidence argument (*RA Fisher*, 1890–1962, statistician, UK).

filtration   (L. *filtrum*, piece of felt used as a filter)
- The passage of molecules through pores. For example, renal glomerular pores are large enough to pass all molecules of molecular weight less than 5000 Da, progressively fewer up to 50 000 Da, depending on their shape and charge, and virtually none above 50 000 Da (examples: albumin, 59 000 Da; heparin, 15 000–20 000 Da; insulin, 5700 Da; penicillin, 372 Da); but haemoglobin (64 500 Da) passes readily (haemoglobinuria).

first-dose effect
- The brisk onset of excessive action of a drug with its first dose, which is not repeated with subsequent doses, e.g. hypotension caused by the first dose of prazosin (probably due to an acute reduction of venous return to the heart consequent on the initial occupation of **adrenoceptors** without compensating tachycardia).

first messenger: second messenger
- A transmitter or hormone, such as noradrenaline, the *first messenger*, combines with a **receptor** on the outside of an effector cell and activates (via a **G-protein**) an enzyme, e.g. **adenylyl cyclase**, on the inside of the cell. This enzyme mediates the formation of the *second messenger*, in this case cyclic-AMP from ATP, which induces the physiological responses. There are many other examples.

first moment (of the concentration)

- In **pharmacokinetics** the product of time (t) and plasma concentration of drug (C) is used in the calculation of the **mean residence time**. This quantity, the product tC, is known as the *first moment* because it is concentration multiplied by time raised to the power of one.

See **area under the (first) moment curve**

first-order (exponential) kinetics   (Gr. *kineo*, move)

- Any process in which the dependent variable (y) is proportionally related to the *first power* of the independent **variable** (x) is said to be *first-order*. If the dependent variable is proportional to the square of the independent variable (or to the product of two variables), then the process is *second-order*, whereas if the dependent variable is constant, irrespective of the value of the independent variable, then the process is described as *zero-order* (i.e. proportional to the independent variable raised to the power of zero):

  Zero-order: $y = kx^0$
  First-order: $y = kx^1$
  Second-order: $y = kx^2$

  where x is the independent variable, y is the dependent variable and k is a constant.

- If y is plotted v. x, the curve is straight with a slope of zero for a zero-order process. For a first-order process, the plot is curved but is rendered straight by plotting $\log_e y$ v. x (slope = k). For a second-order process (rare in biology) a plot of $1/y$ v. x is linear and has a slope of k. (Note: For decay processes k is replaced throughout by $-k$).

- If the pharmacokinetic process for a substance is described as *first order* or *exponential*, the rate of transfer or metabolism of the substance is proportional to the amount (concentration) of that substance present. (Where a reaction proceeds at a rate proportional to the product of the concentrations of *two* substances, then the kinetics are said to be *second-order*, and so on.) For practical purposes the absorption and elimination of drugs conform to first- and/or **zero-order kinetics**.

- Receptor binding is a first-order process, as is passive diffusion.

See **exponential curve/equation/function, exponential kinetics**

first-pass effect

See **hepatic first-pass metabolism, pre-systemic drug elimination**

Fisher's exact test

- A **randomization test** for data in 2×2 **contingency tables** that gives exact probabilities. Fisher's exact test answers the following question: In two-way tables with the same marginal totals as that observed, what is the probability of obtaining the observed frequencies in cells of the table and all frequencies with a greater deviation from the expected? (*RA Fisher*, 1890–1962, statistician, UK.)

'fishing expedition'   See **correlations between variables, data dredging**

fit (of a curve/data)   (Scand. *fitten*, to arrange)
- The closeness (or not) of observed data to a **model** (real or assumed).

fixed-dose combination
- A medicinal formulation containing two or more drugs, generally with the objective of enhancing efficacy (e.g. co-trimoxazole), or enhancing sales (e.g. many antacid and analgesic combinations). They should be used only where all components are necessary for all patients.

fixed-sample trial
- A therapeutic trial in which the number of patients entered is determined before the trial begins, and statistical analysis is done on completion and not before. Disadvantages include a trial that, in the event, is too small (lacks **power**) or that is unnecessarily large (economic and ethical considerations). Choice of sample size requires consideration of the magnitude of effect that is worth detecting and at what level of **probability** or power (taking account of the variability of what is measured); it is an imprecise operation.
                                       See **interim analysis, sequential analysis**

FLAP
- Five-lipoxygenase activating protein. An 18 kDa membrane-associated protein, necessary for the activation of 5-lipoxygenase, the primary enzyme in the synthesis of the **leukotrienes**.

fluorimetry (fluorescence spectrophotometry)   (L. *fluere*, to flow)
- When some chemicals are exposed to light of one wavelength they emit light of another wavelength, i.e. they fluoresce. In fluorimetry the concentration of fluorescent chemicals is measured by the intensity of the emitted light. In biology the most common excitatory and emitted wavelengths are in the ultraviolet part of the spectrum.

fluorocarbons   See **chlorofluorocarbons**

foetotoxic   See **fetotoxic**

Food and Drug Administration (FDA)
- The governmental drug regulatory body of the USA; its regulations have major international impact.

follow-up study   (Old Eng. *folgian*)
                            See **continuation protocol, prospective study**

forced alkaline (acid) diuresis   (Gr. *dia*, through; *ouron*, urine)
- The renal elimination of some drugs, most notably (acidic) **aspirin**/salicylate, can be greatly enhanced by producing an alkaline diuresis with intravenous sodium bicarbonate plus a **diuretic**. The technique was introduced for treating overdose. Its efficacy depends on the properties of salicylate (its pH-

dependent lipid solubility). However, it is now recognized that pH is more important than urine volume and that the diuretic gives little or no benefit and can be hazardous. An acid diuresis for overdose with bases (e.g. amphetamines) is rarely needed in clinical practice.

See **Henderson–Hasselbalch equation, pH and pH partition hypothesis**

formulary (L. *forma*, shape, model)
- A collection of **formulations** and doses of drugs.
- A reference book in which details of formulations and doses of drugs are printed.

formulation (pharmaceutical) (L. *forma*, shape, model)
- The mode of presentation of a medicine, e.g. **tablet, capsule**, cream, solution. Modern formulations are highly sophisticated technical products.
- The composition of a *dosage form* (the completed product).

See **modified-release formulations**

FORTRAN
- *For*mula *tran*slation, one of the earliest programming languages for **computers**.

Fowler
- *Fowler's Modern English Usage*: 1926, 1965, 1996 (Oxford University Press).

fractiles (L. *frangere*, to break)
- Divisions of a data-set into equal parts. See **quantile**

FRAME
- Fund for the Replacement of Animals in Medical Experiments.

fraud in research See **research misconduct**

'free-basing'
- A technique used by the takers, manufacturers and suppliers of illegal drugs to produce the free **base** (nonsalt) form of **cocaine** ('**crack**') from its salt (usually the hydrochloride), which, when heated, forms an **aerosol** and vapour that can be inhaled.

free radical (Old Eng. *freo*, free; L. *radix*, root)
- An atom or molecule that has independent existence with an unpaired electron, that is, without all of its valencies being satisfied (in most molecules all the electrons are paired). The life of free radicals is usually brief (microseconds). They are highly reactive and may play important roles in many biological functions (and pathological processes).

free radical scavenger (Old Eng. *freo*, free; L. *radix*, root; Anglo-Fr. *scawage*, tax on goods offered for sale)
- A chemical that reacts with **free radicals**, thereby inactivating them and pre-

142

venting their effects upon the body. Examples are vitamins C and E, the enzyme system superoxide dismutase (SOD) and **nitric oxide**.

frequency (L. *frequens*, numerous)
— Commonness of occurrence.

frequency distribution (L. *frequens*, numerous; *dis*, asunder; *tribuere*, to give)
— A chart or table showing the frequency with which a value or characteristic occurs in a population or sample by classes or subgroups, e.g. deaths according to age.
— The general position of a frequency distribution on some scale is measured by an **average**: there are *three averages* in common use:
  — *Arithmetic mean*: the sum of all the observations divided by their number.
  — *Median*: the central value when all values are listed in order from lowest to highest.
  — *Mode*: the most frequent value in a series of observations (so long as the shape is not very **skewed**). See **mean, probability distribution**

frequency polygon (L. *frequens*, crowded; Gr. *polus*, many; *gonos*, angled)
— A device that converts a histogram into a continuous line graph. The midpoints of the top of the histogram columns are joined by a line. The area under the graph is the same as that under the histogram columns. Cumulative versions may be prepared.

'freshly and recently prepared preparation' (BP)
— *Freshly prepared*: made not more than 24 h before issued for use.
— *Recently prepared*: deterioration is likely if stored longer than about four weeks at 15–25°C.

Freund's adjuvant See **drugs as tools**

fugu (Jap.)
— Japanese name for the puffer fish, a member of the *Tetraodontidae*. Preparation of this delicacy has become a high culinary art in Japan. Strips of raw fugu are arranged into intricate patterns or pictures. Certain parts of the puffer fish, however, contain high concentrations of *tetrodotoxin* (see **drugs as tools**) as a consequence of which chefs who prepare fugu require a special licence. Nevertheless, several people are fatally poisoned each year in Japan as a result of illicit amateur preparation of fugu.

full agonist
— A full agonist is an **agonist** with high **intrinsic efficacy**, which can therefore elicit a maximal response from a tissue with **receptor reserve** by occupying only a fraction of the receptors (often quite a small fraction). See **efficacy, partial agonist**

functional antagonism See **antagonism**

functional food (L. *functio*, perform; Old Eng. *foda*)
See **nutraceutical**

funnel plot (L. *infundere*, to pour in, as in pouring a liquid
into a truncated cone; Old Eng. *plot*, piece of land)
- Funnel plots are plots of effect estimates against sample size in **therapeutic
trials**. They are useful to assess the validity of **meta-analyses**. "The funnel
plot is based on the fact that precision in estimating the underlying treatment
effect will increase as the sample size of component studies increases. Results from small studies will scatter widely at the bottom of the graph, with the
spread narrowing among larger studies. In the absence of **bias** the plot will
resemble a symmetrical inverted funnel. Conversely, if there is bias, funnel
plots will often be skewed and asymmetrical" (*M Egger et al.*; *British Medical
Journal* 1997;315:629).

Furchgott & Bursztyn method for estimating agonist affinity
- In a system with a **receptor reserve** the **location parameter** (EC_{50}) of the
concentration–response curve is lower than the location parameter (**dissociation equilibrium constant**, K_A) for the drug–receptor binding curve (**Langmuir adsorption isotherm/equation**). Furchgott and Bursztyn developed a
method for measuring agonist **affinity** in a system with spare receptors, which
involves inactivating a proportion of the receptors with an irreversible (insurmountable) **antagonist**. If it is assumed that:
  1. The action of the antagonist does not change the affinity of the drug for the
  remaining receptors;
  2. **Occupancy** of the same number of receptors will generate the same
  stimulus for response; and
  3. The relationship between stimulus and response is unchanged by the
  presence of the antagonist,

then at equilibrium, comparison of equal responses of a tissue when different
fractions of receptors are inactivated (occupied) will allow the affinity to be
determined.

In the absence of an antagonist:

$$S_A = \frac{\varepsilon_A [A][R_t]}{[A] + K_A}$$

where S_A is the stimulus produced by the agonist A; ε_A is the **intrinsic efficacy** of the agonist A; $[A]$ is the concentration of agonist A; $[R_t]$ is the total
concentration of receptors; and K_A is the dissociation equilibrium constant
(1/affinity) of the agonist A.

In the presence of an antagonist, a fraction, q, of receptors remains available
to produce a stimulus. When a second (higher) concentration $[A']$ of agonist is
present, the stimulus is represented by:

$$S_A = \frac{\varepsilon_A [A'][R_t \cdot q]}{[A'] + K_A}$$

In any single piece of tissue, if the responses are the same, then the stimulus is the same, and the number of receptors occupied will also be the same. Consequently, the two equations can be combined. When rearranged,

$$\frac{[A]}{[A]+K_A} = \frac{[A']}{[A']+K_A} \cdot q$$

This can be rearranged further as a double reciprocal equation:

$$\frac{1}{[A]} = \frac{1}{[A']} \cdot \frac{1}{q} + \frac{1}{K_A} \cdot \frac{1-q}{q}$$

When $1/[A]$ is plotted against $1/[A']$ (for the same response after the inactivation of different fractions of receptors), the result is a straight line with a slope of $1/q$ and an intercept of $(1-q)/qK_A$.
Therefore, K_A can be calculated from the relationship K_A = (slope − 1)/intercept (*RF Furchgott & P Bursztyn; Annals of the New York Academy of Sciences* 1967;139:882–899).

  − *Note*: If the two-state **model** applies (see **receptor** (*Two state model*)), the method is not applicable:

$$A + R \xrightleftharpoons{K_A} AR \xrightleftharpoons{K_E} AR^* \longrightarrow response$$

(where A = agonist, R = receptor, AR = the inactive (resting) agonist–receptor complex, AR* = the active agonist–receptor complex, K_A = the dissociation equilibrium constant for binding, and K_E = the dissociation constant for isomerization), whereas the Furchgott & Bursztyn method is based upon a single-step process:

$$A + R \xrightleftharpoons{K_A} AR \longrightarrow response$$

so that the first equation is based upon:

$$y = \frac{[A][R_t]}{[A]+K_A}$$

where y = response. This takes into account the intrinsic efficacy of the agonist only and not the efficacy of the agonist–receptor complex. Therefore the method is only applicable if the agonist–receptor complex is mainly in the inactive state (i.e. it follows the **Langmuir adsorption isotherm**).

furor therapeuticus   (L. *furor*, rage; Gr. *therapeueo*, cure)
  − Fury, craze, uncritical enthusiasm for providing active treatment for any complaint/disorder whenever the opportunity presents itself. A serious (for the patient) occupational disease of the medical profession.

fuzzy logic   (Low Ger. *fussig*, loose; Gr. *logos*, reasoning, discourse)
  − A method of dealing scientifically with vague, inexact (fuzzy) information.
  − It allows degrees of truth between the extreme values of completely true and

completely false; partial truths may be aggregated and developed into higher levels of truth.

- Quantification of value judgements in such a way that they can be processed by a computer. A fuzzy system can, for example, use 500 rules to diagnose the health of people in large numbers and draw up personalized plans to help them prevent disease, reduce stress and stay fit.

GABA
- γ-aminobutyric acid. The most important of the inhibitory amino acid neuro-transmitters in the brain. Its effects are mediated by two major **receptor** sub-types:
  - GABA$_A$ receptors: **ionotropic receptors** (Cl$^-$ channel)
  - GABA$_B$ receptors: **G-protein**-linked receptors coupled to K$^+$ (activation increases **conductance**) and/or Ca^{2+} channels (activation decreases conductance).   See **metabotropic receptors**

Gaddum-Schild equation
- The *Gaddum equation* is the equivalent of the **Langmuir adsorption isotherm/equation** for a system in which two ligands (*A* and *B*) are in equilibrium with a common binding site.

$$p_{AR} = \frac{[A]}{K_A\left(1+\dfrac{[B]}{K_B}\right)+[A]}$$

where p_{AR} is the proportion of binding sites occupied by ligand *A*; [*A*] and [*B*] are the molar concentrations of ligands *A* and *B*; and K_A and K_B are the **dissociation equilibrium constants** for ligands *A* and *B* respectively.
- The *Gaddum-Schild equation* (often called simply the *Schild equation*) is derived from the *Gaddum equation* by equating a version of the *Langmuir equation* and the Gaddum equation for identical receptor occupancies (i.e. occupancy of receptors by a single ligand *A* and the same occupancy by *A* in the presence of a second ligand *B*):

$$r = 1+\frac{[B]}{K_B}$$

where *r* is the **concentration ratio** (sometimes called *dose ratio*); [*B*] is the concentration of ligand *B*; and K_B is the dissociation equilibrium constant for ligand *B*. The beauty of the equation is that it is a **null equation**.
                                        See **Arunlakshana & Schild method**

galenical   (after *Galen*, celebrated 2nd century CE physician,
                                        personal physician to the Roman Emperor Marcus Aurelius)
- A medicine consisting of natural products, i.e. not synthesized in a laboratory.
- Medicine prepared from naturally occurring (herbal) ingredients, e.g. digitalis, to a standard formula.
- Following the methods of Galen.

ganglion-blocking drugs   (Gr. *ganglion*, swelling)
- **Antagonists** that interrupt cholinergic neurotransmission in peripheral autonomic ganglia. Most of these drugs work by **ion channel block** rather than by **syntopic** antagonism.

'garbage in, garbage out' (GIGO)   (*garbage*, etymology unknown)
- Where the input to a computer is of low quality, the output must inevitably

also be of low quality. The *aphorism* encapsulates the concept that, unlike their users, **computers** cannot discriminate between sound and worthless data; they process both types with the same speed, precision and lack of criticality.
- Also applied to **meta-analysis** of nonrandomized or otherwise design-defective therapeutic trials.

gargle   (Old Fr. *gargouille*, throat)
- To exhale slowly and noisily through a volume of medicated liquid suspended in the throat, a peculiarly antisocial form of **placebo** therapy, except it can be practised in total privacy.

gastrokinetic/gastroprokinetic   (Gr. *gaster*, stomach)
                                                                   See **prokinetic**

gastroresistant tablet/formulation   See **enteric-coating**

gating   (O. Frisian *gat*, hole, opening)
- The process controlling the isomerization of an **ion channel** between its open and closed conformations.   See **isomer**

Gaussian or normal distribution   See **normal distribution**

GBH
- 'Street' name for gamma-hydroxybutyrate, one of the so-called *dance drugs*, named because they are popular at nightclubs. Originally developed as an **anaesthetic (general)**, but abandoned due to excessive **toxicity**. Also known as GHB and Liquid E.   See **ecstasy**

GCP/GCResP
- Good clinical practice/good clinical research practice.
- The guidelines/regulations prepared by official regulatory bodies to ensure that **clinical trials** submitted in support of *product licence (marketing) applications* are of adequate standard.
- Because such guidelines have various official origins (e.g. **FDA**, **EU**) and variable content, pharmaceutical companies and contract research companies have devised their own **standard operating procedures** (SOPs).
- An example of a definition (**EU**): GCP is "a standard by which clinical trials are designed, implemented, and reported so that there is public assurance that the data are credible, and that the rights, integrity, and confidentiality of subjects are protected". Detailed guidance for implementation is provided.
                                                                   See **GLP, GMP**

gel   (L. *gelare*, to freeze, so a translucent substance)
- A **colloidal** preparation in which the particles link together to form a jelly-like mass: gels may be **thixotropic**.

-gen/-genic/-genesis (Gr. *gen*, be produced)
– A suffix to describe the effect caused by something, e.g. carcino*genesis* – the process of causing cancer.

gender (L. *genus*, birth, race, stock)
– Gender is nowadays used where it is desired to emphasize the social and cultural differences between the sexes rather than the physiological and anatomical aspects.

gene (Gr. *genea*, race)
– The sequence of DNA bases that codes for a complete protein (or subunit of a protein).

gene product (Gr. *genea*, race)
– A protein (or polypeptide) encoded in a single **gene**.

generations (of drugs) (L. *generare*, beget)
– When, during the development of a class of drugs (e.g. the cephalosporins), the later members have significantly different properties from earlier members (e.g. susceptibility to β-lactamase, or a different range of antimicrobial action), the drugs are sometimes classed as first, second, third generation, and so on.
See **grandfather drug**

generic drug/product (L. *genus*, race, a class of objects)
– When a patent (monopoly of an inventor) on a patented product or **formulation** expires (after 16–20 years in many countries), anyone may make and sell the product in competition with the inventor – as a *generic drug* or *multi-source product*. Pharmaceutical companies complain that so much of the period of the patent life is taken up with expensive development procedures, during which they may not sell the product, that they are unfairly treated in comparison with the makers of most other products.
– A generic drug has the same molecular structure as the proprietary brand, although regulatory authorities may allow variations in the formulation, when it will not be *interchangeable* with the original proprietary product. If the generic drug does not cost less, there is no purpose in making it.
– A generic product may be marketed under a *new* proprietary name, illustrating how perceived commercial advantage may take priority in medicine.
– Plainly it is unacceptably hazardous that there should be formulations labelled as the same dose but with markedly different rate and amount of delivery of active drug. Regulatory authorities therefore require that there be **bioequivalence** studies with the 'parent' proprietary formulation before a licence is granted, e.g. the generic product may be required to deliver a maximum plasma concentration (C_{max}) and **bioavailability (area under the curve or AUC)** within 25 per cent of the 'parent' standard in 75 per cent of cases.
– **WHO** has used the term to mean a pharmaceutical product, usually intended to be interchangeable with the innovator product, which is usually manufactured without a licence from the innovator company, and marketed after expiry

of patent or other exclusivity right. Generic products may be marketed either under the nonproprietary approved name or under a new brand (proprietary) name. They may sometimes be marketed in dosage forms and/or strengths different from those of the innovator products. See **generic substitution, names of drugs, pharmaceutical equivalence, same drug/different drug**

generic name (L. *genus*, race, a class of objects)
See **names of drugs**

generic substitution and generic alternative (drug)
– Substitution by a dispensing pharmacist, without consulting the prescriber, of a **generic drug** for the prescribed **proprietary** formulation. It may be done to save time (if the prescribed formulation is not stocked), but usually to save money. Where pharmacists are not formally authorized to practise generic substitution, they *must* supply the formulation named. In the UK, hospitals practise generic substitution, but community pharmacists do not (unless the prescriber indicates on the prescription that this is acceptable).
See **same drug/different drug, therapeutic substitution**

gene robbery/genetic piracy (Gr. *genea*, race; Old Fr. *robber*, to disrobe, strip; G. *peirates*, one who attempts or attacks)
– Natural products are the basis for many of today's medicines and there can be no doubt that many potential medicines remain undiscovered. Modern technology allows efficient screening and drug developers scour the world for leads amongst microbes, fungi, plants and animals. Developing countries in the tropics, with their luxuriant natural resources, are obvious targets and have justly complained of exploitation (gene robbery). Many now require formal profit-sharing agreements. The arbitrary use of human cell lines is also gene robbery.

gene therapy and genetic medicines (Gr. *genea*, race)
– *Gene therapy* of human genetic disorders is "a strategy in which nucleic acid, usually in the form of DNA, is administered to modify the genetic repertoire for therapeutic purposes" (e.g. cystic fibrosis). "The era of 'the gene as drug' is clearly upon us" (*RG Crystal*).
– *Genetic medicine.* Synthetic **oligonucleotides** are being developed to target defined sites on DNA sequences or genes (double strand DNA; triplex approach) or messenger RNA (**antisense** approach) so that the production of disease-related proteins is blocked. These oligonucleotides offer prospects of treatment for cancers and viruses without harming healthy tissues.
– A major practical problem is the delivery of the nucleic acid to the appropriate cellular site. Current technology includes the use of viruses as vectors, and **liposomes.**

genetic engineering (Gr. *genea*, race)
– The use of **recombinant DNA** technology to alter the structure of **genes** or create new genes. Such techniques have helped to advance our knowledge

of the way **receptors** and **enzymes** function and there is the promise that genetic engineering will lead to treatments for genetic diseases, such as cystic fibrosis and muscular dystrophy. See **biotechnology**

genetic polymorphism   (Gr. *genea*, race; *polus*, many; *morphos*, shape)
- *General*: the existence within a population of two or more forms of a species which are subject to simple inheritance.
- *Pharmacokinetics*: when individuals inherit different forms of drug-metabolizing enzyme, the drugs metabolized by these enzymes will have different pharmacokinetics in different individuals, depending upon the **phenotype** of each person. A common variation is in the ability to acetylate drugs (e.g. isoniazid, hydralazine, and some sulphonamides). Approximately half of some populations are 'fast acetylators' and the other half are 'slow acetylators'. Other examples include variation in the action of plasma cholinesterase (on suxamethonium) and of hydroxylase (on dextromethorphan). In these examples, the atypical enzyme is the result of a single altered gene. Heterozygotes may be partially affected. See **allele, genotype**

genetic prodrug activation therapy
- This technique takes advantage of genetic differences between normal and neoplastic cells. It involves the insertion of a metabolic suicide gene (usually bacterial or viral) selectively into neoplastic cells. The inserted gene leads to the production of an enzyme that converts a prodrug to its active (toxic) form selectively in cancer cells (after *LA Martin et al.; Lancet* 1997;35:1793). See **suicide (enzyme) inhibitor, targeting (of drugs)**

genome   (Gr. *genea*, race)
- The particular set of genes that an individual has, which determines the inherited characteristics exhibited by that person (e.g. eye colour). The term also means the complete set of genes making up the characteristics of a species, i.e. the sequence and location of each gene responsible for each protein. See **pharmacogenomics**

genotoxic/-ology   (Gr. *genea*, race; *toxicon*, arrow poison; *logos*, study)
- A substance is genotoxic if it reacts chemically with DNA, or damages the **genome** in some other way, resulting in heritable consequences.

genotype   (Gr. *genea*, race; *tupos*, image)
- The particular pattern of genes inherited by an individual. If a characteristic is subject to **genetic polymorphism**, the **phenotype** depends upon the *genotype* and the mode of expression, e.g. autosomal dominant, sex-linked.

geriatric   (Gr. *gerus*, old age; *iatros*, physician)
- Age is relevant to pharmacology; people above 65 years of age are deemed *geriatric* for such studies.

geronto-   (Gr. *gerus*, old age, *geron,* old man)
- Prefix for studies of old people, e.g. gerontopharmacology, gerontokinetics.

Gibbs–Donnan equilibrium   (*JW Gibbs*, 1839–1903, mathematician
and physicist, USA; *FG Donnan*, 1870–1956, physical chemist, UK)
- An equation that defines the distribution of diffusible and non-diffusible ions on the two sides of a semi-permeable membrane, or on an ion-exchange resin.

GIGO
- 'Garbage in garbage out'.

gimmick   (USA slang of unknown origin)
- Something designed to attract extra attention or publicity.
- A clever device or stratagem: not unknown in the marketing of drugs or in the practice of academic research.

GIRK
- Gated inward rectifying K^+ channel.

GLP
- Good laboratory practice.
- A code governing the conduct and recording of preclinical tests of new drugs for submission to regulatory authorities.
- The guidelines/regulations prepared by official (generally) regulatory bodies to ensure that laboratory (animal) studies submitted in support of applications are of adequate standards.
- GLP places particular emphasis on the organization of record-keeping, so that claims made in reports to regulatory authorities can be checked, if necessary, by examination of the original laboratory records.
                          See **archiving, audit trail, GCP, GMP**

glutamate
- This is probably the most important of the excitatory **amino acids** in the brain. Effects are mediated by two major subtypes of receptors:
  - **Ionotropic receptors** (nonspecific cation channels) of three types:
    - NMDA-sensitive, agonists at which include glutamate and **NMDA**.
    - AMPA-sensitive (formerly referred to as *quisqualate* receptors), agonists at which include glutamate, **kainate** and **AMPA**.
    - Kainate-sensitive (sometimes grouped with AMPA receptors and referred to as non-AMPA receptors), agonists at which include glutamate and kainate.
  - **Metabotropic receptors** (**G-protein**-linked), agonists at which include glutamate and quisqualate.

glycoside   (Gr. *glukus*, sweet)
- A complex organic molecule having a sugar residue.   See **cardiac glycoside**

GMP
- Good manufacturing practice.

- A code governing the production of medicines, to ensure that they are of consistently high purity and have consistent dispositional characteristics.
- That part of the pharmaceutical **quality assurance** ensuring that products are consistently produced and controlled to the quality standards appropriate for their intended use, and as required by the product specification. Any reference to GMP should be understood as a reference to the current **EC** GMP (*cf. Vol. IV of the Rules Governing Medicinal Products in the European Community*). See **disposition (of drugs), GCP, GLP**

gnotobiology (Gr. *gnotos*, known; *bios*, life; *logos*, study)
- The study of animals that are free from other forms of life: 'germ-free' animals.

gobbledegook (probably derived from the characteristic sound that a turkey-cock makes in its throat when excited)
- The language spoken by pompous officials. See **jargon, officialese**

goitrogen (L. *guttur*, throat; Gr. *gen*, be produced)
- An agent that causes enlargement of the thyroid gland (goitre).

good clinical practice See **GCP**

good laboratory practice See **GLP**

good manufacturing practice See **GMP**

government (L. *gubernare*, to steer)
- Government is the system by which a society is ruled or, preferably, rules itself. It is the intermediate body set up by the people, which is responsible to the sovereign power of the people (parliament in a democracy; a dictator in an autocracy). The functions of government are to execute the laws and to maintain liberty, both civil and political, and to do this by the legitimate exercise of executive power (*J-J Rousseau*, 1712–1778, philosopher, France). The *benefits* of government are:
  - To enable citizens to jointly undertake tasks that they cannot undertake individually, and
  - To protect individual citizens from the actions of others.
- Official *drug regulation* to ensure the quality, safety, efficacy and supply of medicines is an example of government in both roles. The **risks** of government are wrong decisions or policies (caused by ignorance, bad judgement, pressure groups, lobbyists, **regret-avoidance**, timidity).
  See **bureaucracy, policies, regulation (official) of medicines**

G-proteins: guanine-nucleotide-binding proteins (Gr. *proteios*, primary, first)
- Family of **GTP**-dependent, **trimeric proteins** associated with the cell membrane. They link **receptors** on the membrane to an enzyme (which catalyses the production of the **second messenger**) or to an ion channel. If the G-

protein is linked to an enzyme, the receptors are known as **metabotropic receptors**.

- G-proteins are so called because the α-subunit of the G-protein binds GTP and catalyses its hydrolysis to GDP (guanosine 5′-diphosphate). Coupling of the α-subunit to an agonist-occupied receptor causes intracellular GTP to exchange with GDP bound to the α-subunit. The GTP–α-subunit complex dissociates from the receptor and interacts with the effector protein (either an enzyme or ion channel), which causes the GTP to be converted to GDP. Once this hydrolysis has occurred, the affinity of the α-subunit for the effector falls and it reassociates with the β-γ-subunit complex.

- Responses to many external signals (e.g. growth factors, hormones, light, neurotransmitters, physical contact, smell) involve a **transduction** step in which a G-protein is involved. The G-protein is activated by the receipt of the message at the cell surface and, in turn, sets in train a sequence of cytoplasmic biochemical reactions that leads to an appropriate response within the cell.

- G-protein-linked receptors are also known as **slow receptors**, in contrast to **ionotropic receptors**, which are known as **fast receptors**.

grab sample   (Old Eng. *gripe*, grasp)
See **convenience sample**

graded response   (L. *gradus*, a step; *re*, again; *spondere*, to pledge)
- A systematic/consistent relationship between the dose (or concentration) of a drug and the magnitude (or intensity) of its effect such that the response varies smoothly with changing dose (or concentration), being able to assume any magnitude from zero to the maximum of which the system is capable, e.g. endplate potential; changes in blood pressure and blood sugar control are also considered graded responses.   See **all-or-none response**, **continuous variable**, **dose–response curve**, **mass action**, **quantum/quantal response**

'grandfather' drug
- A drug, particularly one still in use, that has been the source of (many) descendants or **generations of drugs**, e.g. morphine, cephalosporin, penicillin, propranolol, chlorpromazine.
- Another definition stipulates that the drug should have been in use before modern rigorous official regulation (*c.* 1960), at least some of the requirements of which, it is often suggested, the grandfather drug might now fail, e.g. **aspirin** as grandfather to **nonsteroidal anti-inflammatory drugs**.

granulocytopenia/neutropenia   (L. *granulum*, small grain;
Gr. *kutos*, vessel, cell; *penia*, poverty; L. *neuter*, neither)
- A decrease in the polymorphonuclear leucocytes in blood, which may be due to drugs. When the count falls below 1×10^9 per litre (1000 per mm^3) (normal 4.4×10^9 per litre), then serious microbial infection is likely to occur.
See **agranulocytosis**

graph: coordinates of (Gr. *graphos*, writing; L. *co, com/cum, con*, with, together, in common, jointly, equally, reciprocally, mutually; *ordinare*, to order)
- The *vertical* axis is the *y axis* (*ordinate*) (L. *ordinare*, to set in order).
- The *horizontal* axis is the *x axis* (*abscissa*) (L. *ab*, off; *scindere*, to cut).
- The *point* at which *x* and *y* axes intersect (originate) is *o* (the *origin*) (L. *origo*, to arise).

GRASE (regulatory **jargon**)
- Generally recognized as safe and effective.

Greek alphabet (Gr. *Graikoi*, prehistoric name of Hellenic peoples (*Aristotle*); from *alpha, beta*)
- The Greek alphabet is used in nomenclature in many sciences, including pharmacology.

A	α	alpha	N	ν	nu
B	β	beta	Ξ	ξ	xi
Γ	γ	gamma	O	o	omicron
Δ	δ	delta	Π	π	pi
E	ε	epsilon	P	ρ	rho
Z	ζ	zeta	Σ	σ, ς	sigma
H	η	eta	T	τ	tau
Θ	θ	theta	Y	υ	upsilon
I	ι	iota	Φ	φ	phi
K	κ	kappa	X	χ	chi
Λ	λ	lambda	Ψ	ψ	psi
M	μ	mu	Ω	ω	omega

green pharmacy (Old Eng. *grene*, green; Gr. *pharmakeia*, the making of drugs)
- Herbal medicines. The modern revival of public interest is largely due to fear of toxicity of synthetic drugs coupled with a (false) belief that plants or herbs are inherently safe because they are 'natural'.
                                                    See **bush teas, drugs as tools**

GRP (regulatory term)
- Good Review Practices. It is good to know from the US **FDA** that it prescribes good practice for itself and not only for others.   See **GCP, GLP, GMP**

GSL
- General sales list.   See **supply of medicines**

GTP: guanosine 5′-triphosphate
- A high-energy phosphate coenzyme formed from guanine, ribose and phosphate groups. Although it functions as a high-energy phosphate transfer medium, it also serves by forming **cGMP**, a **second messenger**, i.e. it is essential in signal **transduction**.   See **G-proteins**

guidelines and regulations (Old Fr. *guide*; L. *regula*, rule)
- Guidelines provide authoritative advice; they guide or advise; they are not mandatory.
- Regulations are mandatory requirements; they rule.
- Official bodies that fear criticism (their usual condition) if they make regulations, may issue guidelines with the intention, conscious or not, of treating them as regulations.

habituation (L. *habere*, to have)
– The regular and often excessive taking of a drug because a person has become accustomed to it rather than psychologically or physically dependent.
See **dependence**

haematinic (Gr. *haima*, blood)
– A loose term for any agent used to treat anaemia or improve the condition of the blood.

haemodialysis See **dialysis, haemoperfusion**

haemolysis (Gr. *haima*, blood; *lusis*, to release)
– The destruction of blood erythrocytes so that the haemoglobin is released into the plasma. It can be caused by disease and by drugs.

haemoperfusion (Gr. *haima*, blood; L. *perfusio*, to pass through)
– A method of extracting poisons from the body, in which the blood is caused to flow over activated **charcoal** or an **ion-exchange resin** (which adsorbs the poison) in an extracorporeal circulation.
– A technique in which isolated organs or tissues are kept alive for pharmacological experimentation *in vitro* by pumping blood into their arterioles. The blood may be from the same animal as the tissue, from another animal of the same species or even from an animal of a different species. Although haemoperfusion of isolated organs may mimic life more closely than perfusion with a physiological salts solution, there are few circumstances in which it is essential. Simpler techniques are usually adequate.
See **dialysis, superfusion**

half-life/half-time ($t_{1/2}$)
– The time taken for a concentration or other measure/**variable** to decline by half. The term is commonly used with reference to the concentration of a drug in blood plasma, the total amount in the body (e.g. radioactive substances), and to biological effects (e.g. pulse rate, gastric emptying time). It is a constant (in the sense that its value is independent of when the timing is started) only for phenomena that have a single exponential time course.
– If an overall process comprises two or more 'sub-processes' which are exponential, then although the overall process cannot be described by a single constant, $t_{1/2}$, each contributory process will have a unique and characteristic $t_{1/2}$. This is so for the elimination of drugs. When a single dose is given intravenously, the plasma concentration almost immediately reaches its peak. It first drops rapidly as the drug distributes outside the vascular compartment (α or *distribution phase*), and then more slowly as the now distributed drug (equilibrated with the tissues) is eliminated by metabolic and excretory processes (β or *elimination phase*). The half-life ordinarily quoted is that measured in the second, or β, phase.
– Where two or more exponential phases of decline (in sequence) of plasma

concentration of a drug are seen, the last (slowest) is called the z or *terminal phase*. See **exponential curve, exponential kinetics, first-order kinetics, time constant**

hallucinogen (L. *alucinari*, to wander in mind)
— A drug that induces hallucinations or illusions, i.e. the apparent perception of external objects, sights, sounds, touch or smells, that are not actually present.

haphazard (Middle Eng. *hap*, to happen, chance; Arabic *al-zahr*, gaming dice and so chance)
— Haphazard selection implies the gathering of a group of experimental subjects without deliberate method or design, in the hope that the selection will be truly random, but without taking steps to ensure that true random selection is achieved. See **random**

hapten (Gr. *haptein*, to fasten)
— A small molecule which by itself cannot stimulate the formation of antibodies, but which, when it is coupled to a large (**carrier**) molecule, e.g. serum albumin, is capable of stimulating antibody production. The antibodies produced will bind either to the hapten or to the carrier. An example of a hapten is the benzylpenicilloyl **moiety**.

haptophore (Gr. *haptein*, to fasten; *phoros*, a carrier)
— The structural element of a protein that allows the molecule to bind to a **hapten**.

harassing agents/short-term incapacitants/antiriot agents
(Old Fr. *harer*, to set a dog on)
See **riot control agents**

'hard' drug: 'soft' drug
— Drugs used/abused for nonmedical/social purposes are sometimes defined as **hard**, i.e. those that seriously disable the individual as a functioning member of society by inducing severe emotional and/or physical dependence (e.g. heroin), and **soft**, i.e. those that are less **dependence**-producing and socially disabling (e.g. cannabis). The terms are plainly unsatisfactory in that alcohol can be used in such a way that, for the individual, it could be put in either class. It is preferable to speak of *hard-use* where the drug is central to the user's life, and *soft-use* where it is merely incidental, i.e. *what is classified is not the drug, but the way it is used*. Precise terminology is lacking in this area.

Hawthorne effect (attention bias)
— The act of studying an outcome can itself change that outcome.
— The occurrence of changes in behaviour or perception in research subjects due to the fact that they are being observed. The name derives from a famous study in the Hawthorne electrical component factory in Chicago (USA) in the 1920s, in which serial changes in working conditions were associated

with increased output. Eventually the investigators reversed these changes and restored the original conditions – and output increased again (*FJ Roethlisberger, J Dickson;* Management and the worker. Harvard University Press, 1939).   See **bias, confounding**

hazard   (Arabic, *al-zahr*, gaming dice, chance)
- "A situation that in particular circumstances could lead to harm" (*Royal Society, London*).

hazard function/rate/ratio   (Arabic, *al-zahr*, gaming dice, chance)
- The *hazard function* is an 'instantaneous' measure of failure at any point in time (t), e.g. the probability of dying in the next small interval of time ($t + 1$), among subjects who have survived to time t.
- The *hazard rate* is the number of outcomes measured, divided by the total follow-up or exposure time. It is often useful to know whether the hazard rate is constant or changes with time.
- The *hazard ratio* is a measure of the relative survival of two groups. (After *MKB Parmar, D Machin*)   See **risk**

health   (Ger. *hal*, whole)
- The World Health Organization demonstrates a noble optimism by defining health as "a state of complete physical, mental and social well-being," and adds its Utopian slogan "health for all by the year 2000". (Utopia is an imaginary ideally perfect, and so boring, place described in a book by Thomas More, 1516; the word derives from Greek, no place).
                    See **just society, psychopharmacology** *(Cosmetic)*

healthy volunteer   See **volunteer**

heat-shock proteins
- A family of closely related proteins produced in response to a rise in body temperature and some other noxious stimuli, such as oxygen deprivation. Heat-shock proteins are found in all species and have amino acid sequences that are the most highly conserved (between species) of all known proteins. For example, the 70 kDa heat-shock protein from *Escherichia coli* is 50 per cent identical to the human 70 kDa heat-shock protein. Little is known of their function, except that they appear to be involved in enabling cells to survive raised temperatures. It is known that some heat-shock proteins can bind to unfolded sections of other proteins that have been denatured by heat, and prevent them from precipitating inside the cell. The heat-shock response is very rapid; transcription of the heat-shock genes begins within minutes of the temperature rise.   See **chaperonins**

hedge   (Old Eng./Ger.)
- A line of things forming a barrier.
- A cautious or evasive statement, being an essential skill in scientific and medical writing for the expression of scientific uncertainty. Five categories are

recognized, as illustrated in an editorial in *Lancet* (1992;340:275–276) thus: "*It seems* [shield] that *most* [approximator] contributors to medical journals find it *extremely difficult* [emotionally charged intensifier] *to be certain which of their conclusions have been proven and which not* [passive voice], *or so one must assume* [(paradoxical) expression of author's personal doubt]".

hedgehog protein   (The hedgehog is a small spiny mammal of genus *Erinaceus*, widely distributed, except in Africa)
- Hedgehog protein (sometimes sonic hedgehog protein) is named after a character in a computer game that has the ability to regenerate after being killed.
- A class of molecule that induces the formation or regeneration of tissues.

hemicholinium   See **drugs as tools**

Henderson–Hasselbalch equation
- This equation relates the proportions of dissociated and undissociated weak acids/bases to the pH of the solution (at equilibrium):
  - For a weak acid:

    $$pH = pK_a + \log([A^-] / [HA])$$

  - For a weak base:

    $$pH = pK_a + \log([B] / [BH^+])$$

  where **pK_a** is the negative log of the **dissociation equilibrium constant** for (ionization of) the weak acid or base, [A^-] is the concentration of anion formed by dissociation of the weak acid, [HA] is the concentration of undissociated weak acid, [B] is the concentration of the weak base and [BH^+] is the concentration of the ionized (protonated) base; pH is the negative log (base 10) of the hydrogen ion concentration. The pK_a is the pH at which half the acid or base is dissociated.

hepatic extraction ratio
- The fraction of a drug removed from the blood during a single passage through the liver. Calculated as the plasma concentration of the drug in the hepatic vein divided by the plasma concentration of the drug in the hepatic portal vein.   See **clearance, extraction ratio**

hepatic first-pass metabolism/clearance
- When a drug is absorbed from the gut all of it must pass through the liver via the hepatic portal vein before it reaches the systemic circulation. A drug that is readily metabolized by the liver may be almost completely altered during this 'first-pass'. Examples of drugs that undergo extensive first-pass metabolism include chlorpromazine and propranolol; aldosterone is unusable by mouth for this reason. Some drugs are cleared in the liver and excreted in the bile without metabolism. Drugs that undergo this are those that are highly

lipid soluble and enter liver cells very readily. Drugs absorbed from the lower rectum may *directly* enter the systemic circulation.

See **enterohepatic recirculation, pre-systemic drug elimination**

heptahelical receptors   See **receptors** *(Heptahelical)*

herbal medicine   (L. *herba,* grass, green crop)
- A medicinal product consisting of a substance produced by subjecting a plant or plants to drying, crushing or any other process, or of a mixture whose sole ingredients are two or more substances so produced, or of a mixture whose sole ingredients are one or more substances so produced and water or some other inert substance (Medicines Act UK).
- Licensing conditions regarding claims for efficacy are similar to those laid down for homoeopathic products.   See **homoeopathy**.
- The term *herbal* is not ordinarily used to refer to the numerous drugs derived from plants that have long had an important role in conventional medicine, having undergone full and rigorous clinical evaluation, e.g. digoxin, quinine, vincristine, morphine, atropine, tubocurarine. Also, the synthesis of some hormones in commercial quantities was made practicable by using plant products, e.g. hydrocortisone from a derivative of soya beans.

Herxheimer reaction   See **Jarisch–Herxheimer reaction**

hetero-   (Gr. *heteros*, the other of two)
- Prefix meaning different, e.g. heterogeneous, heterotrophic.

heterogeneous   See **homogeneous**

heterologous/ly   (Gr. *heteros,* the other of two; *logos*, relation)
- Dissimilar/ity.
- Consisting of different elements.
- Tissue differing from the normal.   See **homologous**

heteromeric receptors   (Gr. *heteros,* the other of two; *meros*, part)
- **Receptors** composed of two or more non-identical subunits.
                              See **homomeric receptors, multimeric receptors**

heteroreceptor   (Gr. *heteros*, the other of two; L. *re*, again; *capere*, to take)
- A presynaptic **receptor** involved in the **modulation** of transmitter release, which is sensitive to a transmitter other than that released by the nerve upon which it resides.   See **autoreceptor**

heteroscedasticity   (Gr. *heteros*, the other of two; *skedasis*, a scattering, dispersion)
- The situation in which the **variance** associated with one **variable** changes according to the magnitude of another variable. For example, in a drug **dose-response** curve, the variance of the concentration of drug that induces a

given response changes according to the size of the response (i.e. the position on the y-axis). Where the variance associated with a variable is constant, irrespective of the magnitude of the other variable, the statistic is *homoscedastic*. This has particular significance when it is necessary to interpolate on a dose-response curve to obtain the concentration that would induce a given response – the variance of the **logarithm** of drug concentration is more nearly homoscedastic.   See **transformation**

heterotrophic regulation   (Gr. *heteros*, the other of two; *trophein*, to feed)
– A form of **allosteric interaction** in which one substance (the allosteric effector or regulator) acts at one site on a macromolecule (regulator site) to modify the characteristics of interaction between a second substance and a different site on the macromolecule.

heuristic   (Gr. *heurisko*, find)
– Method of solving problems for which no **algorithm** exists, involving the narrowing of the field of search by **induction** from past experience of similar problems.
– **Knowledge**, or a solution to a problem, obtained by reasoning from past experience.
– System of education in which the pupils are taught to find out or learn for themselves.

hexamethonium   See **drugs as tools**

HFA
– **Hydrofluoroalkanes**.

hierarchy (evidential value) of therapeutic studies
                        See **evidence-based medicine**

Hill equation/plot   (*AV Hill*, 1886–1977, physiologist, UK)
– A relationship based on the formal scheme

$$n\text{A} + \text{R} \rightleftharpoons \text{A}_n\text{R}$$

where A is a ligand and R is a receptor or other binding site. (In fact the simultaneous binding of n molecules is physically virtually impossible.) The equation gives y, the concentration of receptors occupied (i.e. in the A_nR state), as:

$$y = x^n / (x^n + K^n)$$

where x is the concentration of A and K is a constant (the **location parameter**). For a hyperbolic **dose–response curve**, y can also represent the response. In this case it is preferable to use **EC$_{50}$** instead of K; K is to be preferred for ligand binding experiments, although whether K corresponds to a single **dissociation equilibrium constant** depends upon the experimental conditions and the system under investigation.

- If $n = 1$, the Hill equation is the same as the **Langmuir equation**. If response/occupancy is expressed as a fraction of the maximal response/occupancy, the graph of:

$$\log\left(\frac{p}{1-p}\right) v \log x$$

gives a straight line with a slope of n (often written as n_H), the *Hill coefficient*, where $p = y_x/y_{max}$. This is the *Hill plot*. Slopes greater than 1 are said to indicate positive **cooperativity** and slopes of less than 1 indicate either (a) **heterogeneity** of binding sites or (b) negative cooperativity. At best, the value of n_H (i.e. the slope) places an upper limit on the number of binding sites involved. Often it has no simple physical interpretation at all.
- The *Hill equation* and the **logistic equation** are closely related but not identical.

Hill-Langmuir equation
- For a simple **mass action** interaction between **ligand** L and binding sites R to form a complex LR,

$$p_{LR} = \frac{[L]}{K_L + [L]}$$

where p_{LR} is the fraction of binding sites occupied by ligand L at equilibrium, and K_L is the **dissociation equilibrium constant**.

'hip flask defence'
- The practice of car drivers who have been drinking and who have been involved in road-traffic accidents to quickly drink some alcohol (carried because the 'need' was foreseen) in order to render subsequent breath or blood alcohol measurements useless as evidence of their condition immediately before the accident. It is usual for the drivers to state that they took the drink to steady their nerves, shocked by the experience of the accident.
                        See **backtracking booze, 'cough mixture defence'**

hired gun (slang)
- In litigation: an **expert** witness who is being paid to be partisan rather than objective.

histamine and H-receptors
- Histamine is an **autacoid** derived from the amino acid histidine by decarboxylation. Pharmacologically, at least two major subtypes of histamine receptor have been characterized:
  - H_1-*receptors*, which mediate contraction of the smooth muscle of the bronchioles, ileum and uterus; **syntopic** antagonists include chlorpheniramine.
  - H_2-*receptors*, which mediate positive inotropic and chronotropic responses in the heart and gastric acid secretion; syntopic antagonists include cimetidine.
  There may be more types than this, e.g. H_3.

histochemistry   (Gr. *histos*, web, tissue;
                              khemeia, the art of transmutation, alchemy)
- The use of the differing chemical properties of cells and their components in the study of cells and tissues. For example, selective identification of cell types in micrographs by staining for specific enzymes, glycogen, acids, bases, etc.

histogram   (Gr. *histos*, from *histani*, an upright mast; *gramma*, line)
- A **graph** that displays the relationship between one discontinuous **variable** (ordinate) and another variable (abscissa). It consists of a series of rectangles, or bars, the height of which corresponds to the value of the variable on the ordinate. Often used as a way of displaying the **frequency distribution** of a variable. The frequency with which a particular value, or range of values (indicated by the abscissal position of the bar) is observed is represented by the height (or sometimes by the area) of the bar.

'hit and run' drug
- The effect of the drug outlasts its presence in the blood, e.g. alkylating agents, irreversible monoamine oxidase inhibitors.   See **captive agonist**

Hofmann degradation
- The mechanism by which certain quaternary substances spontaneously break down. The **neuromuscular blocking agent** atracurium was designed to have two unstable quaternary groups so that the molecule cleaves spontaneously in aqueous solutions at pH 7.4, although it is indefinitely stable in the ampoule at acid pH. It therefore has a brief duration of action when injected, and termination of its effect is independent of (a sick person's) metabolic and excretory capacity (*Hofmann*, 1818–1895, chemist, Germany).

'ho-hum' research   (*ho*, exclamation used to attract attention;
                              hum, indistinct sound indicative of embarrassment)
- The term has been applied to trivial studies published for payment in trivial journals, which are often distributed free, and in which there is a paragraph specially written for the purpose of providing a good 'quote' in drug advertising copy, accompanied by an 'impressive' reference.

home medicine
- The term preferred by the pharmaceutical industry for medicines sold directly to the public. Also known as OTC (over the counter) medicines.

homeo-/homo-/homoeo-   (Gr. *homoios*, like, same)
- Prefix meaning *the same*; see below.

homeostasis (homoeostasis)   (Gr. *homoios*, like; *sta*, stand)
- The physiological mechanisms that maintain the chemical and physical properties of the body at a steady state.   See **cybernetics, feedback**

homochiral   (Gr. *homoios*, like; *kheir*, hand)
- A chemical composed of a single **stereoisomer**. Most biological syntheses produce homochiral products. Chemical syntheses generally produce heterochiral products – usually **racemates**.   See **chirality**

homoeopathy/homeopathy   (Gr. *homoios*, like; *patheia*, suffering)
- A system of medicine founded by Dr Samuel Hahnemann (1755–1843, physician, Germany) and expounded in the *Organon of the rational art of healing*. He discovered the 'law': "*Similar symptoms in the remedy remove similar symptoms in the disease*".
    > "Now as experience shows incontestably in regard to every remedy and every disease, that all remedies without exception cure swiftly, thoroughly and enduringly, the illnesses whose symptoms are of the like order with their own, we are justified in asserting that the healing power of medicines depends in the resemblance of their symptoms to the symptoms of disease: or in other words, every medicine which, among the symptoms which it can cause in a healthy body, reproduces most of those present in a given disease, is capable of curing that disease in the swiftest, most thorough, and most enduring fashion.
    > "*This eternal, universal law of Nature, that every disease is destroyed and cured through the similar artificial disease which the appropriate remedy has the tendency to excite, rests on the following proposition: that only one disease can exist in the body at any one time.*" (*Organon*)
- In addition to the above, he 'discovered' that *the effect of drugs is potentiated by dilution*, even to the extent that an effective dose may not contain a single molecule of the drug. AJ Clarke (1885–1941, pharmacologist, UK) pointed out that the '*thirtieth potency*' (1 in 10^{60}), recommended by Hahnemann, provided a solution in which there would be one molecule of drug in the volume of a sphere of circumference equal to that of the orbit of the planet Neptune. That a dose in which no drug is present may be therapeutically effective rests on the belief that there is a spiritual energy diffused throughout the medicine by the particular way in which the dilutions are shaken during preparation ('succussion'), and which affects only the desired molecules, not impurities. "We are asked to put aside the whole edifice of evidence concerning the physical nature of materials and the normal concentration–response relationships of biologically active substances in order to accommodate homeopathic potency" (*AW Cuthbert; Pharmaceutical Journal* 15 May 1982:p.548).
- The dogmas of homoeopathy have incurred ridicule, which is resented by practitioners, who observe that the critics have generally not made a serious study of homoeopathy, and that patients treated according to homoeopathic principles commonly recover. But pharmacologists generally feel that in the absence of *conclusive* evidence from therapeutic trials conducted to the *highest* modern standards (it is not true, as is sometimes alleged, that the individual approach of homoeopathy to patients renders such trials impracticable, and indeed they have been done), there is no point in discussing
    > "...the evidence adduced by the homoeopathists until the latter have succeeded in convincing the physicists that they have demonstrated the exis-

tence of the new form of subdivision of matter. It may be mentioned that the existence of such recognized subdivisions of the atom as electrons, etc., does not help the homoeopathic claims in a significant manner because, to explain the results obtained by Hahnemann, it is necessary to assume that a molecule can be divided into millions of subunits" (*AJ Clarke*; *General pharmacology*. 1937). However, it has been claimed that it has been shown possible experimentally to transmit a 'memory' to water and that this is compatible with modern physics.

– *Homoeopathic products* lack the rigorous evidence of efficacy required by modern **regulation (official) of medicines**. A compromise has been reached whereby they must comply with standards of *quality* and *safety* comparable to those required for licensed conventional medicines, but there is no requirement for evidence of efficacy and the products will not be registered for a specific therapeutic indication.

– To qualify for a licence, a homoeopathic product must contain no more than one part per 100 000 of the mother tincture (below) or – should it contain a prescription-only medicine – the homoeopathic dose should not exceed more than one hundredth of the smallest dose used in conventional medicine (after **WHO**).

– *Mother Tinctures (MT) and potencies*: a *Mother Tincture* is an alcoholic solution or extract of original material. Successive dilutions of the MT are prepared (with *succussion*, above) and are called *potencies*. There is no limit to the number of successive dilutions.

See **complementary medicine, cult, placebo**, ***post hoc ergo propter hoc***

homogeneous, heterogeneous   (Gr. *homoios*, same; *heteros*, other; *genos*, kind)

– Homogeneous: of the same kind.
– Heterogeneous: of different kind.
– Where sampling variation is sufficient to explain differences from a common value within a group, the group is said to be homogeneous. Where sampling variation is insufficient to account for the differences, the group is heterogeneous.
– Anything thoroughly mixed is said to be homogeneous.

homologous/-y   (Gr. *homologia*, agreement)

– Similarity.
– The existence of a common structural feature in molecules, which imparts similar pharmacological properties upon the molecules.
– When sequences of amino acids in proteins (such as receptors or enzymes) are very similar, they are said to have *high homologies*, and it is generally assumed that the greater the homology between two sequences, the closer they are in evolutionary terms.   See **heterologous**

homologous index   (Gr. *homologia*, agreement; L. *indicare*, to show)

– An index in which the main **variable** to be assessed is replaced by a second variable with which it appears to be correlated.

homologous series   (Gr. *homologia*, agreement; L. *serere*, join, connect)
- A family of structurally similar molecules synthesized in such a way that a systematic small change in structure is made between one member of the series and the next. For example, the poly-*bis*-quaternary ammonium series, in which the number of methylene groups between the two nitrogens can be any number from one upwards. There is a systematic change in the pharmacological properties as '*n*' increases. In more complex molecules, such as the benzodiazepines or penicillins, many small modifications to the molecule can be made which make little difference to its pharmacological properties, so that the structures of the active ingredients of different manufacturers' medicines eventually reaching the market may be quite different, although they may well be part of the same homologous series.

homomeric receptors   (Gr. *homoios*, like; *meros*, part)
- **Receptors** composed of two or more identical protein subunits.
                    See **heteromeric receptors, multimeric receptors**

homoscedastic   (Gr. *homoios*, same; *skedasis*, a scattering, dispersion)
                    See **heteroscedastic, transformation**

honorarium   See **fees**

hormesis   (Gr. *hormaon*, to urge on)
- Process whereby low doses of an otherwise harmful agent have beneficial effects. Espoused as the guiding and distinguishing principle behind some systems of **complementary medicine**, but in reality applying to all therapeutic agents used in conventional modern medicine.
                    See **adverse drug reaction, cult, homoeopathy, poison** (*Paracelsus*)

hormone   (Gr. *hormaon*, impel)
- A term devised by Bayliss and Starling (Department of Physiology, University College London) in 1905. Hormones are chemical transmitters produced by endocrine glands, that pass into the blood and act on remote cells/organs.
- Biologically active substances released from cells other than nerve cells and acting locally are called *local hormones* or **autacoids**.
- JW Black has argued that any chemical transmitter can be described as a hormone.   See **autacoid**

host-mediated assay   (L. *hospes*, guest; *mediare*, to be in the middle; *exagium*, a weighing)
- A method of detecting potential carcinogens and mutagens by injecting the substance and bacteria into an animal (often into the peritoneal cavity), re-isolating the bacteria and counting the proportion of mutant forms. It has the advantage that the bacteria are exposed to metabolites of the test substance.
                            See **Ames test**

HPETE
- Hydroperoxyeicosatetraenoic acid. Intermediate in the synthesis of the **leukotrienes**. Produced from **arachidonic acid** by 5-lipoxygenase.

HPLC
– Originally high-pressure liquid chromatography, but now more commonly taken to mean high-performance liquid chromatography. Neither version has any merit over the other as they both are true.   See **chromatography**

5-HT
– 5-Hydroxytryptamine.   See **serotonin**

hybrid drug   (L. *hybrida*, offspring of a tame sow and a wild boar, or of two species or kinds of animal)
– *General*: anything having a mixed character is said to be hybrid.
– A compound having two or more desired (therapeutic) actions, e.g. an antihypertensive with β-adrenoceptor antagonist action plus an additional vasodilator component. If the different actions are due to stereoisomers, the drug is designated *pseudo-hybrid*.

hybrid receptor   See **receptor** (*Cloned receptors*)

hydrofluoroalkanes (HFAs)
– HFAs replace **chlorofluorocarbons** in metered dose inhalers/pressurised **aerosols**.   See **inhalation of drugs**

hydrogen bond   (Gr. *hudor*, water; *genes*, born; Old Norse *band*, fetter)
– A weak electrostatic attraction between an electronegative atom (e.g. oxygen, nitrogen) and a hydrogen atom that is **covalently** linked to another electronegative atom. The structures of ice, proteins and nucleic acids, and the liquid nature of water are dependent on hydrogen bonds. Without hydrogen bonds, ethanol would be an inconvenient gas and unsuitable for social use.

hydrophilic/-phobic   (Gr. *hudor*, water; *philos*, love; *phobos*, fear)
– Having affinity/repulsion for water. The greater (less) the charge separation within a molecule the greater its hydrophilicity (hydrophobicity) The term *hydropathy* embraces the two terms.   See **lipid solubility, solubility**

hydrophobic bond   (Gr. *hudor*, water; *phobos*, fear)
– Attractive forces (**van der Waals bonds**) between nonpolar molecules which cause them to aggregate and exclude water.   See **polar/nonpolar**

6-hydroxydopamine   See **drugs as tools**

hyper-/hypo-   (Gr. *huper*, above; *hupo*, below)
– Prefixes to a large number of words denoting *above* and *below* normal.

hyperbola/-ic   (Gr. *huper*, above; *balein*, to throw)
– A curve that is the locus of a point, the product of the coordinates (x,y) of which is constant (i.e. $x \times y =$ constant).
   See **Black & Leff model, Hill equation/plot, reciprocal plot**

hyperpolarization   (Gr. *huper*, above; L. *palus*, stake, prop)
- The resting **membrane potential** is increased (i.e. is made more negative). It can result from the influx of anions, e.g. Cl^-, the efflux of cations, e.g. K^+, or a reduction in the extracellular concentration of K^+.

hyperreactivity   (Gr. *huper*, above; L. *re*, again; *agere*, to do, to act)
- When the elicited response is greater than normal without there being any change in **sensitivity** (i.e. there is no change in the EC_{50}/ED_{50}).
- The condition when a tissue or organ responds to stimuli that normal tissues or organs do not respond to. For example, in asthma the airways often constrict briskly when exposed to concentrations of air pollutants innocuous to normal airways. In all probability, this is actually due to increased **sensitivity** (in the strict pharmacological sense), but this usage of the term has become a fixed part of the vocabulary of the asthma specialist.

hypersensitivity   (Gr. *huper*, above; L. *sentire*, to feel)
- An allergic reaction to a drug or other **stimulus** (see **delayed h. reaction**).
- A qualitatively normal response that occurs at a lower dose or concentration of the drug than usual (see **sensitivity**).
- An abnormally or unexpectedly strong reaction to a stimulus. In this sense the term **intolerance** is preferred. This use of *hypersensitivity* is less appropriate than the others as it reduces the precision of the term. It should be avoided unless there is evidence that the increased response is because the dose–response curve is shifted to the left.   See **allergy, hyperreactivity**

hypnotic   (Gr. *hupnos*, sleep)
- Sleep-promoting drug.

hypo-   See **hyper-/hypo-**

hyposensitization   (Gr. *hupo*, under; L. *sentire*, to feel)
- To reduce the response to an **antigen** by repeated doses of that antigen (e.g. treatment of allergic rhinitis, hay fever, with pollen extracts).
                                        See **desensitization**

hypothesis/theory   (Gr. *hupothesis*, foundation; *theorein*, to gaze upon)
- A supposition made as basis for reasoning, without assumption of its truth, or as a starting point for further investigations from known facts. Theories should be formulated so as to expose them as clearly as possible to refutation.
- "A first-rate theory predicts: a second-rate theory forbids: a third-rate theory explains after the event" (*Al Kitaigorodskii*, b.1914).
- "...the simple-minded view [is] that a theory is just a model of the universe, or a restricted part of it, and a set of rules that relate quantities in the model to observations that we make. It exists only in our minds and does not have any other reality (whatever that might mean). A theory is a good theory if it satisfies two requirements: It must accurately describe a large class of observations on the basis of a model that contains only a few arbitrary elements, and

it must make definite predictions about the results of future observations" (*S Hawking*, Lucasian Professor of Mathematics, Cambridge, from *A brief history of time*, 1988).

- "A hypothesis is...the obligatory starting point of all experimental reasoning. Without it no investigation would be possible, and one would learn nothing: one could only pile up barren observations. To experiment without a preconceived idea is to wander aimlessly" (*Claude Bernard* 1865).

- "Theories are scientific generalizations or scientific ideas which sum up our present state of knowledge; they are always relative truths, destined to change with the progress of science" (*Claude Bernard* 1865; French physiologist. His *Introduction to the study of experimental medicine* (Eng. Trans. Dover Books) should be read by all intending clinical scientists).

- "The great tragedy of Science – the slaying of a beautiful hypothesis by an ugly fact" (*TH Huxley*, scientist, UK 1825–1895).

See **induction, science/scientific method in pharmacology**

hypothesis of no difference See **null hypothesis**

hysteresis (Gr. *hustereo*, be behind)

- An apparent lag of an effect with respect to the magnitude of the agency causing the effect, e.g. on releasing a *stress* (force per unit area) applied to an object the *strain* (ratio of the dimensional changes induced by the stress to the original dimensions) lags behind.

- In pharmacology, the effect a drug (e.g. alcohol) has may be different for the same plasma concentration during the rising (absorption) phase than during the falling (elimination) phase.

iatrogenic disease   (Gr. *iatros*, physician; *genes*, born)
- Disease caused by the process of medical diagnosis or treatment.
- Any deterioration in the patient's condition due to following medical advice.

IC$_{50}$
- Inhibitory concentration 50 per cent – the concentration of a drug that reduces a response to another drug or a target enzyme by 50 per cent. Under certain conditions it can be used to determine the **affinity** of the inhibitor.

See **Cheng & Prussoff equation**

ICDRA
- International Conference of Drug Regulatory Authorities.

'ice'
- 'Street' name for methamphetamine.

ICH
- **International Conference on Harmonization** of Technical Requirements for Registration of Pharmaceuticals for Human Use.

ICMJE
- **International Committee of Medical Journal Editors.**

idiosyncrasy   (Gr. *idios*, own, personal, individual; *syn*, together; *krasis*, mixture)
- A response that is qualitatively different from that normally seen. Generally due to single gene inheritance (e.g. haemolysis due to primaquine in subjects having a deficiency of glucose-6-phosphate dehydrogenase).

idiotyp/-e/-ic   (Gr. *idos*, private, separate; *tupos*, image)
- That part of an **antibody** that is specific to the **antigen** to which it binds. Antibodies may be made to the idiotypic antibody, i.e. anti-idiotype (or idiotypic) antibody.

IFPMA
- International Federation of Pharmaceutical Manufacturers Associations.

immediate hypersensitivity reaction   See **anaphylaxis**

immediate-release formulation   See **modified-release formulation**

immune effector   (L. *immunis*, exempt from, e.g. military service)
- Chemical **mediators** involved in the body's response to foreign protein; examples include **adhesion molecules, cytokines** and **eicosanoids**.

immunity   (L. *immunis*, exempt from, e.g. military service)
- Resistant or refractory state arising from an adaptive response of an organism to a nonself substance (*PB Medawar*, 1915–1987, zoologist/immunologist, UK).   See **antigen**

immunoadjuvant   See **immunostimulant**

immunohistochemistry   (L. *immunis*, exempt from, e.g. military service;
                    Gr. *histos*, web, tissue; *khemeia*, the art of transmutation, alchemy)
– A technique by which specific parts of cells or tissues can be stained selectively through an antibody–antigen reaction. The antibody, which is linked to a reagent that can be made to undergo a colour or fluorescent reaction, is applied to the tissue and reacts highly selectively with those parts of the cell or tissue that contain the **antigen** against which the **antibody** was raised.
                            See **histochemistry**

immunomodulating agents   (L. *immunis*, exempt from, e.g. military service;
                    modulari, adjust to rhythm)
– Agents that modify immune responses, (as opposed to solely either stimulating or suppressing them), e.g. **cytokines**.   See **modulate**

immunopharmacology   (L. *immunis*, exempt from, e.g. military service;
                    Gr. *pharmakon*, drug)
– The study of the effects of drugs upon the immune system (recognition cells, **antigens, antibodies, mediators, cytokines**, effector systems, etc.)
– "Although immunologists and pharmacologists have not traditionally shared the same experimental approach, the goals of immunology and pharmacology are highly interconnected. Pharmacological science aims to identify agents (generally exogenous) with the capacity to modify biological responses. The goal of immunologists is to define the interactions of the cells and molecules (many of which are natural response modifiers) of the immune system. As understanding of these molecules has increased, so has the realization that they can be used therapeutically in cancer, infectious diseases and autoimmune diseases. In addition to endogenous molecules of therapeutic value, the immune system also presents several targets for pharmacological intervention. The development of synthetic agents that can **modulate** the immune response is the second major area of immunopharmacology; it is already of great value in the control of transplant rejection and is of potential benefit in the treatment of autoimmune disease" (*RB Gallagher, R Brines, D Girdlestone*).   See **biological response modifiers, pharmacology**

immunostimulant   (L. *immunis*, exempt from, e.g. military service;
                    stimulare, to urge on)
– A substance that enhances immunological processes (e.g. levamisole). Also known as an *immunoadjuvant*.

Immunosuppressive   (L. *immunis*, exempt from, e.g. military service;
                    sub, down; *premere*, to press)
– A drug that suppresses immunological responses (e.g. adrenocortical steroids, anticancer drugs). Immunosuppressed patients are particularly at hazard from bacterial and viral infections.

immunotoxicity (L. *immunis*, exempt from, e.g. military service;
Gr. *toxikon*, arrow poison)
– Adverse effects due to interaction of **xenobiotics** with the immune system.

impact factor of a journal (L. *im*, before; *pangere*, drive)
– A ratio obtained by dividing the number of citations of items published in a
journal in one year by the number of papers published in that journal in the
two previous years. "The ubiquitous and sometimes misplaced use of journal
impact factors for evaluation [and ranking of journals] has caused considerable controversy" (*E Garfield*, originator of the procedure). Use in evaluating
publications of university departments and of individual scientists is particularly problematic. See **science citation index**

implant (L. *in*, in; *plantare*, to graft)
– A form of **depot** drug administration in which the solid dosage form is inserted
either intramuscularly (unusually) or subcutaneously, e.g. hormone formulations. See **formulation (pharmaceutical)**

impotent (L. *im-*, not; *potentia*, power)
– The term used to describe a drug which is effective only at high
doses/concentrations. The term does not imply that the maximal effect of the
drug is limited.

IMRAD
– Introduction, Method, Results, Discussion; the classic format of a scientific
research paper/report.

inactivation (L. *in* = *un*, depriving; *actus*, a doing)
– *General*: to render inert.
– *Of the cellular ion channel mechanism*: a phenomenon described for sodium
channels (in squid axons) by Hodgkin and Huxley. Sodium channels normally
respond to depolarization by opening, but if the depolarization is maintained,
the sodium channels do not stay open but enter a refractory (inactivated)
state from which they can recover only if the membrane is repolarized for a
while. Similar properties are exhibited by other ion channels. (*AL Hodgkin*,
b.1914; *AF Huxley*, b.1917: physiologists, UK).

incapacitating agent (L. *in* = *un*, depriving; *capere*, to hold)
See **riot control agent**

incidence rate (L. *in*, in; *cadere*, to fall, hence, to happen; *ratus*, fixed)
– The number of events, e.g. illnesses *beginning* within a specified period (of
time) and related to the average number of persons who experience the event
during that period:

(*no. developing a disease per unit of time*) ÷ (*total number at risk in that time*)

– Incidence describes a *changing* situation: it is *not* the same as **prevalence**.

incompatibility (of medicines)   (L. *in* = *un*, depriving;
                                        compati, to be in sympathy with)
- *Therapeutic incompatibility*: the ingredients of a medicine have mutually an-
  tagonistic pharmacological actions.
- *Physicochemical (or pharmaceutical) incompatibility*:
  - *Unintentional* – the ingredients in a formulation (or mixture of medicines,
    e.g. in a syringe) interact undesirably.
  - *Intentional* – e.g. to retard absorption.

IND
- Investigational new drug (application). Regulatory term (USA).

indicative prescribing amount (IPA) (UK)
- A manifestation of government intervention in prescribing costs in the UK
  National Health Service (NHS). IPA is the sum of money annually allocated to
  general practitioners as a 'benchmark' for their likely expenditure on prescribing for that year. It has been described as a 'bottom-up' process based
  on previous expenditure in practices. The sum is increased annually to take
  account of inflation and local conditions. At its introduction (1991), the implementing medical advisers (NHS) often faced apathy, if not professional hostil-
  ity from general practitioners with whom they sought dialogue. Incentives are
  offered in that underspenders on drugs may use the savings (by agreement)
  to enhance patient care in their practices (*Pharmaceutical Journal* 1993).
                                                        See **PACT**

indirect antagonism   See **antagonism**

individual effective dose (IED)   (L. *in* = *un*, absence of a quality;
                                    dividuus, divisible; *efficere*, to accomplish;
                                    Gr. *dosis*, giving, gift, and so portion of medicine)
- The dose or concentration of a drug required to evoke a response, the nature
  (and magnitude) of which is exactly specified.   See **minimum effective dose**

individual variation   (L. *in* = *un*, absence of a quality;
                                        dividuus, divisible; *varius*, subject to change)
- The range of variation in drug responses, commonly expressed as the **normal distribution curve**, is largely genetically (multigenically) determined; but
  personal habits, environment, etc., also play a role. Single-gene inheritance
  may lead to other forms of variation (e.g. **bimodal**). Variation may be *inter-* or
  *intra*individual.   See **idiosyncrasy**

induction   (L. *in*, into; *ducere*, to lead)
- The method of basing general statements on accumulated observations of
  specific instances. Induction is the normal method of establishing scientific
  '**laws**' or '**truths**'. It is the basic process of experimental science. Unfortunately, the validity of induction cannot be demonstrated since no number of
  singular observations can logically entail an unrestricted general statement.

Despite the probability of this highly purist position, the countless confirming instances, with never a single counter-example, raises the probability of many scientific 'laws' to the highest degree it is possible to conceive, and, in practice if not in theory, this is indistinguishable from certainty.
- "Scientific laws are *in*ductive in origin" (*PB Medawar*).
  See *a posteriori*, *a priori*, **deduction, enzyme induction, hypothesis, law**

inference   (L. *in*, in; *ferre*, bring)
- Forming conclusions from premises, which may be other judgments or direct (experimental) observations.   See **deduction, induction**

influx   (L. *in*, into; *fluere*, to flow)
- The movement of ions, drug molecules, metabolites, etc. into a cell across a diffusional barrier (membrane) or via specific channels or carriers.

information explosion   (L. *informare*, to give shape to, describe;
                                                           ex, out; *plaudere*, to clap)
- The growth of information in the 20th century has been aptly described as an explosion.
- "Pharmacology comprises some broad conceptions and generalizations, and some detailed conclusions of such great practical importance that every student and practitioner [of medicine] should be absolutely familiar with them. It comprises also a large mass of minute details which constitute too great a tax on human memory, but which cannot safely be neglected" (*T Sollman* 1949).
- The development of computers has acted as a life-raft to the scientist and doctor struggling to keep afloat on the ocean of knowledge. Computers have also expanded the total amount of knowledge.
- There are more scientists alive *now*, and writing, than the total of those who existed throughout past ages.
- The number of scientific journals has doubled every 15 years since 1760.
- When an acknowledged premier general scientific journal, *Nature*, was founded in 1869 *most* of its readers could understand or take interest in *most* of the original articles published across the range of natural science. Now *most* of its readers find *most* of the original articles incomprehensible and obtain most of their intellectual profit from the pages of editorial review and comment, and news and views. *Nature* remains a highly influential journal.

information overload (and clinical practice)
- Only a portion of medical knowledge (e.g. of drugs) is ever loaded into the minds of professionals.
- Not all of the knowledge loaded in the minds of professionals is retained.
- Much of the knowledge that professionals retain becomes obsolete, and there is no assurance that they will learn new knowledge relevant to their patients' problems.
- Even with the limited knowledge that it retains, a doctor's unaided mind cannot reliably integrate that knowledge with the infinite variety of data about patients.

- Good medical practice requires tools to extend the human mind's limited capacity to recall and process large numbers of relevant variables.
- Knowledge should be held in tools that are kept up to date and used routinely – not in heads, which are expensive to load and faulty in the retention and processing of knowledge.
- Such information tools would allow fundamental changes in our approach to medical education and practice. (After *LL Weed; British Medical Journal* 1997;315:231–255)

infusion   (L. *in*, in; *fundere*, to pour)
- The continuous administration (**injection**) of a dilute fluid preparation (of a drug) over a period (e.g. hours or days), generally by gravity from a reservoir or by a pump, commonly intravenously.
- A solution of the readily soluble constituents of crude drugs, made, for example, by soaking the crude substance in (hot) water, e.g. tea, coffee.

Ingelfinger rule
- Franz Ingelfinger was editor of the *New England Journal of Medicine* from 1967 to 1977. He formulated the journal's policy to refuse publication of any paper that had been published elsewhere, in whole or in substance. The rule in its original form (1969) stated: "The understanding is that material submitted to the *Journal* has not been offered to any book, journal or newspaper."
- Ingelfinger introduced the rule to protect the commercial profitability of the journal, i.e. by preserving the 'newsworthiness' of the article. The rule has since also been justified on the grounds that the release of research findings before publication of the peer-reviewed scientific paper could lead to the distribution of inaccurate or misleading information to the public. The rule has been adopted in one form or another by many other medical journals of substance. The *New England Journal of Medicine* has abandoned the rule.
- Critics of the Ingelfinger rule have claimed that it has had a chilling effect on the free flow of information. For example, in order to ensure that new discoveries remain eligible for publication, scientists may delay communicating their findings in whole or in part at scientific gatherings. Because most medical research is funded from public funds, the rule has also been criticised on the grounds that it limits or delays public access to the results of research. Another criticism is that of inconsistency. Papers published in journals that apply the rule are not all subjected to the same intensity of rigorous, objective peer review. "Independent analysis is needed to document contentions that the Ingelfinger rule improves and assures the quality of what journals publish. Unless and until supporters provide such evidence, the Ingelfinger rule should be dropped" (*LK Altman; Lancet* 1996;347:1382–1386 & 1459–1463).
                                            See **peer review or refereeing, publication**

inhalation of drugs   (L. *in*, in; *halare*, to breathe)
- Inhalation, except at its most primitive, requires special apparatus:
    - Standard anaesthetic apparatus.
    - *Metered-dose inhalers (MDI)*: these are multidose containers that deliver a

precise **aerosol** dose by actuation of an appropriate metering valve; the propellant is a liquified gas (ozone-sparing) or pneumatic device; they may be breath-actuated. Micronized powders can also be delivered by a breath-actuated device (Spinhaler).

- *Nebulizers* (gas or electricity driven) create a mist of fine particles and can deliver higher doses than a MDI.   See **chlorofluorocarbons, hydrofluoroalkanes, smoking as a route of drug administration**

inhibitory amino acids   See **amino acids**

initial dilution volume
- The (anticipated) plasma concentration at zero time of administration when the whole dose is in the body and none has yet been eliminated (*after Rowland & Tozer*, see Acknowledgements).

initiator (of cancer)   (L. *initium*, beginning)
- A chemical or other stimulus (e.g. radiation) which results in a permanent heritable change in a cell, giving the cell the potential to develop into a tumour (e.g. benzpyrene).   See **carcinogen, tumour promoter**

injection   (L. *in*, in; *jacere*, to throw)
- Introduction of a (sterile) concentrated solution/emulsion/suspension directly into a tissue by needle, tube, jet.   See **infusion, routes of administration**

injuries due to clinical research   See **liability**

INN or rINN
- International **N**onproprietary **N**ame. The **WHO** publishes lists of recommended INNs (rINN).   See **names of drugs**

innocent bystander phenomenon   (L. *in*, into, against; *nocere*, to injure; Old Eng. *be*, at, near; *stand*, to stand; Gr. *phainein*, to show, to be seen)
- A reaction between two molecules, resulting in injury to cells that are not directly or causally involved. For example, in some cases of allergy to drugs, the antigen–antibody reaction has consequences for cells that are not directly involved, e.g. some cases of haemolysis.

innovation, protection of   (L. *in*, in; *novare*, to make new)
- Genuinely innovative pharmaceutical developers spend enormous sums (millions of US$) on research, and it is in the public interest that they should continue to do so.
- If, immediately after initial marketing, competing manufacturers who do no research are allowed to apply to market **copy products** that are **essentially similar**, relying on the originators' research data (deposited in the regulatory authority) to obtain a licence, and so to sell the product at a much lower price, then the simple operation of market forces will prevent the originators from

recovering their research costs and deny them a profit. Successful developers will be driven away from pharmaceutical innovation.
- Governments recognize this and make regulation to provide reasonable (not too little, not too much) protection of socially desirable innovation by granting a period of *marketing exclusivity.*
- Intervention by a second (copy) applicant generally requires:
  - The applicant to have obtained permission (generally by payment) to use the originator's research data, *or*
  - The applicant can rely on published literature (which rarely has sufficient detail), *or*
  - That the originator's product has been on the market for, e.g. 6 or 10 years, *and* is still marketed in the country concerned.

inositol phosphates
- A family of molecules, derived from membrane phospholipids, with important signal **transduction** roles in some cell types. Receptor-mediated activation of certain **G-proteins** leads to activation of phospholipase C, which splits phosphatidyl inositol bisphosphate to yield inositol 1,4,5-trisphosphate (IP_3) and diacylglycerol (DAG). DAG is highly **lipophilic** and remains in the membrane, where it probably has a physiological role, e.g. it is a powerful activator of protein kinase C. IP_3 is **hydrophilic** and passes into the cytoplasm where it acts as a **second messenger**, mediating the release of Ca^{2+} from specialized storage sites in the endoplasmic reticulum via Ca^{2+} channels linked to IP_3-sensitive receptors on the endoplasmic reticulum. There are also mono-, bis-, tetrakis-, and a variety of other inositol phosphates, many of which are synthetic or metabolic intermediates of one another. There is evidence that IP_4 is also a second messenger.

inositol trisphosphate   See **inositol phosphates**

inotropic   (Gr. *inos*, fibre; *tropos*, turning or development in response to stimulus)
- Influencing the **contractility** of muscle (e.g. positive inotropic action on the heart means increased cardiac contractility; negative inotropic action means decreased contractility).

institutional review board (IRB)   See **ethics committee**

in situ hybridization   (L. *in*, in; *situs*, place; *hybrida*, a crossbred animal)
- Technique for localizing within a tissue or organ the mRNA responsible for the synthesis of a particular protein. In pharmacology this is usually a receptor. The probe is a labelled (usually radioactively-labelled) nucleic acid with a sequence that is complementary to the mRNA under study. After the probe has been allowed to penetrate the tissue, determination of its location (e.g. by **autoradiography**) reveals the location of the mRNA for the particular receptor, but this does not necessarily demonstrate the exact location of the receptors themselves.

insufflate/-ion   (L. *in*, into; *sufflare*, to blow)
– To blow into (e.g. to blow a powder into a cavity).

integer   (L. *integer*, intact)
– A whole number.

integrins   (L. *in*, in; *tegere*, to cover)
– A family of cell membrane receptors that mediate cell **adhesion**. These proteins are involved in many key processes, such as cell differentiation and proliferation, embryo development, platelet aggregation, immunity, tissue repair and cancer metastasis.

intellectual property   (L. *intellectus*, comprehension;
                                                    proprietas, something personal)
– The property which the law recognizes in a person's inventions, writings and other intellectual creations.
– A term for intangible kinds of property, such as **copyrights**, trade marks, patents, ideas.
– The skill, learning, expertise and intelligence possessed by an organization by virtue of the staff it employs.
– Intellectual property rights are subject to legal protection against theft.

intention (or **intent**) **to treat**
– Reports of **therapeutic trials** should contain an analysis of all patients entered, regardless of whether they dropped out or failed to complete, or even to start the treatment for any reason. Omission of these subjects can lead to serious **bias**. Subsidiary analyses may, of course, be presented in addition.
                                                    See **observed case**

interaction (drug–drug)   (L. *inter*, between; *agere*, to act)
– The situation in which one drug affects another, whether by a **pharmacokinetic** process or by a **pharmacodynamic** effect.
– Interactions may be *unidirectional*, where one drug affects another but is unaffected itself, or *bidirectional*, where each drug affects the other (*after Rowland & Tozer*, see Acknowledgements).

intercalate   (L. *inter*, between; *calare*, to proclaim)
– To insert between two others.

interchangeable multisource product   See **generic drug**

intercurrent   (L. *inter*, between; *currere*, to run)
– A disease that occurs during the progress of another disease.

interest (conflict of)   (L. *inter*, between; *esse*, to be, make a difference;
                                co, com/cum, con, with, together, in common, jointly,
                                    equally, reciprocally, mutually; *fligere*, to strike)
– A person has a conflict of interest in a matter where there are circumstances

that may, whether consciously or unconsciously, affect his/her judgement or motives to the detriment of impartiality.
- A situation in which professional judgement concerning a primary interest [e.g. patients' health, scientific study] can be influenced by a secondary interest [e.g. personal prestige, financial gain] (*W Nadoolman*).
- The **International Committee of Medical Journal Editors** has made a statement on the subject: "Conflict of interest for a given manuscript exists when a participant in the peer review and publication process – author, reviewer, and editor – has ties to activities that could inappropriately influence his or her judgement, whether or not judgement is in fact affected." Financial interests are the most important, but conflicts can occur involving personal relationships, academic competition and intellectual passion. "Participants in peer review and publication should disclose their conflicting interests, and the information should be made available, so that others can judge their effects for themselves. Because readers may be less able to detect bias in review articles and editorials than in reports of original research, some journals do not accept reviews and editorials from authors with a conflict of interest." Reviewers and editorial staff should not use pre-publication knowledge of work submitted to them to further their own interests (*Journal of the American Medical Association* 1997;277:927).
- Health care institutions, regulatory advisers and investigators having collaborative or advisory relations with pharmaceutical companies may find themselves in conflict of interest situations regarding conduct and publication of research.
- "*Lancet's* simple test, by no means perfect, is this: would a non-disclosed commercial interest, should it be revealed later, prove embarrassing to an author?" (*Lancet* 1996;348:627).
- "Perhaps part of the difficulty with conflict of interest lies in the phrase itself, which has disparaging connotations. The *Annals of Internal Medicine* uses the term 'dual commitment' and asks authors to disclose these to editors. The *Lancet's* policy is much the same" (*Lancet* 1997;349:1112).

See **peer review, scientific misconduct and fraud**

interim analysis   (L. *inter*, between; *in*, in; Gr. *ana*, up; *lusis*, set free)
- Interim analysis allows a formal analysis to be conducted at several *predetermined* intervals during a **therapeutic trial** so that a decision whether to stop or to continue can be made. Designs in which the number of subjects is not decided in advance have been developed in response to the evident need for a design that allows *continuous or intermittent* assessment as the trial proceeds, and stops it *either* as soon as a statistically significant result is reached *or* when such a result becomes unlikely. The essential feature has to be that the trial is terminated when a *pre*determined result is attained and not when the investigator, looking at the results to date, thinks it is appropriate (few investigators would be able to resist picking out the moment when the difference was statistically significant, which inevitably would mean a high rate of false-positive results). Truly continuous monitoring (*sequential analysis*) imposes severe restrictions and a compromise has been attained. *Interim*

analyses reduce the statistical significance of the trial, but not to a serious degree if they are done, say, less than four times in a big trial. Such *modified sequential designs* recognize the realities of medical practice and provide a reasonable trade-off between statistical, medical and ethical needs.

See **fixed-sample trial, sequential analysis**

interleukins (L. *inter*, between; Gr. *leukos*, white)
– One family of **cytokines**.

internalization, of receptors See **receptor** *(Endocytosis)*

International Committee of Medical Journal Editors (ICMJE) (Vancouver Group)
– The ICMJE evolved from a small group of editors who met informally in Vancouver, British Columbia, Canada (Vancouver Group) in 1978. It issues guidance on editorial and on broader biomedical publishing issues which it keeps updated and which are published in several journals. Its *Uniform Requirements for Manuscripts Submitted to Biomedical Journals* are authoritative and over 500 journals have agreed to use them (see *Annals of Internal Medicine* 1997;126;36–47).
– Plainly, prudent authors wishing to be published will acquaint themselves with the current *Uniform Requirements* as well as with other ICMJE statements.
– The committee meets regularly. It establishes guidelines for the format of manuscripts submitted to journals. It also addresses concerns about rights, privacy, descriptions of methods, redundant or duplicate **publication**, **authorship**, editorial freedom and integrity, conflict of interest (see **interest, conflict of**), advertising, supplements, the role of the correspondence column. For a full statement see *Journal of the American Medical Association* 1997;277:927; it will be updated from time to time.

International Conference on Harmonization of Technical Requirements for Registration of Pharmaceuticals for Human Use (ICH)
– The purpose is to minimize the enormous waste of resources caused by the demands of *national* regulatory authorities that *international* drug developers shall adapt their research and documentation to needlessly diverse (national) bureaucratic requirements.

International Pharmacopoeia (Int. P)
– **Pharmacopoeia** published by the World Health Organization.

international system of units See **SI units**

International Union of Pharmacology (IUPHAR)
– IUPHAR is a non-government organization (made up of national societies) that functions under the auspices of ICSU (International Council of Scientific Unions). Its aims and functions include:
  – To facilitate international meetings.

- To facilitate internationally important endeavours, such as its teaching committee, nomenclature committee, etc.
- To strengthen the profession (teaching, continuing education, research and practice) of pharmacology and clinical pharmacology.
- To provide assistance to countries with financial difficulties.
- To create and maintain relationships with international organizations, such as **WHO**.
- To promote public awareness of pharmacological activities.
- To promote IUPHAR activities to the membership of IUPHAR, and to its Divisions and Sections.

International Unit   See **biological standardization**

intolerance   (L. *in* = *un*, depriving; *tolerare*, to sustain)
- A greater than expected quantitative response to a dose of a drug.
- An individual with a qualitatively normal response (to a given dose) that is sufficiently above the average to be of consequence, is described as intolerant. He is at the lower end of the distribution of **individual effective doses**. (An individual with a non-allergic *qualitatively* abnormal response has an **idiosyncrasy**). To describe intolerance as **hypersensitivity** is best avoided as it causes confusion.

intoxication   (L. *in*, in; *toxicare*, to poison)
- A state of being poisoned, now colloquially used in the sense of acute or chronic overdose of alcohol, e.g. detoxi(fi)cation centre – a place where alcoholics are treated.

Int. P
- International Pharmacopoeia (published by the **WHO**).

intra-   (L. *intra*, on the inside)
- Prefix meaning inside, within.

intrathecal   (L. *intra*, within; *theca*, sheath, case)
- Used of injections of drugs into the subarachnoid space.

intrinsic   (L. *intra*, within; *sequi*, follow)
- Belonging naturally to; inherent.

intrinsic activity   (L. *intra*, within; *sequi*, follow; *actio*, from *agere*, to do)
- A measure of the maximum response to an **agonist.**
- The strength of the response produced by occupation of a **receptor** by an agonist.
- The term **maximal agonist effect** (represented by symbol α) is now preferred.   See **efficacy** for a fuller account.

intrinsic efficacy   (L. *intra*, within; *sequi*, follow; *efficere*, to achieve)
- A measure of the ability of a drug to activate a receptor once it is bound to it.
                                              See **efficacy** for a fuller account.

intron
- A segment of DNA that is transcribed, but which is eventually removed from the transcript by **splicing**.   See **codon, exon**

intrinsic sympathomimetic activity   See **ISA**

inverse agonist   (L. *invertere*, to invert; Gr. *agon*, to struggle)
- A drug that possesses **intrinsic** actions opposite in kind to those of the **agonist**, in distinction to a neutral **antagonist**, which has no effect in the absence of an agonist.
- A **ligand** which by binding to receptors reduces the fraction of them in an active conformation. This can occur if some of the receptors are in the active form even in the absence of a conventional agonist...If the ligand combines preferentially with inactive receptors, it will reduce the fraction in the active state (**IUPHAR**, with permission; *Pharmacological Reviews* 1995;47:255–266).
- An inverse agonist is also known as a *contragonist* (L. *contra*, against).
                    See **constitutive activity, receptor** (*Two state model*)

investigational product (regulatory term)   (L. *in*, in; *vestigare*, to track)
- A pharmaceutical formulation of an active ingredient or **placebo**, tested or used as a reference in a **clinical trial**.

in vitro   (L., in glass)
- Used to describe experiments conducted on tissues in an artificial environment, e.g. an organ bath, culture medium.
- *In vitro veritas* (L., in glass lies the truth); an adaptation of the famous proverb of Pliny (*CE 23–79*), *In vino veritas*, the truth comes out in wine. The adaptation implies that pharmacological analysis using tissue *in vitro* (having fewer and more controllable variables) provides a particularly dependable pathway to **truth**.

in vivo   (L., in a living creature)
- Used to describe experiments conducted in a whole living organism.
                                                                    See ***ex vivo***

iodophor   (Gr. *iodes*, violet; *phoros*, a carrier)
- A combination of iodine with a **surfactant** carrier, usually polyvinylpyrrolidine, which slowly releases free iodine. Used as skin disinfectant.

ion channel   (Gr. *ion*, going; L. *canalis*, pipe, conduit)
- A protein structure that spans a membrane, providing a **hydrophilic** pathway that allows small ions (sodium, potassium, chloride) to cross the membrane. Different types of channel are caused to open by different stimuli, for example:
  - Change in membrane potential (*voltage-gated*).
  - A neurotransmitter (*receptor-gated*).

- Intracellular calcium ions (*calcium-gated*).
- G-protein.
- Time.   See **ionophore**

ion channel blocker   (Gr. *ion*, going; L. *canalis*, pipe, conduit;
                                           Fr. *bloquer*, to obstruct)
- An **antagonist** that works by preventing electrical current flow through an **ion channel**, probably by 'plugging' the channel rather than by binding to a **receptor**.   See **ionotropic receptors**

ion exchange/resin   (Gr. *ion*, going; L. *ex*, out of;
                                           cambire, to barter; *resina*, resin)
- General ion exchange is a process in which ions with a positive charge (cation) or negative charge (anion) are exchanged between a solid and a solution. Ion exchange resins are polymers containing ionized groups (cationic, anionic) that can bind anions or cations (i.e. ions of the opposite charge) with which they come into contact (e.g. cation-exchange resins have carboxylic or sulphonic acid (anionic) side-groups).
- In therapeutics resin beads given orally are not absorbed from the intestine and are used to relieve the body of an excess of the cations sodium and potassium. (Some porous resin beads act by **hydrophilic** interaction rather than by ionization.)
- Laboratory use to purify or concentrate substances in mixed or low concentration solutions.

ion trapping   (Gr. *ion*, going; Middle Eng. *trappen*, to ensnare)
- The mounting concentration of a drug in a compartment as a result of the properties of the drug and the particular environment. For example, **aspirin** in the stomach at pH 1 is highly unionized and therefore lipid soluble; it diffuses readily into gastric mucosal cells where it meets a pH near 7, due to which it ionizes and becomes less lipid soluble, so that diffusion out of the cells into the blood is slow. In this way it enters these cells easily and departs with difficulty, so it accumulates (is trapped) within the cell which it may injure.
                        See **Henderson–Hasselbalch equation**

ionic bond   (Gr. ion, going; Old Norse *band*, fetter)
- An ionic bond results from electrostatic attraction between oppositely charged ions. The force of the attraction diminishes as the square of the distance between them. The bond is easily broken, compared with, for example, a **covalent bond**.

ionization constant   (Gr. *ion*, going; L. *constare*, to stand firm)
- The state of ionic equilibrium as described by the law of **mass action**, e.g. acetic acid ionizes in water to hydrogen ions and acetate ions. At the same time hydrogen ions and acetate ions are re-associating to form the electrically neutral acetic acid. At equilibrium the rates of the two reactions (dissociation and association) are equal. The ratio between the concentrations of dissoci-

ated and undissociated acid is the *acidic ionization constant*. The state of ionization of both acids and bases can be described as acidic constants in order to record ionization of both acids and bases on the same scale, just as the pH scale serves to measure both acidity and alkalinity (after *A Albert*).

See **Henderson–Hasselbalch equation**

ionophore (Gr. *ion*, going; *phoros*, a carrier)
— A **lipophilic** molecule (**exogenous**) that forms complexes with ions, the complex then being able to move across lipid membranes. The ion–ionophore complexes may be charged, in which case a potential is generated as the ionophore moves the ion across a lipid membrane; or the complexes may be neutral, when no potential is generated as the ion is transported. Many ionophores (e.g. valinomycin, nigericin) are antimicrobial. (*Note*: molecules that form tubular structures penetrating membranes were not included in the original definition of ionophore but the term now often includes these pore-forming substances, e.g. alamethacin.)
— Membrane-spanning protein molecules, which contain a gated **ion channel**. Such molecules are sometimes also **receptors**.

See **fast receptors, ionotropic receptors**

ionotropic receptors (Gr. *ion*, going; *tropos*, turning; L. *re*, again; *capere*, to take)
— Receptors that are, or form part of, membrane-spanning selective **ion channels (ionophores)**. Activation of the receptor causes the channel to allow the passage of a certain ion. Also known as 'fast' receptors, in contrast to 'slow' receptors (**metabotropic receptors**) which operate by controlling the activity of an enzyme, which in turn produces a **second messenger**.

iontophoresis/ionophoresis (Gr. *ion*, going; *phoresis*, being carried)
— Use of an electrical gradient to cause a net movement of a charged substance.
— A seldom-used method of administering a drug across the skin.
— Used in research to deliver small quantities (micro-iontophoresis) of drugs to discrete areas of, for example, brain or muscle.

IP$_3$
— Inositol 1,4,5-trisphosphate. See **inositol phosphates**

IPA
— **Indicative prescribing amount.**

ipecacuanha (Native Brazilian (Tupi) name meaning small plant causing sickness)
— The dried root of a South American plant (family *Uragoga*); the chief active principle is the alkaloid emetine. Its uses include emesis and the treatment of amoebic dysentery. See **emetic**

IRB
— Institutional Review Board (USA). See **ethics committee**

ISA
– Intrinsic sympathomimetic activity. A term relating to the clinical use of **partial agonists** at β-adrenoceptors. Full β-adrenoceptor **antagonists** may precipitate heart failure in those with little cardiac reserve. **Partial agonists** are thought to carry less risk of this because their **intrinsic activity** at β-adrenoceptors ensures that there is always some stimulation of cardiac β-adrenoceptors, while the heart is protected from excessive sympathetic nerve (noradrenergic) stimulation by the **antagonism** provided by the drug.

iso-　　　　　　　　　　　　　　　　　　　　　(Gr. *isos*, equal)
– Prefix used to mean similar or equal, e.g. isopeptides of the **endothelin** family, ET–1, ET–2 and ET–3 differ structurally by only a few amino acids.

isobologram or isobol　　　　　　　(Gr. *isos*, equal; *bolos*, effect)
– A diagram consisting of lines joining points of equal effect (just as a map contour joins points of equal height); used in drug interaction studies.

isoceptors/isoreceptors　　　(Gr. *isos*, equal; L. *re*, again; *cipere*, to take)
– **Receptors** that are activated by the same class of **agonists**, but with varying **selectivities**, e.g. β_1- and β_2-adrenoceptors are isoreceptors, as are the M_1, M_2 and M_3 subtypes of **muscarinic acetylcholine receptors**.

　　　　　　　　　　　　　　　　　　　　See **isoenzyme**

isoenzyme/isozyme　　　　　　(Gr. *isos*, equal; *en*, in; *zume*, yeast)
– Enzymes with different protein structures which catalyse the same chemical reaction. Isoenzymes may be separated using **electrophoresis**.

　　　　　　　　　　　　　　　　　　　　See **cytochrome P450**

isomer/-ism　　　　　　　　　　(Gr. *isos*, equal; *meros*, share)
– Two or more compounds having almost identical structures and the same **empirical** formula, but having different properties due to a different arrangement of atoms within the molecule.

　　　　　　　See **chirality, optical isomerism, racemic, stereoisomer**

isomeric ballast　　(Gr. *isos*, equal; *meros*, share; Old Ger. *ballast*, useless load)
　　　　　　　　　　　　　　　　　　　　See **chirality**

isometric　　　　　　　　　　(Gr. *isos*, equal; *metron*, measure)
– Of equal length. A device (**transducer**) that allows a muscle to generate force without shortening.　　　　　　　See **auxotonic, isotonic**

isosterism　　　　　　　　　　(Gr. *isos*, equal; *stereos*, solid)
– Isosteric substances (e.g. N_2O and CO_2) have molecules with the same number of atoms and the same total number of electrons. Therefore they have some similar physical properties.
– Groups on complex molecules can also be described as isosteric. Such groups will often be structural equivalents, and molecules in which one struc-

tural group is replaced by different *isosteres* may exhibit similar pharmacology.

isotonic   (Gr. *isos*, equal; *tonikos*, stretching)
- Of equal osmotic strength. When no comparator is mentioned, the term implies osmotic strength equal to human plasma/extracellular fluid. A 0.9 per cent solution of sodium chloride is approximately isotonic.
- Allowing a muscle to contract by shortening without generating any extra force. Devices that allow muscles to perform in this way are called isotonic **transducers**.   See **auxotonic, isometric**

isotope   (Gr. *isos*, equal; *topos*, place)
- Atoms of the same element, differing only in the number of neutrons in their nuclei. They have the same atomic number but different mass number. Some isotopes decay spontaneously into lighter elements by emitting atomic particles – radioactive decay. These *unstable isotopes* are known as **radioisotopes** and can be detected, and their amounts estimated, by analyzing the emitted particles, which are characteristic for each isotope. The relative amounts of *stable (nonradioactive) isotopes* (abundance) can only be assessed by measuring their masses, e.g. by **mass spectroscopy**.

IU
International unit.   See **biological standardization**

IUPHAR
- **International Union of Pharmacology**.

jackknife method (statistical)   (A convenient, general purpose, folding knife,
and, by extension a convenient **pragmatic** statistical method)
- A method of linear regression analysis which involves finding the straight lines
that join all possible pairs of points and then taking the resulting median as
the best **fit** to all the points.

jargon   (Fr. corruption of a Dutch–Yiddish word *bargoens*,
used in the criminal underworld of Amsterdam
in the 16th century and itself a corruption of Old Fr. *argot*)
- A mode of speech familiar only to a group or profession: its sole justification is
to enhance communication, although it is often used to parade superior
learning, to conceal ignorance and to mystify.
- Unintelligible talk, gabble, gibberish (*S Johnson*, 1755).
- *Jargon as verbal shorthand*. For those who understand it, jargon is a kind of
shorthand that makes long explanations unnecessary and it can then be an
efficient and effective language (Oxford Companion to the English Language).
A kinder term for this class of jargon is *terminology* (L. *terminus,* a limit; Gr.
logia, study)   See **officialese**

Jarisch–Herxheimer reaction
- A brisk illness occurring within hours (and lasting a few hours) of initiating
effective antimicrobial therapy (e.g. in neurosyphilis, typhoid fever), and
thought to be due to the release of endotoxins from destroyed bacteria. It is
variously characterized by fever, muscle and joint pains, and hypotension (*A
Jarisch*, 1850–1902, Austria, and *K Herxheimer*, 1861–1944, Germany: der-
matologists).

John Henry effect
- The John Henry effect is a source of experimental **bias.** It occurs where research subjects acting as controls see the experimental treatment (groups) as
a challenge to which they rise competitively. This negates the purpose of
having a control group (after *P Vogt*).
- John Henry was a legendary railroad constructor in 19th century USA. When
confronted with a steam drill (which could replace his labour), he challenged
it. The steam drill tunnelled nine feet (2.74 m) and broke down. John Henry
tunnelled fifteen feet "an' he lied down his hammer an' he died" (American
Folk Song).   See **Hawthorne effect**

joro spider toxin   See **drugs as tools**

J-shaped curve   See **U-shaped curve**

judicial execution/capital punishment (drugs and)
- Judicial execution, employed by some legal systems, often uses drugs; usually a combination of intravenous barbiturate, neuromuscular blocker and
potassium chloride to provide prompt loss of consciousness, respiratory pa-

ralysis and cardiac arrest. A similar combination may be used in countries where physician-assisted suicide is legally permitted.　　　　See **euthanasia**

just society　　　　　　　　　　　　　　(L. *jus*, right; *socius*, companion)
- A just society is one, the principles of which we would all accept, if we did not know in advance what position or state of health we would have in it. It would include access to **essential drugs**.

K

K_a
- Acid **ionization constant**. The negative log (base 10) of K_a is the **pK_a**.

K_A, K_B, K_d
- There is considerable confusion about the terms used to describe **association/dissociation equilibrium constants** of drugs. The most commonly used forms are:
  - K_A – this is the **IUPHAR**-preferred term for the dissociation equilibrium constant for an **agonist**. Other similar terms (now obsolete) that have been used, and their interpretation, include:
    - K_a – dissociation equilibrium constant for an agonist.
    - K_A – dissociation equilibrium constant for drug 'A' in a two-drug mixture.
    - K_A – association equilibrium constant (**affinity** constant).
  - K_B – this is the **IUPHAR**-preferred term for the dissociation equilibrium constant for an **antagonist**. Other similar terms (now obsolete) that have been used, and their interpretation, include:
    - K_b – dissociation equilibrium constant for an antagonist.
    - K_B – dissociation equilibrium constant for drug 'B' in a two-drug mixture.
    - K_B – association equilibrium constant for an antagonist.
  - K_d (sometimes K_D) – dissociation equilibrium constant for an agonist. In this notation, (now obsolete) K_d' (or K_D') is used to designate the dissociation equilibrium constant for an antagonist.

kainate/kainic acid   See **drugs as tools**

Kaplan–Meier survival curve
- A plot of cumulative survival (or other outcome) probability against the number of patients alive immediately before the intervention (event); a life table or curve.

keratolytic   (Gr. *keratos*, horn; *lusis*, loosening)
- Dissolves keratin (the protein that forms the basis of the skin surface and nails).

khat
- A plant (*Catha edulis*) of Arabia and East Africa. It is chewed as a **psychostimulant**. The active principles are an **alkaloid** (cathinone) and norpseudoephedrine (cathine).

kindling   (Old Norse: *kindill*, a torch)
- A phenomenon in which repeated subconvulsive electrical stimulation of the brain leads to an epilepsy-like state in which a previously subconvulsive shock now causes a fit. Kindled animals are used as a laboratory **model** in the development of antiepilepsy drugs. The phenomenon can also be described as *inverse tolerance*.

kinetics   (Gr. *kinein*, to move)
                                   See **pharmacokinetics**

kinins (Gr. *kinein*, to move)
– Polypeptide mediators, e.g. **bradykinin, substance P.** See **tachykinins**

knockout mutant (Old Norse, *knoka*, to hit; Old Eng. *ut*; L. *mutare*, to change)
– Genetically engineered animal lacking a specific gene (i.e. a 'null' mutation) and therefore unable to express the protein coded for by that gene. For example, the 5-HT$_{2C}$ knockout mouse cannot manufacture 5-HT$_{2C}$ receptors and, among other abnormalities, never stops eating.

knowledge (Middle Eng. *knavlege*)
– Knowing: to know is to feel certain of the truth or accuracy of a fact or opinion.
– At no stage are we able to prove that what we now 'know' is **true**, and it is always possible that it will turn out to be false. The popular notion that the sciences are bodies of established fact is entirely mistaken. Nothing in science is permanently established, nothing is unalterable and, indeed, science is quite clearly changing all the time.
– Knowledge is built up by the correction of mistakes, by trial and error problem-solving.
– "Knowledge is of two kinds. We know a subject ourselves or we know where we can find information upon it" (*S Johnson*, 1709–1784).
– "Half of knowledge is knowing where to find knowledge"; inscription on the wall of the library at Florida State University, USA.
– "Knowledge is one. Its division into subjects is a concession to human weakness" (*HJ Mackinder*, 1861–1947, geographer, UK).
– We think so because other people all
    think so;
Or because – or because – after all, we do
    think so;
Or because we were told so, and think we must
    think so;
Or because we once thought so, and think we still
    think so;
Or because, having thought so, we think we will
    think so.
        (*H Sidgwick*, 1838–1900, philosopher, UK).

L

label (radioactive) (Old Fr. *label*, ribbon)
- A 'label' may be attached to a drug molecule by replacing an atom with a radioactive atom or with a stable **isotope** to enable identification of the drug and/or its metabolites in tissues or body fluids. See **radioactivity**

labelling (of drugs/medicines) (Old Ger. *Lappa*, a rag)
- In some countries this term is used synonymously with **data sheet,** in particular it records licensed uses. See **unlabeled (off-label) use**

labile (L. *lapsus*, to slip)
- Unstable, liable to change.

lachrymator (L. *lachryma*, tear)
- A substance that causes the flow of tears. Used as antiriot or **harassing agent**.

laetrile
- A preparation of apricot seeds (pits, kernels), containing principally amygdalin, and called laetrile, was introduced in 1952 as a cancer 'cure'. By the 1970s "Laetrile completely eclipsed any other unorthodox therapy ever used for any disease in our time". The hypothesis of action was that in the presence of the enzyme β-glucuronidase (in cancer cells), enough hydrogen cyanide would be released to kill the cancer cells selectively. There is no evidence that this actually occurs, but the product is certainly hazardous. Commercial exploitation has been enormous. Attempts by the USA regulatory authority (**Food and Drug Administration**; FDA) to control laetrile resulted in smuggling from Mexico, with indictments of doctors and others, bills in State Legislatures legalizing laetrile, etc. Eventually, properly conducted (phase II) **therapeutic trials** failed to show efficacy and a randomized controlled trial (phase III) was not considered ethically justified. "The whole amazing brouhaha goes to show that victims of serious diseases who believe in miracles and seek the philosopher's stone are open to manipulation in ways far more subtle than used by travelling medicine men of the last century" (*British Medical Journal* 1977;1:3): see also *New England Journal of Medicine* 1982;306:201,236,1482; 1983;307:118–120).
See **phases of clinical studies of new drugs**

lag time (*lag*, origin uncertain; Old Eng. *tima*)
- The delay between the administration of a drug and the commencement of absorption (*Rowland & Tozer*, see Acknowledgements).

Langendorff preparation
- A technique for performing experiments upon an isolated heart *in vitro*. A cannula is tied into the aorta just above the aortic valves. A suitable oxygenated physiological salts solution is passed into the cannula under sufficient pressure to close the valves. The solution passes into the coronary arteries (L. *corona*, a crown) and nourishes the myocardium so that the heart, which

has minimal capacity for anaerobic work, will beat for many hours. Drugs are added to the perfusing solution and the force of contraction and heart rate can be recorded by attaching levers or **transducers** to the ventricles and/or atria (*Langendorff*, 1895, pharmacologist, Germany).

Langmuir adsorption isotherm/equation
- The **hyperbolic** relationship between the fraction (*p*) of binding sites occupied by a **ligand** at equilibrium and the concentration, *x*, of the ligand:

$$p = x/(x + K)$$

where *K* is the **dissociation equilibrium constant** for the binding of the ligand. Usually attributed to Langmuir (1918) but actually first derived by AV Hill (1909) in his final undergraduate year at Trinity College Cambridge (see also **Hill equation**). The derivation depends upon the assumption that there is a finite number of binding sites and that they are identical and independent (*I Langmuir*, 1881–1957, chemist, USA).

language   (L. *lingua*, tongue)
- Any systematic or nonsystematic means of communication, including spoken systems and gesture.
- *A computer language* is a system for coding instructions to a computer, e.g. **FORTRAN, ALGOL**.
- "Language is the dress of thought" (*S Johnson*, 1709–1794).   See **computer**

language of science
- The language of international science is "broken English spoken slowly" (*A Kaldor*, physician, Hungary).
- In 1992 a French scientist claimed he was denied promotion (in France) because none of his work was published in English (*Nature*).
- In 1989 there was a national outcry (France) when the Pasteur Institute decided to publish its journals in English (*Nature*). A French scientist stated that researchers "are not only there to work but to diffuse their discoveries", and that the latter is more efficient in English (*Nature*).
- Native anglophone scientists should recognize that "a considerable percentage [of scientists] have to rely on a foreign language (known as basic English, scientific English or simply poor English)" (*U Trendelenburg*, pharmacologist, Germany) and therefore they have a duty of courtesy to minimize the disadvantage by avoiding colloquialisms or slang at meetings and in writing, e.g. dialogue heard at an international meeting on adrenergic mechanisms:
  - English speaker: "That is a red herring."
  - Scandinavian: "What is a red herring and what has it to do with this subject?"
  - *Answer. The English speaker was saying "That is an irrelevant diversion"* (*Oxford English Dictionary*). A red herring is a form of smoke-cured fish. It has a strong smell and has therefore been used to make a trail for exercising hunting hounds, and for sport, instead of an animal quarry.

lanthanides   See **drugs as tools**

last observation carried forward (LOCF)
– Method of assessing the **mean** effect of a treatment in a **clinical trial** in which not all the subjects in the group completed the treatment as laid down in the protocol. The mean value of the measure being assessed is calculated by including the last recorded value (the value at endpoint) in all the subjects in each treatment group, whether or not they completed the treatment, irrespective of the reason for their dropping out of the study.

See intention to treat, observed case

latent period　　　　　　　　(L. *latere*, to lie hidden; Gr. *periodos*, circuit)
– The interval between stimulus and response, or between infection and clinical manifestations (of a disease).

Latin square design　　　　　　(*Latium*, district of Italy including Rome)
– Arrangement of *n* items, each occurring *n* times, in a square array on *n* compartments, so that each item appears once, and only once, in each row and each column:

    A   B   C   D
    B   C   D   A
    C   D   A   B
    D   A   B   C

– Although this kind of arrangement works well for agricultural research, it is less useful in pharmacological research because the order in which drugs are given may modify the response. In the Latin square given above, dose B always follows dose A, except in row 2; dose C always follows dose B, except in row 3, etc. It is better to try to arrange that every dose is given once after every other dose, and to try to avoid repeating the same sequence of doses. With a four-dose design this is not possible; one repeat must be made:

    A   B   C   D
    B   D   A   C
    D   C   B   A
    C   A   D   B

In the second square the sequences CD, DB and AC each repeat, but the square is still balanced (i.e. each row and each column contain all four treatments) and can be used as the basis of, for example, a 2 + 2 doses **analytical dilution assay**.　　　　　　See **random/-ization**

law　　　　　　　　　　　　　(Old Eng. *lagu*, law; L. *lex*, law)
– *In society*, law tells us what we may or may not do; it can be broken. It is concerned mainly with external conduct and standards deemed to be essential to the functioning of society. Its rules, whether by formal enactment or by custom, are binding and are enforceable by external coercion. It may or may not have a moral basis. **Ethics** and law, often overlapping, have a common concern – justice. See **just society**
– *In science (nature)*, a law is descriptive, it tells what happens, it cannot be 'broken', for it is not a command, although it may be found imperfect (falsified/refuted) and so require revision. The origin of this ambiguity (peculiarly

unfortunate in that it has misled many), is that in pre-scientific times it was believed that the events and uniformities of nature were in fact commanded/prescribed by gods).

- *In logic* a scientific law may be conclusively falsified but it can never be conclusively verified since the experiment or observation that would falsify it may simply not have been made. But man-made law may be changed when it no longer serves its purpose. See **hypothesis, induction, liability, right, science in pharmacology, proof/prove**

law of initial value
- The magnitude of the response is related to the prestimulation level: proposed in neurophysiology by Wilder. Wilder's interpretation of this law implies that the magnitude of response is related to base-line (initial) levels, e.g. blood glucose, blood pressure, and that apparently equal responses are not equal if their initial values differed. Thus responses should be looked at both in relation to *absolute* and *percentage* change.
  See **regression to the mean, statistical regression**

laws (various)
- *Anon*: Easy to read, damned hard to write; easy to write, damned hard to read.
- *Anon*: If there is a 50:50 chance of it going wrong, it will go wrong nine times out of ten.
- *Anon*: The light at the end of the tunnel is that of an oncoming train.
- *Bernard Shaw's rule*: The golden rule is that there are no golden rules.
- *Bowie's theorem*: If an experiment works you are using the wrong equipment.
- *Carson's consolation*: No experiment is ever useless: it can always be used as a bad example.
- *Clark Kerr's dictum*: A university is a collection of disparate **academic** entrepreneurs united only by a common grievance over [car] parking.
- *Crossley's approximation*: The quality of documentation of a clinical study (commissioned by a pharmaceutical company) is inversely proportional to the reputation of the principal investigator.
- *Darwin's observation*: Nature will tell you a direct lie if she can.
- *Deng Xiaoping's dicta*: 1) Seek truth from facts; 2) It does not matter whether the cat is black or white; so long as it catches the mouse, it's a good cat (a peasant saying from Anhui Province, China); 3) It's the economy, stupid.
- *Falkland's rule*: When it is necessary to make a decision, it is necessary not to make a decision.
- *Fetridge's law*: Important things that are supposed to happen do not happen, especially when people are looking.
- *Feynman's admonition*: In science it is easy to be fooled and the easiest one to fool is yourself.
- *Finagle's creed*: Do not be misled by facts.
- *Golden principle*: Nothing will be attempted if all possible objections must first be overcome.

- *Hall's law*: The means justifies the means; the approach to a problem is more important than its solution.
- *Jukes' law*: To every complex question there is a simple answer – and it's wrong.
- *Kafka's law*: In the fight between you and the world, back the world.
- *Kilroy's dogma*: If Murphy had not discovered Murphy's law(s), someone else would have.
- *Lasagna's law*: The number of patients actually available for a clinical trial is inevitably only a small percentage of the patients estimated to be available for such a trial during the planning stage.
- *Law of augmented complexity*: There is nothing so simple that it cannot be made difficult.
- *Leahy's law*: If a thing is done wrong often enough, it becomes right.
- *Levy's law*: Eternal boredom is the price of constant vigilance.
- *Lowney's law*: If it jams – force it: if it breaks, it needed replacement anyway.
- *Mandy Rice-Davies's dictum*: He would [say that] wouldn't he? (*MR-D*, UK courtesan and popular philosopher; giving evidence at a trial relating to a political scandal in 1963, in response to an aristocrat's denial of her version of events at his house parties).
- *May's mordant maxim*: A university is a place where men of principle outnumber men of honour.
- *Murphy's law(s)*: If anything can go wrong it will: Nothing is ever as simple as it seems: Everything takes longer than you expect: Left to themselves all things go from bad to worse: If you play with anything long enough you will break it: Whatever you want to do you have to do something else first: Enough research will confirm your conclusions: If a student has to study he will claim the course was unfair.
  (These variants are all derived from: "If there are two or more ways of doing something, and one of them can lead to catastrophe, then someone will do it", said by captain EA Murphy, US Air Force, in 1949, when an immaculate test run on his newly designed pilots' safety harness failed to provide data because the monitoring electrodes had all been wired incorrectly: *Scientific American* 1997;276:72).
- *Murphy's Law* is itself subject to Murphy's law so that it cannot ensure that everything that should go wrong actually does so; which accounts for the observation that things occasionally go right.
- *Nelson Bunker Hunt's dictum*: If you can count it, you ain't got much.
- *O'Brian's law*: If an editor can reject your paper, he will.
- *Osborn's law*: Variables won't, constants aren't.
- *Paradox of selective equality*: All things being equal, all things are never equal.
- *Parkinson's law (1955)* originally consisted of two maxims: an official wants to multiply subordinates, not rivals; and, officials make work for each other. These have spawned a number of variants, such as: work expands so as to fill the time available for its completion; expenditure rises to meet income. In 1992 *The Economist* (which published the original, then anonymous, article) added a coda, arising from the proliferation of computers since 1955, thus:

because data expand to fill the hard disks available, and officials proliferate to process the data available, technology is the ally of bureaucratic expansion, not its foe (as had been optimistically predicted).

– *Parsimony, law of*. See **Occam's razor**.

– *Parson's law(s)*: A meeting lasts 1½ hours however short the agenda: The place you want to get to is always just off the edge of the map.

– *Paul principle*: People become progressively less competent for jobs they were once well equipped to handle.

– *Peer's law*. The solution to a problem changes the problem.

– *Peter principle*: In every hierarchy each employee tends to rise to his level of incompetence: every post tends to be filled by an employee incompetent to perform its duties. This should cause civilization to end, but *Heggie's objection* explains; there is a vastly insufficient number of slots above any given level in the hierarchy for everyone to rise to his Level [of incompetence].

– *Pieron's law*. If you're coasting you're going downhill.

– *Popper's law*. Statements can never be shown to be true – only falsifiable.

– *Principle of opposite effect*. Most new policies contain something unexpected that tends to offset the original intention.

– *Sod's law or la loi d'emmerdement maximum*: The degree of failure is in direct proportion to the effort expended and to the need for success.

– *Tom Sawyer's definition*: Work consists of whatever a body is obliged to do, and play consists of whatever a body is not obliged to do.

– *Uhlmann's corollary*. It seemed the right thing to do at the time.

– *Uhlmann's razor*. See **Occam's razor**.

– *Unexpected consequences*: When one thing is made better, something else goes wrong.

– *Weisman's college exam law*. If you're confident after an exam its because you don't know enough to know better.

– *Wittgenstein's dictum*: Everything that can be thought at all can be thought clearly. Everything that can be said can be said clearly. (Sadly, Wittgenstein himself was not able to put this into practice in his own writings).

– *Wolf's law*. If you can't beat them, have them join you.
(Many of the above are taken, by permission, from *P Dickson; The official rules*, Arrow Books, 1978.)

laxative   (L. *laxare*, loosen)
– A medicine that induces bowel emptying.   See **purgative**

LC–API/MS
– Liquid chromatography–atmospheric pressure interface/mass spectroscopy. Analytical tool in which a liquid **chromatography** system is connected to a mass spectrometer through an atmospheric pressure interface.
See **mass spectroscopy**

LD$_{50}$ See **lethal dose**

lead compound   (Old Eng. *laeden*; L. *com*, together; *ponere*, to put)
– A compound chosen for detailed study (often from among thousands) as par-

ticularly likely to lead to the development of a potential medicine. It is often the first compound to have marked **potency** (or **selectivity**) at the therapeutic target. See **combinatorial chemistry**

leaders and managers (Old Eng. *laeden*; L. *manus*, a hand)
– *Leaders* do the right things; *managers* do things right (*W Bennis*).
See **management and administration**

learned intermediary (Mid. Eng. *lernen*, learner/teacher;
L. *inter*, between; *medius*, middle)
– Where, for example, a manufacturer of a **medicinal product** fulfils its **duty of care** by providing prescribers with all necessary information, it becomes the professional responsibility of the latter to ensure that patients are adequately informed, e.g. about adverse reactions. The professional prescriber is, in fact and in law, a *learned intermediary*, and may be held responsible in law for any failure in duty of care that results in injury. See **liability, negligence**

least squares (Old Eng. *laessa*, less)
– A criterion for getting the 'best' estimate of parameters from data. The **parameter** values chosen are those that minimize the sum of squared deviations, the deviations in question being the differences between observed points and the fitted points that are calculated from the parameter values. Each item in the sum may be multiplied by an appropriate **weight**.
See **maximum likelihood**

least squares mean
– In a clinical trial, the value of the mean of any class or subclass that would be expected from a balanced design, involving the class variables with all **covariates** set at their mean values. For example, in an **analysis of variance**, subclasses could be the different centres participating in the study. Covariates could include age, length of illness, gender etc. If the covariates are influential, they must be identical at each centre for a balanced comparison. If a simple mean is calculated, there is no way of knowing how much its value has been influenced by imbalance in the covariates between centres. The least squares mean is calculated using an equation which includes the average values for the covariates. The least squares mean in this example is thus the mean value for the centre, adjusted for any imbalances in covariates. It therefore allows an unbiased estimate of the difference in the measured characteristic between groups at each centre and which can be ascribed entirely to the influence of that centre (as far as can be judged). The term **least squares** arises from a widespread technique in statistics for estimating the best **fit** to experimental data in which the individual differences between the data and the fitted equation are first squared to remove negative values.

length constant (Old Eng. *long*; L. *com*, with; *stare*, stand)
– In the general exponential equation $y = e^{-kx}$ (which is a solution of the equation $-dy/dx = ky$), k is the **proportionality constant**. The reciprocal of k has

the same units as x, and is known as the length constant if x represents distance; or **time constant** if x represents time. In the former case, for example, the length constant is the distance over which the function falls to a fraction $1/e$ (= 36.788%) of its initial value at $x = 0$. It is a characteristic of the exponential process that the length constant is independent of where the initial value is taken. The dissipation of an electric charge down a conductor such as an axon can be described by its length constant (the distance over which the charge falls to 36.788% of its starting value i.e. its value at distance zero).

See **exponential curve, half-life/half-time**

lethal dose (LD) (L. *lethum*, death)
- LD$_{50}$: the dose of a substance lethal to 50 per cent of animals; a measure of acute toxicity that is now discarded in new drug development.
- MLD: minimum lethal dose See **EC$_{50}$, toxicity tests**

lethal synthesis (L. *lethum*, death; Gr. *syn*, with; *tithenai*, to place)
- The metabolic conversion of a substance to a toxic form, e.g. fluoroacetate to fluorocitrate, which inhibits the enzyme aconitase, essential in the Krebs cycle: fluoroacetate is used as a rat poison and occurs in certain plants.

See **prodrug, suicide (enzyme) inhibition**

Letheon (Lethe, a river in Hades in ancient Greek mythology, the water of which induced forgetfulness)
- The name under which William Morton (USA) hoped to *patent* ether anaesthesia, which he introduced in 1846; but hospital officials would not let him use it again until he revealed its chemical nature (*RJ Wolfe*).
- A *patent* is a grant of a monopoly, i.e. the exclusive right to exploit an *invention* (the *process* of anaesthesia in this case).

leucopenia (Gr. *leukos*, white (cell); *penia*, poverty)
- This condition exists when the level of leucocytes in the blood falls below 5×10^9 per litre. It may be due to drugs.

See **granulocytopenia, immunosuppressive**

leukotrienes
- A family of inflammatory mediators formed from **arachidonic acid** as a result of the action of 5-lipoxygenase. The slow-reacting substance of anaphylaxis (SRS-A) is now known to be a mixture of several leukotrienes, principally LTC$_4$ and LTD$_4$.

levamisole See **drugs as tools**

level (L. *libella*, diminutive of *libra*, scales)
- Horizontal line or plane. The following two usages are undesirable:
  - Plasma level (to mean plasma concentration).
  - Significance (or confidence) levels (to mean the value of a probability, which should simply be stated).

liability/liable   (L. *ligare*, to bind)
– Legally bound, answerable for. There are various forms of legal liability, in-
  cluding:
  – *Liability in tort* (L. *tortus*, twisted): this is the familiar concept of **negli-
    gence**; a failure to use reasonable care doing, or omitting to do, some-
    thing is an essential element in the modern test of negligence. The simple
    idea of liability for negligence can be expressed: "If a person by rash or
    careless conduct causes injury to another, the wrongdoer has, or ought
    to have, a feeling of guilt which needs to be expiated and the victim has
    a feeling of indignation which needs to be appeased and that expiation
    and appeasement are achieved by a payment of compensation" (*Royal
    Commission on Civil Liability and Compensation for Personal Injury
    1978*).
  – *Strict liability* is *not* concerned with *fault*; it imposes the cost of compensa-
    tion on the person who causes an accident or is responsible for something
    that causes it (e.g. a pharmaceutical company might be liable for an un-
    avoidable adverse effect of a drug it produced).
  – *No-fault liability (scheme)* provides for compensation (without proving fault)
    from some central fund (in the case of drugs, not from the producer). It re-
    moves the necessity of the injured person to proceed against the producer.
    The central fund may make a levy on producers in general to provide the
    means of compensation.
  – *Market-share liability*: the principle or device whereby liability to compen-
    sate for injury due to a drug is shared amongst the manufacturers currently
    in business (according to the share each has of the market). It is applied
    where the injured person cannot prove the identity of the manufacturer of
    the product that caused the injury (or if the manufacturer has gone out of
    business, perhaps long ago). Market-share liability is unnecessary where a
    no-fault scheme for drug injury is in place. The principle has been applied
    in the case of injury due to **stilbestrol**, where daughters of women who
    had been given that synthetic oestrogen in the belief that it would prevent
    miscarriage, developed vaginal carcinoma in adult life. Legal actions have
    succeeded in at least two countries (including the USA), but the principle is
    not yet recognized in UK law.
  – All systems of liability are (must be) based on initial proof of a causal rela-
    tionship, which can be difficult, indeed impossible, where, for example, ad-
    verse drug reactions mimic spontaneous disease (e.g. fetal deformity,
    thromboembolism).
  – *Research*: in the case of healthy volunteers the reasonable inference
    should be that any unexpected injury or harm suffered during or shortly
    after the study is due to participation in the study. In marginal cases the
    benefit of the doubt should be given to the volunteer (*Royal College of
    Physicians of London*), i.e. the burden of proof of causation should be re-
    versed. The situation for patients is more complex, particularly with regard
    to acceptance of risk.   See **causation of injury, compensation,
                       contract, product liability, science in pharmacology**

ligand (L. *ligare*, to bind)
- A structural group on a bioactive substance **(endogenous** or **exogenous)** that contributes to **receptor** binding.
- An atom or molecule that binds to another atom or molecule, usually applied to the smaller of the interacting species.
- A radioactively **labelled** drug (agonist or antagonist) used in experiments to measure the extent of binding to receptors (radio**ligand-binding assay**).

ligand-binding assay (L. *ligare*, to bind)
- Several techniques have been developed for assessing the characteristics of either **receptors** or drugs **(ligands)** by using radioactively **labelled** drug molecules. There are two main techniques:
  - *Saturation analysis*: the amount of radioactivity that accumulates in a tissue in the presence of a known concentration of labelled drug (under equilibrium conditions) is measured for a number of nonsaturating concentrations of the drug. The data are then fitted to a **hyperbolic** function (or the **logistic equation**) and from this the **dissociation equilibrium constant** of the drug (K_A) and the density of binding sites/receptors (B_{max}) can be found. A convenient way of displaying such binding data is the *Scatchard plot* (see **reciprocal plot** for problems associated with Scatchard analysis).
  - *Displacement or competition analysis*: the characteristics of an unlabelled drug can be determined from its ability to interfere with the binding of a radioactively labelled drug with known binding properties (usually an antagonist with relatively slow dissociation characteristics). The interaction follows the **Gaddum–Schild equation** and analysis reveals the dissociation equilibrium constant for the unlabelled drug. If only a few concentrations of the unlabelled drug can be used, its dissociation equilibrium constant can be estimated using the **Cheng & Prusoff equation**.
- In both techniques, care must be taken to account for *nonspecific* binding, i.e. binding of radioligand to binding sites of types other than those under analysis.
- By using ligands with known binding properties, ligand-binding assays can be used to classify the receptors in tissues.
- **Radioimmunoassays** are a form of ligand-binding assay.

likelihood (Old Norse *likligr*)
- The condition of being likely or probable.
- Likelihood is a measure of the plausibility of a hypothesis. It is defined by a number that is proportional to the probability of getting the observations that have, in fact, been made, if the hypothesis in question is indeed **true**.
- The relative frequency with which different causes would produce a given outcome. See **probability**

linctus (L. *lingere*, to lick)
- A viscous liquid preparation used for cough.

linear kinetics See **first-order kinetics**

Lineweaver–Burk plot   See **reciprocal plot**

liniment   (L. *linire*, to smear)
- A liquid or semi-liquid preparation intended to be applied to unbroken skin with friction.

lipid mediators   (Gr. *lipos*, fat; L. *mediare*, to be between)
- **Mediators** formed from membrane phospholipids through the action of phospholipase enzymes (e.g. **prostaglandins**, **leukotrienes**, **PAF**, diacylglycerol).
- Some of these, especially the **eicosanoids**, have potent inflammatory effects and are likely to have important roles in inflammatory diseases. Others act by modifying the function of intracellular enzymes (e.g. diacylglycerol activates protein kinase C).

lipid solubility   (Gr. *lipos*, fat; L. *solvere*, to loosen, release)
- Pharmacologists' **jargon** meaning **oil:water partition coefficient**. Thus a drug described as 'lipid soluble' may dissolve very well in water, but when shaken (to equilibrium) in a mixture of equal volumes of water and oil, a higher concentration will be found in the oil.
- Since **compartments** of the body are composed of cells bounded by phospholipid bilayer membranes, through which drugs must pass if they are to enter the body, distribute throughout it and enter cells, the capacity of drugs to dissolve in and **diffuse** through lipid is evidently important – lipid soluble substances (hydrophobic) cross lipid membranes better than water soluble substances (hydrophilic).
- Lipid solubility is influenced by:
  - The presence of charged group(s) (the more charged groups the less lipid soluble).
  - The environmental pH (if the molecule has an ionizable group with a pK_a in the relevant range). If the pH is such that the molecule is *charged (ionized)* it will have *low lipid solubility*; if the molecule is *uncharged (unionized)* it will be *lipid soluble*.
  - The characteristics of the remainder of the molecule (large hydrophobic regions on a molecule confer lipid solubility).
                                    See **hydrophilic/-phobic, polar/nonpolar**

lipophilic/-phobic   (Gr. *lipos*, fat; *philos*, love; *phobos*, fear)
- Having affinity (or no affinity) for lipids (esters of fatty acids):
  - *Lipophilic*, lipid soluble or hydrophobic.
  - *Lipophobic*, water soluble or hydrophilic.
- In pharmacologists' jargon, a lipophilic drug is one with a high oil:water partition coefficient.   See **hydrophilic/-phobic, lipid solubility**

liposomes   (Gr. *lipos*, fat; *soma*, body)
- Small vesicles of phospholipid-protein bilayer membrane with an aqueous interior which may carry a drug. They are prepared by sonicating (exposing to

high frequency sound wave energy) **amphipathic** phospholipid molecules in a medium containing a drug. Liposomes can be used to:
- Allow absorption from the alimentary tract of substances that would otherwise be digested (e.g. insulin).
- Study ion fluxes across membranes.
- Reduce the toxicity of drugs given intravenously.
- Enable the delivery of nucleic acid in **gene therapy**.

'litogen'   (L. *litis*, lawsuit; *generare*, to beget)
- A drug/medicine, the principal effect of which is to generate litigation.

loading/priming dose   See **dose**

location parameter   (L. *locus*, place; Gr. *para*, alongside; *metron*, measure)
- The term in an equation for a curve (usually a **hyperbola**) that determines the position of the curve on the *x*-axis. For a ligand–receptor binding curve, the location parameter is the **dissociation equilibrium constant**, equivalent to the concentration at which half the receptors are occupied by ligand.
                   See **Black & Leff, Furchgott & Bursztyn, Hill equation/plot**

Locknet
- The international **peer review** research network; named after Stephen Lock, a past editor of the *British Medical Journal*.

LOEL
- Low-effect dose level.

logarithm   (Gr. *logos*, reckoning, ratio; *arithmos*, number)
- Power to which a fixed number (the *base*) must be raised to produce a given number, e.g. the logarithm of 1000 to base 10 is 3, i.e. $10^3 = 1000$. (At one time – before the pocket calculator – logarithm tables were used to facilitate multiplication and division, allowing these to be done by addition and subtraction which are easier to get right.)

logarithmic transform(ation)   (Gr. *logos*, reckoning, ratio;
                                            L. *trans*, across; *formare*, to give shape to)
- In nature most phenomena have a **log-normal distribution**, i.e. the distribution is only **normal** (Gaussian) when the **variable** is plotted on a logarithmic scale. Consequently, for a log-normally distributed variable, indicators of **variance** (e.g. **standard deviation**) or of precision (e.g. **standard error of the mean**) will be asymmetric about the **mean**. The arithmetic mean of that variable will also be a distortion of the true population value. This is one reason for pharmacologists' preference for plotting semilogarithmic **dose–response curves**; the response is plotted v. the log of the dose (concentration) of drug inducing that response. In addition to rendering the curve **homoscedastic**, this transformation also turns the **hyperbolic** curve into a sigmoid (S-shaped) curve. All **full agonists** acting at the same **receptor** will produce

curves with the same shape and midpoint slope, and their maxima will differ only in their location on the log-concentration axis. Similarly, for a single **agonist**, increasing concentrations of a *competitive antagonist* (see **competition**) will cause rightward displacement of the agonist curve without changing its shape or maximum. The horizontal distance between each curve and the control curve is the log of the **concentration ratio** (equieffective concentration ratio, also previously called *dose ratio*). The logarithmic transformation also compresses the concentration axis so that dose–response curves of drugs differing in potency by many orders of magnitude can be displayed on the same graph between the same axes; drugs differing in potency by a million-fold (or a million-fold antagonism) can be represented on a graph with only six units on the *x* axis ($\log_{10}10^6 = 6$). The logarithmic transformation used by pharmacologists should properly be called a **semilogarithmic transformation**. See **mean (arithmetic, geometric), transformation**

logic   (Gr. *logike*, art of reason)
– Science or art of reasoning.
– Chain of reasoning by which a specific conclusion necessarily follows from a set of general premises.   See **deduction, induction, inference**

logistic equation/function
– An equation that can be used to **fit** a **hyperbolic** curve to a set of data points, for example a concentration–response curve or concentration–occupancy curve.
– The logistic function is defined by the equation:

$$y = \frac{1}{1+e^{-(a+bx)}}$$

where *a* and *b* are constants. The constant *b* is referred to as the slope constant, and is normally 1 for simple law of **mass action** processes. For pharmacological applications, *a* is redefined as $-\log_e(K^b)$, and *x* is redefined as $\log_e Z$, which produces an equation of the same form as the Hill equation:

$$y = \frac{z^b}{K^b + z^b}$$

where *z* is the concentration of ligand and *K* is the **dissociation equilibrium constant**. The constant *b* is now equivalent to n_H, the slope of the Hill plot, or the Hill coefficient (after **IUPHAR**; *Pharmacological Reviews* 1995;47:255–266).
– The logistic equation can be used to fit binding data or dose–response curves directly without using a transformation to a linear form, e.g. Scatchard plot, Lineweaver–Burk plot (see **reciprocal plot**), as these transformations introduce statistical distortions.

logistic regression analysis   (Gr. *logos*, word, reason:
                                                              see **regression analysis**)
– Type of **regression analysis** used when the *dependent variable* can only

have two values – either 0 or 1 (e.g., dead or alive, success or failure, infected or not infected). In logistic regression analysis the *independent variable* can be either *categorical* (i.e. one of a fixed set of values or steps) or *continuous* (i.e., capable of having any value within the experimental range). The technique uses **maximum likelihood** *estimation* on the natural logarithms of the data (which reduces nonlinearity), rather than the **least squares** method. It gives an estimate of the probability of an event.

See **variables and analysis of variables, variable (scales for)**

logit
– Acronym for logistic probability unit. See **logistic regression analysis**

log-normal distribution
– A distribution of **data** that is **skewed** and which can be rendered more nearly symmetrical (i.e. made into a **normal distribution**) by the device of taking logarithms of the data. Examples include **dissociation equilibrium constants** and K_M.

See **logarithmic transformation, mean (arithmetic, geometric), transformation**

logrank test
– A test used to compare two or more groups of (life) survival data. It is a test of the **null hypothesis** (that the groups come from the same population).

longitudinal study
(L. *longus*, long; *tudo*, a suffix for abstract nouns)
– A prolonged **cohort study** in which individual subjects are repeatedly observed.

loop diuretic (high-ceiling d.)
(Middle Eng. *loop* unknown origin; Gr. *dia*, through; *ouron*, urine)
– Diuretic acting on the ascending limb of the loop of Henle (of the renal tubule), e.g. frusemide. These are the most highly **efficacious** diuretics.

See **aquaretic, diuretic, natriuretic**

lotion
(L. *lotus*, participle of *lavare*, to wash)
– Liquid preparation for application to unbroken skin.

lozenge
(Old Fr. *lauze*, flat stone)
– Medicaments contained in a hard, solid, usually flavoured base to provide slow **dissolution** for medication in the mouth.

LSD
– **Lysergic acid diethylamide.**

luciferin/luciferase
See **drugs as tools**

luck
(Old Dutch *luk*)
– Chance as bestower of good or bad fortune; fortuitous events affecting a per-

son's interests; an important element in pharmacological research and development. See **chance**, **serendipity**

lusitropic (Gr. *lusis*, to release or loosen; *tropos*, turning)
- Pertaining to the rate of muscle relaxation. For example, catecholamines have a *positive lusitropic* effect on the heart, as well as positive **inotropic** and **chronotropic** effects, whereas digoxin has a positive inotropic action only and alters the rate of neither contraction nor relaxation of heart muscle.

lymphokines See **cytokines**

lyophilization (Gr. *lyo*, loosen; *phileo*, love)
- A freeze-dried product, e.g. a powder or vaccine (which is too unstable to be presented as a solution); it is dissolved or suspended in liquid for use.

lysergic acid diethylamide, lysergide, LSD
- A semi**synthetic** hallucinogen derived from **ergot**. Its hallucinogenic effect was discovered in 1943 by a Swiss chemist who absorbed enough while working with it in his laboratory to induce fantastic images of extraordinary plasticity and colour. The popular, or 'street', name is 'acid'.

lysis/-lytic (Gr. *lusis*, to release or loosen)
- A suffix meaning:
    - The destruction or disintegration of cells (e.g. haemo*lysis*).
    - An agent producing a gradual reduction in severity (e.g. anxio*lytic*).
    - The breakdown of a biochemical substance by the action of an **enzyme**.

lysosome (Gr. *lusis*, to release or loosen; *soma*, body)
- A subcellular membrane-bounded structure containing a variety of hydrolytic enzymes. Lysosomes are important in destroying invading organisms, although some organisms are resistant to lysosomal destruction because they possess thick, hydrophobic coats. The disruption of lysosomes releases the enzymes into the cytoplasm, resulting in cell damage or death. Some remodeller cells, such as osteoclasts, release lysosomal enzymes into their extracellular environment.

MAb
- Monoclonal antibody.

'magic mushroom'
- *Psilocybe mexicana*, which contains the alkaloid hallucinogen psilocybin. Psilocybin also occurs in other fungi.

magistral formula (regulatory term)   (L. *magister*, master; *forma*, form)
- Any medicinal product prepared in a pharmacy in accordance with a prescription for an individual patient (**EU**).   See **officinal formula**

magnetic resonance imaging (MRI)   (Gr. *magnes*, ancient mineral-rich area;
                                                            L. *resonare*, to resound)
- Originally an analytical technique in chemistry, but now adapted to form an imaging system in medicine. Subatomic particles spin on their axes. If placed in a strong magnetic field, they will align themselves with this field because the spin turns them into dipoles. If a brief pulse of electromagnetic radiation (high-frequency radio waves) is passed through the body, the dipoles are perturbed and as they 'relax' back to their previous orientation they emit their own characteristic electromagnetic radiation. This can be amplified and used to identify the particles. By tuning the excitant radio signal to an appropriate frequency, accumulations of particular atoms can be visualized.
- In *functional* MRI of the brain, local changes in neuronal activity while the brain is engaged in particular tasks can be detected by the signal from the oxygen atoms in haemoglobin – the signal changes when the blood becomes deoxygenated. This is being used to investigate the effect of **antipsychotic** drugs on different aspects of brain function in schizophrenia, for example.

MaLAM
- Medical Lobby for Appropriate Medicine, a consumer body that monitors the conduct of multinational pharmaceutical companies, in particular their activities in developing countries.

malinger   (Old Fr. *mal*, bad; *haingre*, feeble)
- To exaggerate or pretend illness to obtain sympathy or to avoid unpleasantness, especially work, military service. Some malingerers show enormous ingenuity, and drugs (e.g. anticoagulants) have been used to simulate natural illness.   See **factitious**

mammillary model   (L. *mamma*, breast, teat)
- **A model** used in **pharmacokinetics** that consists of a large central compartment with several smaller compartments connected to it but not to one another, supposedly resembling a mother sow suckling a litter of piglets.

management and administration   (Ital. *maneggiare*, to control;
                                          L. *manus*, hand; *ad*, to; *ministerium*, service)
- A *manager* controls.

- An *administrator* provides a service.
- "Management is often confused with administration. Administration is a necessary skill and a part of management...Administration is essentially about the *status quo* and ensuring that the machine runs smoothly, [it] is not about change or improvement. Management is about continuous change... Management in practically every field is about the creation of more, or better, from less" (*J Harvey-Jones*).   See **bureaucracy, leaders and managers**

Mann–Whitney test
- A nonparametric test for comparing data from two independent groups.
                    See **analysis of variance, parametric and nonparametric statistics**

Mantel–Haenszel method
- A statistical method for estimating the pooled **odds ratio** and its **confidence interval** across a number of studies or across several strata within a single study.   See **Cochrane plot**

MAO(I)
- **Monoamine oxidase (inhibitor).**

margin of safety   See **therapeutic index**

marketing exclusivity   (L. *mercari,* trade; *ex,* out of, *cludere,* to shut)
                    See **innovation, protection of**

masking (in clinical trials)   (Arabic *maskara,* buffoon)
                    See **double-blind**

mass   (Gr. *maza,* a barley cake; L. *massa,* that which forms a lump)
                    See **SI units**

mass action (law of)   (L. *massa,* that which forms a lump)
- The rate of a chemical reaction is proportional to the concentration (mass) of the reacting substance (or the product of the concentrations or masses of the reactants if there are more than one). Since drug–receptor interactions are chemical reactions, the law of mass action is relevant to the analysis of drug–receptor kinetics.   See **competition**

mass media and scientists
- Scientists ought to take the trouble to communicate with the general public on whose goodwill their careers ultimately depend. But their relationships with the mass media are fraught with danger.
- It is essential that the basis of any conversation with a journalist be agreed at the outset, *before* anything else is said. You should *assume* that you are being interviewed and will be quoted by name unless it is agreed otherwise, and agreement may not be possible *after* you have spoken.

- Bernard Ingham, press secretary to a former UK Prime Minister, gives these definitions:
  - *On the record*: any information and remarks can be quoted and attributed to the informant;
  - *Unattributable*: the information can be freely used but the source must not be disclosed;
  - *Off the record*: nothing that is said may be imparted or broadcast: "It is extremely risky to say the least, to give any journalist anything you do not wish to be made public. And fastidious journalists refuse anything off the record, for their hands would be tied if they got the same information elsewhere."
- When journalists *explicitly* agree not to reveal you as a source, they are making a profound commitment of honour of a profession not noted for such, and you should be safe (but see above) – after all, journalists are always hoping for more, and do not wish to frighten all those who may leak private information in the future.
- One way of deflecting journalists without seeming rude is to say that you want to help but are too busy right now, so would they please write to you; or tell them the name of a book where they can find the information they want. Journalists do not engage in either of these activities – they want oral, quotable information *now*.
- If you really want to 'mount the elephant of publicity', let it be known that you are always ready for an 'on the record' conversation at short notice and at any hour, and that you will always return a journalist's telephone call. Another way of getting your public career started is to write a few letters to newspapers condemning your fellow scientists, the medical profession and the pharmaceutical industry for unethical conduct individually and in conspiracy. But remember that it may not be as easy to dismount from the 'elephant', at your convenience and unscathed, as it was to mount.

mass spectroscopy (L. *massa*, that which forms a lump; *spectrum*, image; Gr. *skopeo*, to look at)
- When an ion passes at high velocity through an electrical field at right angles to its motion, its trajectory will deviate from a straight line in a manner determined by both its charge and its mass. An array of detectors set across the path of the particles and aligned with the electrical field will show that the heaviest particles deviate least from a linear track, whereas the lightest particles will deviate most. This forms the basis for *mass spectroscopy*. The technique can be used to distinguish between *stable isotopes* (see **isotopes**) and can be used to help determine the structure of complex chemicals by identifying fragments of the chemical formed when it is degraded under controlled conditions.

matched or paired observations/data (Old Eng. *gemecca*, spouse, mate; L. *par*, equal)
- When making a comparison of two treatments it is plain that if pairs of patients alike in all material features (age, sex, duration and severity of disease,

etc.) can be chosen, and one of each pair (chosen at **random**) is given the treatment under test and one the current standard treatment, then the accuracy of the evaluation of a new treatment may be enhanced. The reason that matched pairs of patients are seldom used is that they are extremely difficult to form for multiple criteria and contemporaneously.

Matthew effect
– "The frequent misallocation of credit to the more eminent author of co-authored papers" (*E Garfield*, after *RK Merton*; *Science* 1968;159:55). The term derives from a cryptic passage in the Gospel According to Saint Matthew: "For unto every one that hath shall be given, and he shall have abundance: but from him that hath not shall be taken away even that which he hath."
– The effect also extends to the citation of high impact factor journals in preference to others as well as to the allocation of scientific resources, and the attraction of staff.   See **impact factor of a journal**

maximal agonist effect (α)
– The maximal effect that can be elicited by an **agonist** (conventional or **inverse**), expressed as a fraction of that produced by a **full agonist** acting at the same receptors under the same conditions. The term *maximal agonist effect* is preferred to the older term *intrinsic activity* (after **IUPHAR**; *Pharmacological Reviews* 1995;47:255–266).   See **efficacy, intrinsic activity**

maximum likelihood   (L. *magnus*, great; Old Norse *likligr*, likely)
– A criterion for getting the 'best' estimate of parameters from data by maximizing their **likelihood** (see **Bayes' theorem**), i.e. the **parameter** values chosen are those that maximise the probabilities of the observed data. For data that follow a **normal distribution** this criterion of 'best' estimate is the same as the **least-squares** criterion.

maximum residual level (MRL)
– The concentration of a medicinal or non-medicinal (e.g. growth promoting) agent in a food producing/source animal that is deemed safe for human consumer.

MCA
– Medicines Control Agency: part of the UK regulatory machinery.

MDA
– Methylenedioxyamphetamine or tenamfetamine, a hallucinogen, also known as 'mellow drug of America' and 'love drug'.   See **designer drugs**

MDMA
– Methylenedioxymethamphetamine, better known as **ecstasy**.
                                        See **designer drugs**

'me-again' drugs   See **'me-too' drugs**

mean (arithmetic, geometric, harmonic, weighted) (L. *medianus*, mean; *medius*, middle; Gr. *arithmos*, number)

- *Of a population*: the expected ('true') mean $\bar{Y}$ of a continuous **variable** Y is the point on the abscissa of the plot of the **probability density function** through which a vertical line divides the curve into two equal areas, i.e. the central point of a population.
- *Of a sample*: the term 'mean' is often (but by no means exclusively) used loosely, to imply the *arithmetic mean* (the sum of all observations divided by the number of observations), i.e. the **average**. The *sample mean* is an unbiased estimate of the population mean.
- If the variable is not normally distributed (see **normal distribution**), the arithmetic mean distorts the calculated central point of a population. In pharmacology, as in biology generally, **log-normal distributions** are more common. For example, **affinity** (or K_A) and **EC$_{50}$** are log-normally distributed. To obtain an unbiased estimate of the mean of such variables, the *geometric mean* of Y (GM$_Y$) must be calculated:

$$GM_Y = \text{antilog}\frac{\sum \log Y}{n}$$

where Y is the variable and n is the number of observations.
- For quantities that are reciprocals, e.g. volumes of distribution, the central position is distorted if arithmetic means are used. The *harmonic* mean of Y (HM$_Y$) is the arithmetic mean of the reciprocals of the original measurements:

$$HM_Y = 1\Big/\sqrt{\frac{\sum(1/Y)}{n}}$$

$$= \frac{n}{\sum(1/Y)}$$

- The *weighted mean* is the average of two or more means, each of which is weighted by the number of observations upon which it is based:

$$\bar{Y}_w = \frac{\left(n_1 \times \bar{Y}_1\right) + \left(n_2 \times \bar{Y}_2\right) + \cdots + \left(n_j \times \bar{Y}_j\right)}{n_1 + n_2 + \cdots + n_j}$$

where n_j is the number of observations in each group and $\bar{Y}_j$ is the arithmetic mean of each group. See **median**, **mode**

mean channel life-time
- The average/**mean** duration for which an **ion channel** remains open.

mean residence time (MRT)
- The average (**mean**) time that drug molecules reside within the body after a single dose. It is the same as the **turnover time** for endogenous substances. It is most easily measured after a single intravenous **bolus** tracer dose of (radio)labelled drug, from urinary excretion or plasma concentration.

- It can be shown that:

MRT = AUMC/AUC

where AUMC is the area under the **first moment** v. time curve, and AUC is the area under the concentration v. time curve. As it is not possible to continue collecting plasma concentration data until infinity, approximations are applied to allow extrapolation to infinity.
- This method of calculating MRT is said to be 'model independent' as no assumptions are made about the process by which drug molecules leave the body.   See **area under the curve (AUC), area under the (first) moment curve (AUMC), statistical moment**

meaning   (Old Saxon *menian*, to intend)
- Sense or significance of a word; **semantic** content; underlying purpose.
- If language is not correct, what is said is not what is meant (*Confucius*, 551–479 BCE; philosopher, China).
- In 1923 CK Ogden, linguist, psychologist and inventor of *BASIC English* (**B**ritish, **A**merican, **S**cientific, **I**nternational, **C**ommercial: 850 words), published (with IA Richards) a classic book entitled *The meaning of meaning*.

mechanism   (Gr. *mekhare*, machine)
- System of mutually adapted parts working together.
- How a process functions.

MedDRA
- *Medical Dictionary of Drug Regulatory Activities* is a medical terminology prepared by an international working party for use by regulatory authorities, pharmaceutical companies and other relevant groups. It is developed by **ICH.**

median   (L. *medius*, middle)
- *Of a sample:* the central or middle value when all observations are listed in order from lowest to highest, i.e. the number of values equal to and below the median and those equal to and above the median are equal.
- *Of a population:* the value that bisects the area under the distribution curve.
                                                                             See **mean**

mediate   (L. *mediare*, to divide into two equal parts)
- *In politics, society:* to act as the agent for bringing about reconciliation between apparently irreconcilable groups or individuals.
- *In physiology:* in modern usage mediate means to cause. It is wrong to use the word to mean to control (**modulate**), or to lessen (*moderate*).

mediated transport   (L. *mediare*, to be in the middle;
                                                                     trans, across; *portare*, to carry)
                                            See **diffusion (facilitated), transporter**

mediator   (L. *medius*, middle)
— A chemical released or formed by cells in response to a stimulus that causes responses from that and/or other cells. A mediator can be physiological, e.g. **hormones, second messengers** and **autacoids**, or pathological.

medical student (on graduation)
— Uncommitted iatroblast (*AC Dornhorst*) (Gr. *iatros*, physician; *blast*, immature precursor cell), i.e. someone who has the attitudes and intellectual equipment to benefit from postgraduate experience in any speciality.   See **education**

medicinal product (regulatory term)   (L. *mederi*, to heal; *pro*, before; *ducere*, to lead)
— Official regulation of medicines requires definitions that will withstand legal challenge. It must be clear what is regulated and what is not. A European Community Directive (65/65EEC) (which member states are obliged to incorporate into their national law) defines a medicinal product as: "Any substance or combination of substances presented for treating or preventing disease in human beings or animals, or which may be administered to human beings or animals with a view to making a medical diagnosis, or to restoring, correcting or modifying physiological functions in human beings or animals". The European Court in 1992 clarified (by request) the definition, stating that it extends to any product recommended or described as having **prophylactic** or **therapeutic** properties, even if it is generally regarded as a foodstuff and has no known therapeutic effect. Individual member states may extend the EC definition provided that the result is not unlawfully to inhibit the free movement of goods within the Common Market.
— Medicinal products commonly contain numerous substances in addition to the therapeutically active drug (see **excipient**).
— For *licensing purposes* a medicinal product that is deemed **essentially similar** to an existing licensed product (i.e. is a **copy product**) may be the subject of an **abridged application**.
— A *proprietary medicinal product* is a ready-prepared product in a special pack marketed under a special (proprietary) name.
                    See **cosmeceutical, nutraceutical, medicinal purpose**

medicinal purpose (regulatory term)   (L. *mederi*, to heal; *pro*, before, *ponere*, to place)
— This means "any one or more of the following purposes:
    — Treating or preventing disease;
    — Diagnosing disease or ascertaining the existence, degree or extent of a physiological condition;
    — Contraception;
    — Inducing anaesthesia;
    — Otherwise preventing or interfering with the normal operation of a physiological function, whether permanently or temporarily, and whether by way of terminating, reducing or postponing, or increasing or accelerating, the

operation of that function or in any other way" – example from UK Medicines Act, 1968.　　　　　　　　　　　　　　See **medicinal product**

medicine　　　　　　　　　　　(L. *medicus*, physician; *mederi*, to heal)
- *General*: the whole art and science of diagnosing, managing and treating disease.
- The practice of the above, but excluding surgery and obstetrics, and relying heavily on the use of **medicinal products** or **drugs**.
- *Specific*: a substance or mixture of substances used in restoring or preserving health.　　　　　　　　　　　　　　　See **drug or medicine**

Medicines Commission (UK): as an example of a statutory advisory regulatory body
- The Medicines Act 1968 states: "There shall be established a body to be called the Medicines Commission", appointed by the Ministers of Health after consultation with appropriate organizations. It shall comprise at least one person having wide and recent experience of, and to have shown capacity in:
  - The practice of medicine (other than veterinary medicine).
  - The practice of veterinary medicine.
  - The practice of pharmacy.
  - Chemistry other than pharmaceutical chemistry.
  - The pharmaceutical industry.
- Its function is to advise (government) Ministers (the Licensing Authority) on matters relating to the execution of the Medicines Act, and on medicinal products where the Commission thinks it expedient, or it is requested by the Minister. It is thus the government's principal source of independent advice on medicines. It hears appeals regarding adverse decisions of the Licensing Authority/Medicines Control Agency.
　　　　　See **FDCA, Committee on Safety of Medicines, QUANGO**

membrane potential　　　　　　　　(L. *membrana*, skin; *potentia*, power)
- The electrical potential difference that exists across excitable cell membranes by virtue of the selective permeability of the membrane to ions, and the different concentrations of ions maintained inside the cell by the operation of selective ion pumps, such as Na^+/K^+-ATPase.　　See **equilibrium potential**

membrane-stabilizing effect　　　　　　(L. *membrana*, skin; *stabilis*, steady)
- A nonspecific decrease in membrane excitability. It is not clear that this represents a definable category of drug action, and the term is generally used to cloak ignorance rather than to impart understanding. *Membrane labilizing* effect (L. *lavi*, to slide) may be regarded as the opposite.

mescaline　　　　　　　　　　(Mexican Indian *metl*, agave plant; *ixcalli*, stew)
- Hallucinogen obtained from a Mexican cactus *Lopophora williamsii* (*Anhalonium lewinii*) known as mescal or peyotl.

messenger　　　　　　　　　　　　　　　See **first messenger**

meta- (Gr. *meta*, with, after; sharing, joint action; behind, hindmost; as a prefix in chemistry, *ortho, meta, para*)

– Prefix denoting chiefly sharing, change: used freely (and not always in accordance with Greek analogy) in scientific terms since about 1850.

– In *chemistry*, a term used to denote the relative position of two or more substituents on a benzene ring. If hydrogen atoms on two adjacent carbons are replaced, the resulting compound is the *ortho* **isomer**; if the substituents are on alternate carbons, the compound is the *meta* isomer; and if hydrogen atoms on opposing carbons are replaced, the compound is the *para* isomer.

– In *philosophy*, it is used for a description, analysis or examination of the original body of knowledge or practice, e.g. meta-ethics (*O'Grady*).

See **meta-analysis**

meta-analysis (Gr. *meta*, with, after; *analusis*, unloose, undo)

– Meta-analysis is a technique for grouping the results of many different, including contradictory, therapeutic or safety studies. A major problem is defining the minimum standards of quality for admitted studies, e.g. competent, **randomization, (double) blind, intention-to-treat analysis**. Although controversial, it provides an objective way of extracting a consensus answer from studies that are individually inconclusive, often because they are individually small. Reliance on published studies is convenient, but this can introduce an important bias (**publication**) and, ideally, unpublished studies should also be sought – no easy task. Investigators are also faced with translation problems in reviewing world literature. Although used widely for drug trials, meta-analysis can be used in other situations (using different study selection criteria), e.g. the health consequences of living close to electric power lines.

– A variant technique involves the collection and re-analysis of detailed *individual patient data* from the chosen trials. This procedure enhances reliability, but it takes more time and resources than do studies involving only what is published because it is liable to involve worldwide collaborations, since full individual data are seldom published in journals for reasons of space.

– Inevitably, meta-analyses have themselves been subject to meta-analysis.

– The existence of a large body of unpublished (usually negative) clinical trials and of duplicate publication have a serious adverse effect on the precision (and therefore the value) of meta-analyses. See **clinical trials, unreported; systematic review**

metabolism of drugs (Gr. *metabole*, change)

– *Metabolism*: general term for chemical transformations (usually catalysed by enzymes) that occur in the body. The products are *metabolites*.

– *Metabolism of drugs* occurs in many tissues – the gut mucosa, lung, etc. – but principally in the liver.

– BB Brodie (biochemical pharmacologist, USA) suggests that since drug metabolizing enzymes are not the usual enzymes of intermediary metabolism, they were developed in evolution to permit the organism to dispose of lipid soluble substances – hydrocarbons, alkaloids, etc. – ingested in food. If such

metabolism to water soluble, and so excretable, compounds did not occur, lipid soluble substances would accumulate in the body and remain for years.
- It is broadly divided into two phases (see **phases of drug metabolism**).

metabotropic receptors (Gr. *metabole*, change; *tropos*, turn; L. *re*, again; *cipere*, to take)
- Membrane-associated receptors which are **G-protein**-linked, i.e. they activate a **GTP**-binding protein when agonist is bound, which in turn activates or inhibits an intracellular enzyme leading to production (or inhibition of production) of a **second messenger**. Members of this **superfamily of receptors** are made up of a single, continuous polypeptide (i.e. *monomeric*; see **homomeric**) with seven membrane-spanning regions (**domains**).
See **ionotropic receptors, G-proteins, slow receptors**

metameter (Gr. *meta*, with, after; *metron*, measure)
- The measure of response used for calculations is called a *response metameter*. It may be that a transformation of the response is actually measured. The transformed concentration or dose is called the *dose metameter*.
See **parameter**

metaphor (Gr. *metapherein*, transfer)
- An aid to vivid speech in which a descriptive term is used of an object to which it is not properly or strictly applicable. For example:
  - His communication to the meeting opened the *flood-gates* of controversy (or put the *cat among the pigeons*).
  - The administration of **stilbestrol** to pregnant women in the hope of preventing miscarriage planted a *biological time-bomb* in their daughters.

metered-dose inhalers (Gr. *metron*, measure)
See **inhalation of drugs**

methaemoglobin (metHb) (Gr. *haima*, blood; *globin*, a protein)
- Haemoglobin (Hb) in which oxidation of iron (II) to iron (III) has occurred.
  - It is useless for carrying oxygen.
  - It can be produced by drugs, e.g. nitrates, nitrofurantoin.

method/-ology (Gr. *methodos*, a going after)
- A way of doing something, especially a regular or systematic way.
- An orderly doing or arranging.
- The techniques of a particular field of study.

methonium compounds See **drugs as tools** (*Methonium compounds*)

metirosine See **drugs as tools** (*Metirosine*)

α-methyl-L-tyrosine See **drugs as tools** (*Metirosine*)

'me-too' drug

- *Slang* for a drug developed to allow a pharmaceutical company to gain a share of the existing market. Any gain to therapeutics is purely incidental. *Slang* (18th century, unknown origin) is not the same as **jargon**. Slang is not appropriate to formal use. Much of this book is jargon, in the useful sense of the word.
- The process of systematic search for such molecules has been described as "methyl, ethyl, propyl, butyl, futile" (*JW Black*).
- Where a company introduces a drug very similar to one of its own existing drugs, this has been called a *me-again* drug.
- Products which fail to offer clear advantages over existing therapies.

See **seeding trial, switch campaigns**

Meyer–Overton
See **Overton–Meyer**

MHW

- Ministry of Health and Welfare (Koseisho) (Japanese medicines regulatory authority).

micelle
(L. *micella*, a little crumb)

- Molecular aggregates occurring in high concentrations of solutions of surface-active substances (**surfactants**).

Michaelis–Menten equation
(L. *aequalis*, level)

- The Michaelis–Menten equation (published in 1913) describes, for some enzymes, the relationship between the initial rate of the reaction (v) and the substrate concentration (C).

$$v = V_{max}C \div (K_m + C)$$

- Initial rate (mol s^{-1}) is the rate measured over a time period during which C is essentially constant, where C is the concentration of substrate, and V_{max} is the maximum rate (velocity) of appearance of products of the reaction (rate as C approaches infinity), supposed to be directly proportional to the total amount of metabolizing enzyme. K_m (the Michaelis–Menten constant) is the value of C at which the initial rate of reaction is 50 per cent of maximum. (*LVS Michaelis,* chemist, USA; *M Menten*, chemist, Canada; 1913).
  Note: a similar equation may describe the rate at which a membrane carrier works. The equation is formally the same as the Langmuir binding equation, but the **Langmuir equation** applies only at equilibrium and K is an equilibrium constant whereas K_m is not. See **reciprocal plot**

Michaelis–Menten kinetics

- The therapeutic concentration of most drugs is such that, if they are eliminated by enzymatic transformation, the process follows **first-order (exponential) kinetics**. However, some drugs, e.g. phenytoin and ethanol, saturate the enzymes responsible for their metabolism at very low concentrations. As a result, the rate of elimination of these drugs is first-order at very low plasma concentrations, but does not continue to increase proportionately as the plasma concentration rises. At therapeutic concentrations the rate of elimination is constant, irrespective of the plasma concentration. This pattern of elimination is known as *Michaelis–Menten kinetics* because the rate of drug metabolism in relation to the plasma concentration can be represented by the **Michaelis–Menten equation**.   See **saturation kinetics, zero-order kinetics**

Mickey Finn
– An alcoholic drink to which chloral hydrate has been maliciously added. Mickey (Michael J) Finn ran a bar named The Lone Palm Saloon in 19th century Chicago (USA). He employed girls to ensure that the customers consumed drinks to which chloral hydrate had been added. When the customers became unconscious they were taken into an alley and 'rolled'. The lone palm was a sickly potted palm in one corner of the saloon.

microsomal fraction   (Gr. *mikros*, small; *soma*, body)
– When liver cells are homogenized and subjected to high-speed centrifugation, one of the sedimentation layers is rich in **microsomes**. This fraction is useful for investigating the metabolism of drugs *in vitro*.

microsomal oxidation   (Gr. *mikros*, small; *soma*, body; *oxus*, sharp, acid)
– Liver cells contain a specialized system of **isoenzymes** known as the **mixed-function oxidase system**, capable of carrying out a variety of oxidation reactions. Because these enzymes are especially abundant in **microsomes**, the process is often called *microsomal oxidation*. These isoenzymes are forms of **cytochrome P450**, a haem protein that binds molecular oxygen as well as the substrate, and forms part of the electron transport chain. Several chemical groups on a variety of foreign molecules are substrates.

microsomes   (Gr. *mikros*, small; *soma*, body)
– The endoplasmic reticulum of cells rolls up into small, dense bodies when the cells are homogenized. These can be isolated by high-speed centrifugation and are called microsomes. When prepared from liver, these microsomes contain the enzymes responsible for **microsomal oxidation** (*microsomal enzymes*). Microsomes are *in vitro* artefacts.

milk (drugs in)   (Old Eng. *milc*, Old Saxon *miluc*)
– Unionized lipid soluble drugs diffuse easily from the blood into the milk, but since the pH values of blood (7.4) and human milk (7.2) differ, the concentration of the drug will not be the same in both fluids. Breast-fed babies may be adversely affected by drugs given to the mother. Allergic reactions to penicillin (used to treat bovine mastitis) have occurred in humans due to penicillin in milk when the farmer has failed to allow the legally prescribed time to pass before selling the milk from that cow.

mimetic   (Gr. *mimesis*, imitation)
– Suffix meaning to mimic or imitate, e.g. **sympathomimetic** – a drug that causes responses resembling those produced by activity in the sympathetic nervous system.

minimum alveolar concentration (MAC)   (L. *minimus*, least; *alveus*, cavity; *cum*, with; *centrum*, sharp point)
- A measure of the potency of inhalation **anaesthetics**; the minimum concentration of the agent in the pulmonary alveoli at one atmosphere pressure that induces a defined effect, e.g. suppression of response to a painful stimulus or immobility in 50% of subjects (animal or man); it allows prediction of brain concentrations (which are difficult or impracticable to measure).

minimum effective dose (MED)   (L. *minimus*, least; *efficere*, to work out; Gr. *dosis*, giving, gift, and so portion of medicine)
- The smallest dose needed by any individual to produce some specified response. This term is fairly obviously meaningless as it stands. Unless every individual in the population is tested, the answer must depend on the size of the sample that is taken, because the **individual effective dose (IED)** always varies from one individual to another. The usual way to avoid this problem is to specify the proportion of individuals. For example, the **median** effective dose is the dose that causes the specified effect in 50 per cent of individuals (**ED$_{50}$**) (i.e. in that section of the population with IEDs equal to, or less, than the ED$_{50}$).

minimum publishable units   See **publication** (*Salami p.*)

miotic   (Gr. *muein*, to shut the eyes; *osis*, process or state)
- A drug that constricts the ocular pupil by contracting the iris (e.g. **parasympathomimetic** agent).

mitogen   (Gr. *mitos*, a thread)
- A substance that induces cell mitosis, e.g. cholera toxin which increases the production of **cyclic-AMP**.

mixed-function oxidase system
- Substrates for **microsomal oxidations** include a wide range of substances. Consequently, the microsomal oxidase enzymes have been named mixed-function oxidases. There are approximately 100 **isoenzymes**.
See **cytochrome P450, microsomes**

mixture   (L. *miscere*, to mix)
A liquid drug **formulation** (solution, suspension) for swallowing.

MLA (regulatory term)
- Medicines licence application **(EU).**

MLD
- Minimum lethal dose.   See **lethal dose**

modality   (L. *modus*, measure, manner)
- A method or procedure including use of a therapeutic agent such as a drug.
- Relating to statistical **mode**.
- Forms of sensation, heat, touch, pain etc.

mode (L. *modus*, measure, manner)
- *Of a sample*: the most frequently occurring value in an observed series.
- *Of a population*: the value corresponding to the maximum on the distribution curve. See **bimodal distribution, frequency distribution, mean, median**

model (L. *modellus*, model)
- Person or thing proposed for imitation.
- Representation of a structure.
- A simplified representation designed to facilitate prediction and calculation.
- It is not practicable to conduct the early development of new medicines on patients having the target disease. Therefore, predictive *models* are necessary. Initially these may be *in vitro* preparations involving **receptors**, cell cultures and isolated animal and human tissues. Then follow studies in intact animals (which may have been genetically or physiologically or chemically modified to constitute what is hoped to be a model for the target human disease), and eventually in patients having carefully chosen uncomplicated (model) disease, until the final test in the naturalistic conditions of everyday medical practice. See **therapeutic trial**
- Mathematical (algebraic equation) and computer models are used for predictive or explanatory purpose in experimental bioscience, including pharmacokinetics and pharmacodynamics.

modified-release (MR) drug delivery systems/dosage forms/formulations
(L. *modus*, measure)
- These are designed to modify or control the rate or the place at which active ingredients are released in the body.
- They comprise:
  1. *Delayed-release*, i.e. release at a time other than immediately after administration.
  2. *Repeat-action*, i.e. released at intermittent intervals after administration.
  3. *Sustained-release*, i.e. released slowly.
  4. *Controlled-release*, i.e. released at a constant rate.
  5. *Enhanced-release*, i.e. increased speed of release, e.g. by reduction of particle size.
- *Extended-release* comprises 1–3 above.
- Other terms include prolonged-action, timed-release (after Pharmaceutical Codex).
- Techniques to delay release include the use of multiple small, coated, spheres (microencapsulation), chelates, resins, porous plastic matrices and cellulose derivatives. Generally oral preparations, but also by other routes, e.g. **transdermal, implantation**. Sometimes a proportion of the formulation is in *immediate-release* form to provide an initial priming dose (see **dose**).
See **depot formulation, formulation (pharmaceutical)**

modify/-ication (L. *modus*, measure)
- To cause change.
- When applied to normal physiological functions, it often implies an **exogenous** agency.

- The term **modulate** is increasingly misused where *modify* is meant (neuro-transmission across synapses may be *modulated* by a transmitter acting at presynaptic receptors, but a drug (exogenous) acting at those receptors *modifies* transmission).

modulate/-ion   (L. *modulare*, to regulate)
- To change, regulate, adjust or control (e.g. by **feedback** mechanisms). The term generally, but not always, implies an **endogenous** mechanism.
- [A modulator is a] **ligand** that increases or decreases the action of an **agonist** by combining with a distinct (**allosteric**) site on the receptor macromolecule (**IUPHAR**, with permission; *Pharmacological Reviews* 1995;47:255–266).
                              See **modify/-ication, receptor** (*Modulatory site*)

moiety   (L. *medius*, middle)
- One of two parts into which a thing is divided.
- A chemical group on a molecule.

mole/molar/molal   (L. *molus*, pile, heap)
- One *mole* of a substance is the mass of that substance in grams that is numerically equal to its relative molecular mass (relative to the mass of an atom of carbon). This is the *gram mole*; the millimole (mmol) is one thousandth part of one mole (0.001 mol; 10^{-3} mol).
  - A *molar* solution contains one mole of substance per litre of *solution**.
  - A *molal* solution contains one mole of substance per 1000 g of *solvent**
    (*molar* or *molal* may be used according to convenience and circumstances).
- *The molar and molal concentrations in plasma differ because some of the volume of plasma is occupied by protein, and one litre of plasma therefore contains appreciably less than 1000 ml of water.

molecular biology   (L. *molecula*, diminutive of *molus*, pile, heap;
                                                                          Gr. *bios*, life; *logy*, study)
- The study of biological phenomena at the molecular level.
- More recently the term has been hijacked to mean exclusively the study of genes and gene products.

molecular design/modelling
- *Molecular modelling* aided by three-dimensional computer graphics (including virtual reality) allows the design of structures based on new and known molecules to enhance their desired, and to eliminate their undesired, properties to create highly selective targeted compounds. In principle all molecular structures capable of binding to a single high-affinity site can be modelled.
- The modern approach to the invention of new drugs is to use objective, quantitative techniques to determine the structural features needed to give the drug the desired pharmacological properties. This is done by the identification of **descriptors** (characteristics based on some property unique to the molecule). When all the descriptors for a number of structures are plotted in multi-dimensional space by a computer, structures with similar properties will, theoretically, cluster near one another. This approach offers ways of defining the

features common to different drug molecules that cause them to bind to the same receptor, for example. See **molecular pharmacology**

molecular imprinting
- A method for creating **selective** recognition sites in synthetic polymers which mimic **antibodies**. The polymer ('antibody') is made by joining functional monomers in the presence of molecules of the substance it is eventually intended to detect (target or 'print molecule' – equivalent to the antigen). When polymerization is complete, the print molecules are removed, leaving sites on the rigid polymer that are complementary to the print molecule. When exposed to a test sample containing target molecules ('antigen'), the polymer ('antibody') will bind these molecules for which it has highly selective **affinity**. The technique has been used, like **radioimmunoassay**, to measure minute amounts of drugs and hormones.

molecular pharmacology
- The study of the properties of drugs at the molecular level.
- More recently the term has been rediscovered and applied to the study of drugs using methods of **genetic engineering**. This is a shame because it limits the scope of a useful term. For example, the new use of the term excludes the study of drug molecules by other technologies.

See **pharmacogenomics**

monitor
(L. *momere*, to advise)
- To maintain regular/continuing surveillance over, as in drug monitoring, e.g. for adverse reactions.

monitored dosage systems (MDS) or customized patient medication packages (patient med-packs)
- Devices, e.g. boxes with labelled compartments, that may be filled by an appropriately qualified person as an aid to patient **compliance** with (**adherence to**) prescribed **regimens**. Their use poses problems of formulation stability, particularly regarding moisture penetration and duration of stay of the formulation in the device.

monoamine oxidase inhibitors (MAOI)
- Inhibitors of the MAO enzymes (which inactivate monoamines such as noradrenaline, dopamine and serotonin, by oxidative deamination) have beneficial effects in some cases of depression. The inhibitors are famous for their interaction with cheese (containing the monoamine, tyramine, preservation of which can cause a severe, even fatal, hypertension).

monoclonal antibody
(Gr. *monos*, alone, single; *klon*, twig, shoot; *anti*, against; Old Eng. *bodig*, body, corpse)
- When an animal is exposed to a foreign protein (**antigen**) its immune system mounts a response in which lymphocytes are recruited to make **antibody** to the antigen. If a sample of these antibody-producing cells is removed from the

animal and cultured, the antibody can be produced *in vitro*. If the culture is diluted sufficiently, and samples taken and recultured, it is possible to produce a colony of antibody-producing lymphocytes which have all derived from a single cell. This is a **clone**. The antibody that a clone produces is **homogeneous**, i.e. all the protein molecules are identical, and is called a monoclonal antibody. The antibody therefore has very high **specificity**. Monoclonal antibodies are useful in **radioimmunoassay** and **histochemistry**, and *humanized* monoclonal antibodies, prepared in animals, are appearing in **therapeutics**, targeted, for example, against certain classes of T cells in the suppression of rejection after organ transplantation.

Monod–Wyman–Changeux 'induced-fit' model of drug–receptor interaction
- The concept of 'induced-fit' was introduced to enzymology by DE Koshland, and it may be applicable to drug–receptor interactions. The central idea is that the **receptor** only adopts the conformation suitable for interacting with the drug in the presence of the drug. In the Monod–Wyman–Changeux model, the receptor is envisaged to be an **oligomeric** protein which can exist in two (or more) conformational states, the conformation of each subunit depending upon the conformation of the next. The drug induces a change in the conformation of the binding subunit, which alters the conformation of the next subunit and facilitates drug binding (positive **cooperativity**) (*J Monod, J Wyman, J-P Changeux*; On the nature of **allosteric** interactions: a plausible model, *Journal of Molecular Biology* 1965;12:88).

monotonous/-y
(Gr. *mono*, single; *tonos*, tension)
- A curve that increases (or decreases) continuously (i.e. has no maxima or minima) is described as a monotonic curve.

Monte Carlo techniques
(The name symbolizes gambling, luck, probability)
See **random**

morbidity
(L. *morbus*, illness)
- Diseased state: usually expressed as morbidity **rate**.

mortality or fatality
(L. *mors*, death; *fatum*, that which is spoken)
- Death: usually expressed as mortality or fatality **rate**.

moxibustion
See **acupuncture**

MPPP
- 1-Methyl–4-phenyl–4-propionoxypiperidine. A **designer drug** with **opioid** activity. Easily contaminated with **MPTP** and consequently responsible for the spate of cases of Parkinson's disease among Californian drug users in the 1980s.

MPTP
- *N*-methyl–4-phenyl–1,2,3,6-tetrahydropyridine. A compound structurally related to pethidine (meperidine). A contaminant of **MPPP**, a **designer drug**

intended to be a heroin substitute. In 1982 a number of Californians suddenly developed a severe form of Parkinson's disease. The cause of the disease was traced to the contaminant MPTP in the MPPP they had all used. It is now known to cause irreversible damage to dopaminergic fibres in the nigrostriatal system, and has been used in models of Parkinson's disease in experimental animals. The neurotoxicity is due to the formation of a toxic metabolite by the enzyme monoamine oxidase-B.

MR or **m-r**
− **Modified-release (formulation).**

MRT
− **Mean residence time.**

mucoadhesive   (L. *mucus*, slimy substance; *ad*, towards; *haerere*, to stick)
                                                    See **bioadhesive polymer**

mucolytic   (L. *mucus*, slimy substance; Gr. *luien*, to release)
− A substance that reduces viscosity of mucus by, for example, depolymerization of mucopolysaccharide-protein fibres.

multidrug resistance   (L. *multus*, much, many; see **drug**; *re*, again; *sistere*, stop)
− Organisms that have acquired resistance to several antimicrobial agents, each with a different mechanism of action, are said to be multidrug resistant. Primarily the result of indiscriminate drug use.

multi/location/centre clinical trial
− A study conducted at two or more locations; the term location may be preferred to centre as being more precise, since a multilocation trial can be coordinated from a single centre.

multimeric receptors   (L. *multus*, much, many; Gr. *meros*, part;
                                                    L. *re*, again; *capere*, to take)
− **Receptors** composed of two or more protein subunits. The subunits may be identical (*homomultimeric*) or different (*heteromultimeric*).
                                                    See **heteromeric, homomeric**

multiple looks (in clinical trials)   See **interim analysis**

multipotent drugs   (L. *multus*, much, many; *potentia*, power)
− Drugs with low selectivity.   See **'dirty' drugs, hybrid drug,**
                                    parallel pharmacology, promiscuous drugs

multisource pharmaceutical product   See **generic drug/ product**

multivariable analysis   See **variables and analysis of variables**

muramyl dipeptide   See **drugs as tools**

224

murexide   See **drugs as tools**

murine   (L. *murinus*, of mice)
− Pertaining to, or derived from, any animal of the family *Muridae*, which includes rats and mice.

muscarine   (L. *muscarinus*, of flies)
− An **alkaloid** from various fungi, but named after *Amanita muscaria* (fly agaric)
  which was used as a fly (*Musca domestica*) killer, although the alkaloid is not,
  in fact, the active agent for this effect. The alkaloid forms a basis for the classification of **acetylcholine** receptors.

muscarinic acetylcholine receptors/cholinoceptors
− **Acetylcholine** receptors that respond to **muscarine** and its **analogues**.
  Genes that code for five subtypes of muscarinic **receptor** have been identified; they are designated m1 through m5. (*Note*: the lower-case 'm' denotes
  cloned receptors; numbers are not subscripted). However, only four types
  have been defined pharmacologically on the basis of functional assays and
  ligand-binding assays. They are designated M_1 through M_4. (*Note*: the up-
  per-case M; numbers are subscripted).

muscle relaxant   (L. *musculus*, a little mouse; *laxus*, loose)
− Drugs that relax a contracted voluntary muscle and/or prevent its contraction.
  They may act centrally (spinal cord, e.g. baclofen) or peripherally (at the vol-
  untary neuromuscular junction, e.g. tubocurarine).   See **curare**

mustard gas
− A **vesicant** poison developed for warfare. It was first used in 1917.

mustards   (L. *mustus*, must, i.e. prefermentation pressed
                                grape juice, used in an ancient Roman *condiment*)
− Family of **vesicants**, usually short-chain sulphur-containing aliphatic molecules with reactive halogens (usually Cl) on each terminal carbon.
− The seeds of the black mustard plant (*Brassica nigra*) liberate allyl iso-
  thiocyanate when crushed. This is a powerful vesicant. White mustard (*B.
  alba*) seeds release the less powerful quaternary ammonium vesicant,
  sinapine.
− Agents in which the sulphur is replaced by nitrogen are much more reactive
  alkylating agents, known as **nitrogen mustards**; these have a place in cancer therapy.

mutagenesis/-ic   (L. *mutare*, to change; Gr. *gignesthai*, to be born)
− Causation of abnormalities of the genetic material (genes, chromosomes) of
  cells, so that a permanent change in hereditary constitution (mutation) occurs.
                                                          See **Ames test**

mydriatic   (Late Latin from Gr., origin obscure)
− Drug that dilates the ocular pupil by relaxing the iris (e.g. **sympathomimetics**
  or **antimuscarinics**).

n = 1 clinical trial   See **single-patient clinical trial**

NAC
- **New active compound.**

nachschlag   (Ger. *nach*, after; *schlag*, stroke, second helping,
                                          grace or unnecessary note (music), serial publication)
- The occurrence of two (or more) openings of an individual **ion channel** in
  quick succession, even when the overall opening rate is low. Originally applied to the second of a pair of openings, it is now used to describe the whole
  phenomenon, or sometimes to describe the short gaps between such openings. It may result from repeated openings during a single **receptor** occupancy.

nadir   (Arabic *nazir as-samt*, opposite the zenith)
- The lowest point, e.g. used in clinical oncology where the lowest point to
  which the blood leucocytes fall during chemotherapy provides an indication of
  the amount of bone marrow suppression experienced, and so allows monitoring of the safety of the course of treatment.

named-patient exemption   See **compassionate drug use**

names of drugs
- A drug may have names in each of three classes. For example, for *pro-
  pranolol*
  - *Full chemical name*: (±)-1-isopropylamino–3-(naphthyloxy)propan–2-ol
    HCl.
  - Nonproprietary (official, approved, generic) name: propranolol.
  - *Proprietary (trade) names*: Inderal, Bedranol, Efektolol, Pylapron, Tesnol,
    and about 38 more. An initial capital letter is conventional for proprietary
    names.
- Standardisation of drug nomenclature is plainly desirable. Numerous bodies
  recommend names, including national and international **pharmacopoeias**,
  IUPHAR (receptors and drug classification), the World Health Organization
  (recommended International Non-proprietary Names, **INN** or rINN).
- The term **generic** has gained widespread acceptance as synonymous with
  non-proprietary name. This is a pity because it misuses a word already having a useful meaning – characteristic of a genus or class, applied to a large
  group or class. For example, barbiturate and sulphonamide are true generic
  names, embracing classes of substance, whereas the nonproprietary names
  of the individual barbiturates or sulphonamides are not truly generic, they are
  specific. But, as always, the way a word is used in practice is what carries the
  day, even though it originates in misuse; see *Leahy's law* in **laws (various)**.
- Some substances are named after their supposed principal or useful action.
  This is undesirable (e.g. emetine has its principal use in amoebiasis, not as
  an emetic: vasopressin is the antidiuretic hormone rather than being useful as
  a vasoconstrictor).

- Many multiple-ingredient fixed-dose formulations have *only* a **proprietary name**; they do not deserve the recognition conferred by an official, nonproprietary (generic) name.
- **WHO** states two primary principles used in devising International Nonproprietary Names (INN):
  1. International Nonproprietary Names (INN) should be distinctive in sound and spelling. They should not be inconveniently long and should not be liable to confusion with names in common use.
  2. The INN for a substance belonging to a group of pharmacologically related substances should, where appropriate, show this relationship. Names that are likely to convey to a patient an anatomical, physiological, pathological or therapeutic suggestion should be avoided.

  Secondary principles include:
- The use of an isolated letter or number should be avoided: hyphenated construction is also undesirable.
- To facilitate the translation and pronunciation of the INN, 'f' should be used instead of 'ph', 't' instead of 'th', 'e' instead of 'ae' or 'oe', and 'i' instead of 'y'; the use of the letters 'h' and 'k' should be avoided.
- Provided that the names suggested are in accordance with these principles, names proposed by the person discovering or first developing and marketing a pharmaceutical preparation, or names already officially in use in any country, should receive preferential consideration.
- Group relationship in INNs (see Primary Principle 2) should if possible be shown by using a common stem. The following list contains examples of stems for groups of substances, particularly for new groups. There are many other stems in active use. Where a stem is shown without any hyphens it may be used anywhere in the name.

Latin	English	
-acum	-ac	Anti-inflammatory agents of the ibufenac group
-actidum	-actide	synthetic polypeptides with a corticotropin-like action
-adolum	-adol	analgesics
-adol-	-adol	analgesics
-astum	-ast	antiasthmatic, antiallergic substances not acting primarily as antihistaminics
-astinum	-astine	antihistaminics
-azepamum	-azepam	diazepam derivatives
-bactamum	-bactam	β-lactamase inhibitors
bol	bol	steroids, anabolic
-buzonum	-buzone	anti-inflammatory analgesics, phenylbutazone derivatives
-cain-	-cain-	antifibrillant substances with local anaesthetic activity
-cainum	-caine	local anaesthetics
cef-	cef-	antibiotics, cefalosporanic acid derivatives
-cillinum	-cillin	antibiotics, derivatives of 6-aminopenicillanic acid

-conazolum	-conazole	sytemic antifungal agents, miconazole derivatives
cort	cort	corticosteroids, except prednisolone derivatives
-dipinum	-dipine	calcium channel blockers, nifedipine derivatives
-fibratum	-fibrate	clofibrate derivatives
gest	gest	steroids, progestogens
gli-	gli-	sulfonamide hypoglycaemics
io	io	iodine-containing contrast media
-ium	-ium	quaternary ammonium compounds
metacinum	-metacin	anti-inflammatory substances, indometacin derivatives
mycinum	-mycin	antibiotics, produced by Streptomyces strains
-nidazolum	-nidazole	antiprotozoal substances, metronidazole derivatives
-ololum	-olol	β-adrenoceptor antagonists
-oxacinum	-oxacin	antibacterial agents, nalidixic acid derivatives
-pridum	-pride	sulpiride derivatives
-pril(at)um	pril(at)	angiotensin-converting enzyme inhibitors
-profenum	-profen	anti-inflammatory substances, ibuprofen derivatives
prost	prost	prostaglandins
-relinum	-relin	hypophyseal hormone release-stimulating peptides
-terolum	-terol	bronchodilators, phenethylamine derivatives
-tidinum	-tidine	histamine H_2-receptor antagonists
-trexatum	-trexate	folic acid antagonists
-verinum	verine	spasmolytics with a papaverine-like action
vin-	vin-	vinca alkaloids
-vin-	-vin-	vinca alkaloids

NANC
– Non-adrenergic, noncholinergic, as applied to some efferent neurons in the peripheral, nonsomatic nervous system. As the term implies, such neurons release a transmitter other than acetylcholine or noradrenaline. When the transmitter in such nerves has been identified, the nerves will be described in terms of that transmitter by the use of the **-ergic** suffix. For example, some NANC nerves are known to be NO-releasing or **nitrergic**; **ATP**-releasing nerves are described as **purinergic**.

NANCE
– Non-adrenergic, noncholinergic excitatory fibres.   See **NANC**

NANCI
– Non-adrenergic, noncholinergic inhibitory fibres.   See **NANC**

narcotic   (Gr. *narkosis*, state of being benumbed)
– A drug that induces drowsiness, sleep or stupor (dazed state) especially with analgesia (e.g. morphine). The word is used loosely in some legal systems to include other drugs of abuse, e.g. cocaine, which are, strictly, not narcotics.

NAS/NBAS/NCAS
– **New active substance,** new biological active substance, new chemical active substance.

natriuretic (Gr. *nitron*, soda; *ouron*, urine)
– Causing the excretion of Na⁺ ions in the urine. See **aquaretic**, **diuretic**

natural justice/rights
– The term 'natural justice' derives from the ancient concept of 'natural' law (or **rights**) binding on all human beings *independent* of any laws laid down by human organizations. For example, in the case of drug licensing (appeal) hearings the Medicines Commission (UK) is adjured to ensure that its proceedings are consistent with natural justice, i.e. *fairness*. This involves appellants knowing the objections to their application in sufficient detail to answer them if they can; giving them adequate facilities and time to present their case; ensuring that members of the Commission do not read newspapers or engage in private conversations during the hearing, and so forth; and giving the reasons for an unfavourable decision in writing. See **law**
– Natural rights include the right to **consent** knowingly to participate in clinical research.

naturalistic research (L. *natura*, be born)
– Research in naturally occurring settings; it may be qualitative or quantitative; observational study or by experiment.
See **science in pharmacology, therapeutic trial**

NCE
– **New chemical entity.**

ND
– Not determined/done: used in tables of experimental **data**.

NDA
– New drug application (for marketing) (USA); variants include *accelerated, supplemental, abbreviated* NDA.
– *NDA Phase*: time from NDA submission to **FDA** marketing approval.
See **new drug development**

NDGB
– Non-departmental governing body; a poor substitution for **QUANGO**.

nebulizer (L. *nebula*, mist, cloud; Gr. *nephele*, a cloud)
– Device for creating an **aerosol** or spray.

'need' clause
– A clause in medicines regulatory law that specifies that the applicant has to demonstrate to the authority that a drug is *needed* medically or socially. Mere

demonstration of efficacy and safety are not considered (as is usual) sufficient to gain regulatory approval. The objective of a 'need' clause is to avoid the proliferation of '**me-too**', or unessential, drugs. The 'need' clause (for licensing, although not necessarily for government reimbursement) tends, not surprisingly, to be confined to countries that lack a significant research-based pharmaceutical industry, although this could change. But at the time of licensing it is not practicable to require completed comparative studies with (all) other drugs for the same use, which can take years; see **oculomucocutaneous syndrome**.

negative efficacy See **inverse agonist**

negligence (L. *neg*, not; *legere*, choose)
– Failure to exercise reasonable care.
– A plaintiff seeking to obtain compensation from a defendant (via the laws of tort or negligence) must prove three things:
  – that the defendant owed a **duty of care** to the plaintiff
  – that the defendant failed to exercise reasonable care
  – that the plaintiff has suffered actual injury as a result.
– **Compensation for injury** due to negligence: the aim in quantifying damages is to place the injured person, as far as is possible, in as good a position financially as if the negligence had not occurred, but in no better position (*Lord Justice Butler-Sloss*).
– In some countries, additional *punitive* (L. *punire*, to punish) damages may be awarded when the defendant's conduct is judged to be particularly disgraceful. Such awards have been made against pharmaceutical companies.
See **liability**

NEL
– No effect dose level. See **NOAEL**

neonatal period (Gr. *neos*, new; *natus/nasci*, to be born)
– The first 4 weeks of life (human). See **paediatric**

Neosalvarsan See **Salvarsan**

nephropathy (Gr. *nephros*, kidney; *patheia*, suffering)
– Any disease of the kidney, but especially chronic disease, e.g. analgesic nephropathy.

Nernst equation (*HW Nernst*, 1864–1941, chemist, Prussia)
See **equilibrium potential**

'nerve gas'
– Irreversible (acetyl)cholinesterase inhibitors, usually organophosphorus compounds, used as war gases and insecticides. They are distributed as liquids and deployed as **aerosols**.

neurocrine   (Gr. *neuron*, nerve; *krinein*, separate)
- A nerve cell that also releases a **hormone**. The word was invented by analogy with **endocrine**, to imply the same function as a ductless (endocrine) gland, but carried out by a nerve.

neurokinins   (Gr. *neuron*, nerve; *kinein*, to move)
- Types of **tachykinin**.

neuroleptanalgesia   (Gr. *neuron*, nerve; *lepsis*, seizure; *an*, without; *algesis*, sense of pain)
- The patient is in a state of analgesia but is cooperative. It is obtained by combined use of a **neuroleptic** (e.g. droperidol) and an **analgesic** (e.g. fentanyl).

neuroleptic   (Gr. *neuron*, nerve; *lepsis*, seizure)
- A loose term generally used for the more therapeutically effective (major) **tranquillizers**, having also selective **antipsychotic** action, e.g. phenothiazines.

neuromuscular-blocking agent   (Gr. *neuron*, nerve; *musculus*, little mouse: from the creeping appearance of some muscles when moving)
- Drugs that interfere, by a variety of mechanisms, with chemotransmission at the junction of voluntary motor nerves with striated muscle. Those in clinical use (to facilitate tracheal intubation and to assist the surgeon by providing muscular relaxation) act by **competitive antagonism** or **depolarizing block(ade)**, or a combination of the two (*dual block* by **partial agonists**).

neuroplegic   (Gr. *neuron*, nerve; *plege*, stroke, and so paralysis)
- Causing paralysis of the emotions. Obsolete term for **antipsychotic**.
       See **neuroleptic**

neuronal uptake   (Gr. *neuron*, nerve)
- An active **transport** mechanism by which neuron terminals that are depleted of their transmitter regain it by (re-)uptake of released transmitters or by repletion from exogenous administration.

neurotransmitter   (Gr. *neuron*, nerve; *trans*, across; *mittere*, to send)
- A substance released from a nerve terminal following the arrival of an action potential, and which induces a change in the membrane potential of the postsynaptic cell.   See **false transmitter**

new active substance (NAS) (regulatory term)
- A new, previously unlicensed (or not tested in humans), active substance, produced from any source and put before a regulatory authority for approval as a **medicinal product**. It is classed as either a *new chemical active substance* (NCAS), or *a new biological active substance* (NBAS).

new chemical entity (NCE)
- The term **new active substance** is now preferred.

new drug development
- "Care in choosing a target is the most critical decision point in pharmaceutical research" (*JW Black*).
- The personal approach of one scientist who has been particularly successful in the field (*JW Black*, Nobel Laureate, 1988, for research on β-adrenoceptor blockers and histamine H_2-receptor blockers) is to seek answers to six questions:
  - Is the project purged of wishful thinking regarding desire and the means to satisfy it?
  - Is there a chemical starting point?
  - Are there relevant bioassays?
  - Will it be possible to confirm laboratory-defined specificity in humans?
  - Is there a clinical condition relevant to this specificity?
  - Does the project have a champion? (a person who has the passion and conviction to keep the project going during lengthy periods of stalemate).

  (By permission, after *JW Black; Receptors as pharmaceutical targets*, in *Textbook of receptor pharmacology*. JC Foreman, T Johansen (eds), 1996, CRC Press.)   See **phases of clinical studies of new drugs, post-marketing/licensing surveillance, regulation (official) of medicines, toxicity tests, model**

new molecular entity (NME) (regulatory term)
- A compound that can be patented, which has not previously been approved **(FDA)**.

nicotine
- A liquid alkaloid from tobacco named after *Jean Nicot* (1530–1600), a French diplomat who introduced tobacco into France. The alkaloid is an agonist at **nicotinic**, but not at **muscarinic acetylcholine receptors**.

nicotinic acetylcholine receptors/cholinoceptors
- Acetylcholine **receptors** that respond to **nicotine**. They belong to the ligand-gated (**ionotropic**) receptor superfamily, i.e. they are hetero**multimeric** proteins with an integral **ion channel**.
                    See **acetylcholine, superfamilies of receptors**

NIH
- National Institutes of Health (USA).

NIR
- Near-infrared spectroscopy.

nitrergic
- Nerves having **nitric oxide** as a neurotransmitter, e.g. some **NANC** nerves.

nitric oxide (NO)
- Nitric oxide is a potent vasodilator and a neurotransmitter. It is **endothelium-derived relaxing factor** (EDRF).

- Nitric oxide carries an unpaired electron and is therefore highly reactive, consequently its life-time, once synthesized (from L-arginine), is only a few seconds.
- It acts by activating one form of guanylyl cyclase to produce the **second messenger** cyclic-GMP.
- Inhibitors of the enzyme nitric oxide synthase may have clinical use.
- Some nerves (e.g. some **NANC** nerves) are now thought to be **nitrergic**.

See **free radical scavenger**

nitrogen mustards
- Substances related to **mustard gas**, having two reactive chloroethyl chains attached to an alkylated nitrogen, i.e. R-N-*bis*-(2-chloroethyl). In aqueous solution the chlorine atoms are lost and two reactive ethyleneiminium (aziridinium) groups are formed, which can interact covalently with DNA and other molecules. Nitrogen mustards such as mustine, cyclophosphamide and chlorambucil have a place in cancer chemotherapy.

nitrosamines
- Substances with the structure:

$$\begin{array}{c} R_1 \\ \diagdown \\ \diagup \\ R_2 \end{array} N - N = O$$

where R_1 and R_2 are alkyl or aryl groups. Formerly an intermediate in organic chemistry, but found to be toxic and carcinogenic to all vertebrate species tested. Formed in nature by the reaction of nitrite and amines in food (e.g. bacon) and in the gut. Synthesized by some bacteria and moulds.

NMDA
- *N*-methyl-D-aspartate. A synthetic selective **agonist** used to classify **receptors** for excitatory **amino acids** in the CNS.   See **AMPA, glutamate, kainate**

NME
- **New molecular entity.**   See **NAS, NCE**

no-adverse-effect level (NEL)
- A measure used in the evaluation of hazard from environmental chemicals. It assumes that there is a threshold below which the body can safely dispose of a **xenobiotic**. It is now recognized that this is naïve, and simple NEL estimations are being replaced by more sophisticated toxicological profiles made up from the full spectrum of biological and biochemical events induced by xenobiotics.

NOAEL
- No adverse effect dose level.   See **NOTEL**

nocebo (L. I shall injure)
See placebo-reactor/responder

nociceptors (L. *noxa*, injury)
- Sensory **receptors** that detect pain due to physical or chemical tissue injury.

NOEL
- No-effect dose level.

noise (Old Fr., outcry, disturbance: from L. *naus*, a ship, and so inclination to vomit, nausea)
- A signal (voltage, tension, etc.) that varies in a more or less random way. Frequently undesirable because noise (e.g. from amplifiers) obscures the signal of interest. But sometimes noise may itself be of great interest, e.g. when it arises from the random opening and shutting of **ion channels** in a membrane. See **spectral density**

nomogram (Gr. *nomos*, law, custom; *gramma*, a line)
- A chart from which it is possible to find the value of one **variable** if two others are known. It consists of three lines, each of which is graduated and numbered. When a straight edge is laid between known variables on two of the lines, the third variable can be read from the point on the third line where the edge intersects it.

noncompetitive antagonism (L. *non*, not; *cum*, together; *petere*, to seek; Gr. *anti*, against; *agon*, to struggle)
- **Agonist** and **antagonist** can be bound [to different sites on the same **receptor** macromolecule] simultaneously: antagonist binding reduces or prevents the action of the agonist. (**IUPHAR**, with permission; *Pharmacological Reviews* 1995;47:255–266).
- **Antagonism** in which the maximal response to the agonist is decreased but the **potency** or **EC$_{50}$** is unchanged. One possible mechanism is for the antagonist to combine only with the agonist–receptor complex, rather than with the unoccupied receptor, and by so doing inactivate the receptor. This is an example of **allotopic** antagonism.
- The term is sometimes used loosely (and inappropriately) to describe **antagonism** by any mechanism that is *not* **competitive**, for example **ion channel block**, **depolarization block**, *chemical* or *functional* antagonism. Antagonism that is not competitive is not necessarily noncompetitive in a strict pharmacological sense.
- The term was once popular to describe **antagonism** caused by irreversible **antagonists (nonequilibrium antagonism)**. By analogy with biochemical terminology, this usage is inaccurate and should be avoided.
See uncompetitive antagonism

nonequilibrium antagonist (L. *non*, not; *equi*, equal; *libra*, balance; Gr. *anti*, against; *agon*, to struggle)
- A term introduced by M Nickerson for antagonists that combine chemically and irreversibly with **receptors**, e.g. 2-halo-alkylamines. Because the **an-**

tagonist dissociates from the receptors at a negligible velocity (if at all), the reaction between antagonist, agonist and receptors never comes to equilibrium within a practicable period of time. Consequently, classical receptor kinetic approaches cannot be applied. The degree of antagonism produced by these drugs is a function not only of concentration and the avidity* with which they react with receptors, but also of time. The classic feature of nonequilibrium antagonism is a reduction in the maximal response to an agonist without any rightward shift in the concentration–effect curve. If there is a **receptor reserve** in the system, and the agonist is a **full agonist** (with high **intrinsic efficacy**), there will be an initial irreversible rightward shift before the fall in maximal response.

*The term *avidity* is used here in its normal, nontechnical dictionary sense. The term **affinity** is wrong for such drugs, as affinity is a value that applies only to systems at thermodynamic equilibrium.

nonlinear kinetics See **Michaelis–Menten kinetics, saturation kinetics**

nonparametric analysis See **parametric and non-parametric statistics**

nonselective/nonspecific (L. *non*, not; *se*, apart; *legere*, to choose)
- Nonselective describes drugs that produce effects at many **receptor** types at similar doses/concentrations. Alternative terms include **multipotent, promiscuous** and **'dirty'**.
- *Nonspecific* means that the properties of a drug are not due to its precise three-dimensional chemical structure, but result from some physicochemical property of the drug.

nonshivering thermogenesis
- Substances that induce *energy expenditure without accompanying muscle movement* attract interest for possible clinical use (e.g. in the treatment of obesity); induction of shivering excludes clinical application.

nonspecific antagonism See **antagonism, nonselective**

nonstarch polysaccharide (NSP)
- Dietary fibre is an imprecise term and fibre is difficult to measure precisely in the laboratory. Its major component is NSP which is easy to measure and can be used as an index of fibre content, e.g. 20 g of dietary fibre contains 12 g NSP.

nonsteroidal anti-inflammatory drugs (NSAID) (L. *non*, not; Gr. *stear*, tallow, fat; *oides*, like)
- Drugs, not (adrenocortical) steroids, that relieve inflammation, usually by inhibition of prostaglandin synthesis, and including **aspirin** (a **grandfather drug**), ibuprofen and indomethacin. Some drugs used in the treatment of rheumatoid arthritis, e.g. gold, penicillamine, are not generally regarded as NSAIDs.

nootropic   (Gr. *noos*, mind; *tropos*, turning)
- Agents that enhance vigilance and the acquisition (learning) and retrieval (memory) of information. Also known as **'smart' drugs** (slang).

noradrenaline/norepinephrine   (*nor*, see below; L. *ad*, at; *renes*, kidneys)
- The principal neurotransmitter of postganglionic sympathetic neurons. **Adrenaline** was identified in the body and characterized many years before noradrenaline was recognized as the sympathetic transmitter. Consequently, noradrenaline obtained its name from adrenaline. 'Nor-' is a chemical term meaning without substitution; adrenaline is synthesized from noradrenaline by *N*-methylation. (It has been suggested that 'nor-' stands for the German *'N-ohne Radikal'*, N(itrogen) without a substituent. This is probably not true.) *Norepinephrine* has been designated the r**INN**.

noradrenergic-neuron-blocking agent/drug
                              See **adrenergic-neuron-blocking agent/drug**

norepinephrine   See **noradrenaline**

normal   (L. *norma*, carpenter's rule or square)
- Usual, typical, common, conventional, average.
- Constituting a standard.
- Chemistry:
    - A solution containing 1 gram-equivalent per litre (obsolete).
    - An isomer with a straight chain of atoms.
- Normal distribution: see below.
- *Normal range*: it is usual to agree that values falling within two **standard deviations** on either side of the **mean** constitute the normal range (this comprises 94.63 per cent of the observed values). But the word *normal*, applied to the human condition, is contentious: "Show me the normal man and I will cure him" (attributed to *Sigmund Freud*).

normal distribution curve   (L. *norma*, carpenter's rule or square;
                              dis, apart, reversal of previous state; *tribuere*, to give)
- A symmetrical, bell-shaped distribution curve (i.e. **probability density function**). This form of distribution is often assumed in the absence of evidence because it is statistically convenient. It is often said that statistical methods making this assumption work well: but this is wishful thinking, not science; there is no real evidence to this effect. In principle, the means of several sets of observations will tend to have a normal distribution, whatever (almost) the distribution of the original observations (the central limit theorem). The normal distribution is also known as the *Gaussian* distribution (*KF Gauss*, 1777–1855, mathematician, Germany).

normal equivalent deviate (NED)   (L. *norma*, carpenter's rule or square;
                              equi, equal; *valere*, to be strong; *de*, away from; *via*, way, road)
- A Gaussian **normal distribution curve** resembles the profile of a classical

bell. If the frequency is plotted as a cumulative frequency on the ordinate the curve becomes sigmoid ('S'-shaped). If the curve is a *standard* Gaussian curve (i.e. one with a mean of 0 and a **standard deviation** of 1.0), it can be rendered straight by converting the ordinate to a **probability scale**. If the probability scale on the ordinate is graduated in standard deviation units instead of percentages, the standard deviations equivalent to cumulative percentages are known as *normal equivalent deviates* (NEDs). The relationship between cumulative frequency and normal equivalent deviate is the same for any normal distribution curve – i.e. the same proportion of a population will always be included in 1, 2 or 3 standard deviations, irrespective of the **mean** or the **variance**. When these cumulative frequencies are calculated, expressing deviations from the mid-point of the curve, a line drawn at −2 standard deviations from the mid-point will correspond to a cumulative frequency of 2.27%. At −1 standard deviation from the mid-point, 15.87% of the values will be included; a cumulative frequency of 50% corresponds, by definition, to 0 standard deviations. As the normal distribution curve is symmetrical, +1 standard deviation from the mid-point will include 84.13% of values and +2 standard deviations will encompass 97.73%. Normal equivalent deviates can be rendered more convenient by conversion into **probits**, which are simply NEDs coded by the addition of 5.0. The number 5.0 is chosen because it is the smallest convenient number sufficient to convert all but the most extreme (and rare) deviates to a positive value. Thus the probit value of 5.0 corresponds to a cumulative frequency of 50 per cent, 3.0 corresponds to 2.27 per cent, 4 corresponds to 15.87 per cent, 6.0 corresponds to 84.13 per cent and 7.0 corresponds to 97.73 per cent.

norms and protocols (**EU** regulatory term)

(L. *norma*, carpenter's rule or square)

– The term is used to define the *documents and particulars* that shall accompany an application for marketing authorisation. The requirements are updated/amended in subsequent **EU** Directives according to technological advances.

nosocomial disease   (Gr. *nosokomeian*, hospital, from *nosos*, disease; *komeo*, to take care of)

– A new disease, contracted in hospital (i.e. not what the patient entered hospital to have treated).   See **iatrogenic disease, opportunistic infection**

nostrum   (L. *noster*, our)

– A **quack** medicine.

NOTEL

– No toxic effect dose level.   See **NOAEL**

N-protein

– The old term for some classes of **G-proteins**.

NSAID

– **Nonsteroidal anti-inflammatory drug.**

null equations/methods (L. *nullus*, none; *equatio*, to make equal, to balance)
- Equations intended to allow the determination of properties of drugs, particularly **antagonists**, by making the minimum number of assumptions about the relationship between receptor **occupancy** and response. The prototypical null equation is the **Gaddum–Schild equation**, which led to the **Arunlakshana & Schild method** for determining the **dissociation equilibrium constant** of an antagonist. In both cases the assumption is that, whatever the relationship between receptor occupancy and response, it is reasonable to assume that when the same number of receptors are occupied by an agonist, the same response will occur, irrespective of the number of receptors occupied by antagonist molecules. See **receptor**

null hypothesis: hypothesis of no difference (L. *nullus*, none; Gr. *hupothesis*, foundation)
- **Hypothesis** that there is no relationship between two or more variables, for example, two drug treatments proposed as a basis for therapeutic comparisons. If an observed difference is sufficiently great it renders the null hypothesis unlikely at a standard level of **probability**, i.e. it is *un*likely that there is *no* real difference between the treatments; in other words, there is a difference (probably) (the *alternative hypothesis*).
- The null hypothesis is the basic idea underlying general hypothesis testing.

null mutation See **knockout mutant**

number needed to treat (L. *numerus,* number)
- The number of people who must be treated to prevent one adverse (or produce one desired) outcome, or the numbers of events prevented per 100 people treated. It can be expressed as the reciprocal of absolute risk reduction. See **risk** (*Relative and absolute*)

Nuremberg Code See **Declaration of Helsinki**

nutra(i)ceutical
- A blend word of *nutrition* and *pharmaceutical*, for a substance that may be considered a food or part of a food and that provides medical or health benefits, including the prevention or treatment of disease. These substances pose problems for official medicines regulators. Japan legislated in 1992 to regulate foods engineered to have special medical benefits, e.g. rice from which globulin allergen has been removed. Such products have been designated as 'physiologically *functional foods*' or *pharmafoods*. See **cosmeceutical, medicinal product**

nyctohemeral (Gr. *nux*, night; *hemera*, day)
- Both daily and nightly. See **circadian**

objective   (L. *ob*, against; *jacere*, to throw)
- Existing independently of perception.
- Undistorted by emotion or **bias**; value-free.   See **subjective**

observational study/research   (L. *ob*, towards; *servare*, to watch)
- Study in which there is no active intervention by the investigator; a non-experimental study.   See **science/scientific method (in pharmacology), Hawthorne effect, experiment**

observed association and causality   See **science in pharmacology**

observed case (OC)
- Method of assessing the mean effect of a treatment in a **clinical trial** in which some subjects in a treatment group fail to complete the treatment as laid down in the protocol. Unlike the **last observation carried forward** method, in which the mean value includes the last recorded values in subjects who withdraw, the *observed case* method calculates the mean effect size by including **data** from only those subjects who complete the treatment as intended. In cases where the drop-out rate is very high, the observed case method gives a **biased** estimate of the effect of the treatment, especially if one of the valid reasons for withdrawal is failure of treatment. In cases where the drop-out rate is low, the observed case method could be argued to give a better estimate of the average effect of the treatment. This is because subjects who drop out prematurely, for example due to an **adverse event**, may not have received the treatment for long enough for a full response to have been reached, and inclusion of their responses will dilute the average value.

observer drift   (L. *ob*, towards; *servare*, to watch; Old Norse *trift*, movement of cattle)
- The tendency of observers to become inconsistent over time.   See **observer variation**

observer variation   (L. *ob*, towards; *servare*, to keep)
- This may be *inter-* (between different observers) or *intra-* (the same observer at different times) variation.

obstruction to change   (L. *ob*, against; *struere*, to build)
- When seeking needed change in an organization or department, or to a long-standing practice, the prudent proposer should have prepared in advance responses to objections that:
  - The proposed change will establish a dangerous precedent, or open the door to unforeseen eventualities.
  - The time is not ripe.
  - The proposal is change for the sake of change.

obtund   (L. *ob*, against; *tundere*, to belabour)
- To dull or blunt sensation, especially of pain.

Occam's (Ockham's) razor   (L. *radere*, to scrape)
- "William of Occam (*c*. 1295–1350, philosopher, England) is best known for a
  maxim which is not to be found in his works, but which has acquired the name
  of 'Occam's razor'. This maxim says: '*Entities are not to be multiplied without
  necessity*' [law of **parsimony**]. Although he did not say this, he did say
  something which has much the same effect, namely: '*It is vain to do with
  more what can be done with fewer*'. That is to say, if everything in some science can be interpreted without assuming this or that hypothetical entity,
  there is no ground for assuming it" (*Bertrand Russell*, 1872–1970, philosopher, UK).
- In more practical terms, it means that the minimum number of explanations or
  arbitrary **parameters** that can adequately explain or fit the observations
  should be used: or, if one explanation is sufficient to account for a group of
  facts, multiple explanations should not be invoked. Though not invariably true,
  this is good general advice.
- *Davenport's dictum*: God does not shave with Occam's razor.
- '*Esquire's*' *variant* of Occam's razor: cut the crap (Middle Dutch *crappen*,
  chaff, break off; *crap* is also a taboo word for faeces).
- *Uhlmann's razor*: when stupidity is a sufficient explanation there is no need to
  have recourse to any other.
- The philosopher was known as *Doctor invincibilis* (in logic).
- Ockham (Occam) is a village 35 km south west of London, where there is a
  memorial.

occlusive dressing   (L. *ob*, against; *claudere*, to close)
- Impermeable plastic sheets fixed to the skin at the edges by adhesive tape.
  By preventing evaporation they allow hydration of the horny layer of the skin
  so that drugs applied under the dressing can penetrate more readily. Substantial absorption, with systemic effects, can occur. Babies' plastic pants are
  virtually occlusive dressings.

occupancy   (L. *occupare*, to seize hold of)
- The number (or fraction, in which case *fractional occupancy*) of **receptors**, or
  other **binding sites**, having a bound **ligand** molecule. (In some cases the
  term is used with the restricted meaning of occupancy at equilibrium.)

occupation theory   See **receptors**

occupational disease (of scientists)
- The occupational disease of scientists (and of academics in general) is intellectual arrogance: in its most advanced form it includes the belief that scientists have the right to do whatever they please and to be provided, where
  necessary, with public funds (salaries, grants) to do it. In justifying their position, sufferers from the disease will describe their stance as being a defence
  of academic freedom. The disease is virtually incurable.

oculomucocutaneous syndrome (L. *oculus*, eye; L. *mucus*, slime, from Gr. *musethsai*, nose, nostril; L. *cutis*, skin; Gr. *sun*, together; *dromos*, running)
- A clinical **syndrome** comprising principally keratoconjunctivitis (*oculo*), sclerosing peritonitis (*muco*) and skin rash (*cutaneous*). It was first caused by *practolol*, the first cardioselective β-adrenoceptor blocker to be marketed (1970). The syndrome was not recognized, despite widespread use of the drug in common cardiovascular disease (particularly angina pectoris), until four years later. Because of the seriousness of the immunologically-mediated syndrome practolol is no longer used. Its history illustrates the difficulty of operating a **need clause** in **regulation (official) of medicines.**

odds ratio (Old Norse *odda*, third man; L. *ratus*, reckon; *testu*, earthen pot)
- A nonparametric statistical test in which changes in subjects are not graded but are recorded as present or absent, e.g. benefit:no benefit.
- The odds of an event in an active treatment group divided by the odds of the event in the control group.
- A way of estimating the *relative risk* for a given disease associated with exposure to the factor under study, e.g. treatment. If the **incidence** or frequency of some outcome is assessed in two groups of individuals defined by the absence or presence of some characteristic (such as exposure to a certain factor), the outcome probabilities in exposed and unexposed individuals are $A \div (A+C)$ and $B \div (B+D)$, respectively, where A is the incidence of the outcome in individuals with the group characteristic, B is the incidence of negative outcome in individuals with the characteristic, C is the incidence in those without the characteristic and D is the incidence of negative outcome in those without the characteristic. The *relative risk*, or *risk ratio*, is the ratio of these proportions:

$$R = [A \div (A+C)] \div [B \div (B+D)]$$

- The *odds ratio* is an approximate estimate of the relative risk. In a **case-control study**, the odds ratio (OR) is given by the expression:

$$OR = \frac{\text{No. of exposed cases with characteristic}}{\text{No. of exposed cases without characteristic}} \times \frac{\text{No. of unexposed cases without characteristic}}{\text{No. of unexposed cases with characteristic}}$$

See **parametric and nonparametric statistics/test, risk**

OED
- *Oxford English Dictionary.*

official formula or substance (L. *officium*, performance of a task)
- A substance or formulation identified as a standard in an official **pharmacopoeia.**

officialese (L. *opus*, work; *facere*, do)
- A pejorative term for a style of writing marked by peculiarities supposed to be characteristic of officials. Its chief feature is circumlocution, caused by a feeling that this gives dignity and politeness, by avoiding the blunt statement, and, above all, that vagueness is safer than precision. It results in a stilted and verbose style, not readily intelligible (after **Fowler**). *Legalese* is a dialect of officialese.

officinal formula (L. *officina*, shop; *forma*, form)
- A drug or **formulation** kept in stock. See **magistral formula**

off-label drug use See **unlabeled drug use**

Ogston effect
- The enzymatic transformation of one enantiotropic group on substances that contain a plane of symmetry (*AB Ogston*). See **optical isomerism**

oil:water partition coefficient
- The ratio of concentrations of a substance in the oily layer and the aqueous layer of a biphasic mixture at equilibrium. In such a biphasic mixture, *hydrophobic* or *lipophilic* substances will tend to *partition* into the oily layer, whereas *hydrophilic* or *lipophobic* substances will tend to partition into the aqueous layer. **Lipid solubility** is a short-hand expression meaning oil:water partition coefficient.

ointment/cream (L. *unquere*, to anoint; *cramum*, cream)
- Semisolid preparations for application of drugs to surfaces. They are usually oil-in-water or water-in-oil emulsions in which drugs are dissolved or suspended. An ointment is 'stiffer' than a cream, and a *paste* is stiffer than an ointment.

oligo- (Gr. *oligos*, small, few)
- Prefix meaning few, e.g. oligospermia.

oligomeric (Gr. *oligos*, small, few; *meros*, part)
- Composed of relatively few subunits.

oligonucleotide (Gr. *oligos*, small, few)
- A sequence of DNA composed of only a few nucleotides, and therefore only a few **codons**.

oligoprobe See **oligonucleotide**

oncogene (Gr. *onkos*, tumour; *genes*, born)
- A gene, either of mammalian or viral origin, which, when activated, leads to cell proliferation and tumour development. See **oncoprotein**

oncogenesis/-ic (Gr. *onkos*, tumour; *genesis*, birth)
- Causing tumours, whether benign or malignant (cancer).

242

oncoprotein (Gr. *onkos*, tumour; *proteios*, primary)
- A protein produced as a result of activation of an **oncogene**, which is responsible for tumour development.

one-tailed statistical test: two-tailed test
- *One-tailed*: the testing of the **null hypothesis** relates to one side of a **confidence interval** (e.g. *x* is no greater than *y*).
- *Two-tailed*: the testing of the null hypothesis relates to both sides of a confidence interval (e.g. *x* is no different from *y*, i.e. neither greater than nor smaller than).

ontogenesis (Gr. *on*, being, part; *genesis*, birth)
- The origin and development of an individual. See **phylogenesis**

open clinical trial/open label trial
- A clinical investigation in which investigators, observers and subjects are allowed to know the identity of treatments, so that **bias** due to this knowledge is uncontrolled. See **double-blind**

operational instructions (L. *opus*, work; *in*, in; *struere*, build, teach)
- A framework standardising the way in which an investigation will be conducted, defining conditions, end-points etc.; an essential part of the **protocol**.

operational model See **Black & Leff model**

operationalism and operational approaches (L. *operare*, to work)
- *Operationalism*, as a term of philosophy, is the definition of concepts by specifying the procedures (operations) that are employed to validate them.
- *Operational approaches* to pharmacology mean treating drug targets as binding and responding units having a myriad of mechanisms. Such approaches to quantifying molecular activity in biologic systems do not require precise knowledge of molecular mechanisms (after *TP Kenakin*). See **Black and Leff model, receptor**

opiate/opioid (Gr. *opos*, juice of a plant)
- *Opiate* (noun) any directly acting (agonist or antagonist) substance derived from opium (and semisynthetic **congeners**) having effects that are mediated through the same class of receptors as are acted on by morphine.
- *Opioid* (adjective) as in opioid receptor/analgesic/peptide.
- *Opioid* (as noun, considered an improper use by purists) embraces all agonists and antagonists of any origin, including endogenous opioid peptides, e.g. **endorphins**.
- Non-purists think the above are distinctions without differences and use *opioid* indiscriminately as noun or adjective.
- The term *opiate* has been used to mean pharmacologically morphine-like substances that *also* have a close structural similarity to morphine i.e. phenanthrenes. Thus, codeine (a phenanthrene) is classed as an opiate (and is

also opioid), whereas fentanyl (a phenyl piperidine) although opioid is not an opiate.

opium   (Gr. *opos*, juice of a plant)
- The dried juice (latex) of the opium poppy, *Papaver somniferum*. The juice is usually obtained by scoring the ripening seed heads with a sharp knife.

opportunistic infection   (L. *opportunus*, coming to harbour for protection, and so, to take advantage of favourable circumstances)
- An infection occurring in the immunosuppressed (by disease or drugs) patient, or as a consequence of having freed a drug-resistant organism from the competition of drug-sensitive organisms. Often due to organisms of low intrinsic pathogenicity that normally inhabit the body or environment.

opportunity cost   See **economics**

opsin
- A primary member of the family of light-sensitive pigments that include the mammalian visual pigment, rhodopsin. Coded for by the same **superfamily of genes** as code for the **metabotropic receptors**, and having a similar seven transmembrane **domain** structure to that of, for example, β-adrenoceptors.

optical isomerism (enantiomorphism)   (Gr. *optos*, visible; *isos*, equal; *metron*, measure)
- A kind of **stereoisomerism**: a compound has two structures that are mirror images (enantiomers – Gr. *enantios*, opposite) of each other and so are not superimposable.   See **isomer, chirality**

order of magnitude   (L. *ordo*, row, rank; *magnitudo*, size, from *magnus*, great)
- A class determined by progressive steps (multiples) in size, usually ×10. For example, a number between 100 and 999 is one order of magnitude greater than a number between 10 and 99, and three orders of magnitude less than a number between 10^5 and 9.9×10^5.

order of reaction   (L. *ordo*, row, rank; *re*, against; *agere*, to do, to act)
- The 'order' of a reaction is the sum of the powers of the concentration terms appearing in the equation that relates rate of reaction to concentration. If the rate (R) of elimination of a drug is directly proportional to its concentration (C), i.e. R proportional to C^1, then the elimination is said to show first-order kinetics, i.e. **exponential kinetics**. When, however, the rate of elimination of a drug remains constant, regardless of changes in concentration, i.e. R proportional to C^0, then it is said to show **zero-order kinetics**.

ordered and unordered array   (Gr. *an*, not; L. *ordo*, row, array: Old Fr. *areer*, well-ordered series)
- *Ordered array* or *ungrouped frequency distribution*: observations are ranked from lowest to highest.

- *Unordered array*: observations are listed regardless of their magnitude or frequency of occurrence.

organoleptic   (Gr. *organon*, tool; *lambanein, lepsomai*, to seize)
- Capable of being perceived by a sense organ, e.g. taste, smell.

ORI
- Office of Research Integrity (USA).   See **research misconduct and fraud**

original (patient) pack dispensing
- The medicine is dispensed in an original manufacturer's package, unopened after leaving the factory. Its advantages are the reduced likelihood of **dispensing** error or contamination, and ensuring that each patient receives an information leaflet (*patient package insert*) each time a new supply is dispensed. Its disadvantage is that it is more expensive than dispensing from a large stock-container.   See **packaging and safety**

orphan drug/disease   (Gr. *orphanos*, bereaved)
- A free-market economy is liable to leave unresearched or untreated, *rare diseases*, e.g. some cancers (in all countries), and *some common diseases*, e.g. parasitic infections (in poor countries). When a drug is not developed into a useable medicine because the costs will not be recovered by the developer, it is known as an *orphan drug*, and the disease is an *orphan disease* (as are rare diseases that are unresearched); the sufferers are *health orphans*.
- The **FDA** (USA) permits a drug to be designated under the Orphan Drug Act (which encourages development) where a patient population for use has a ceiling of 200 000 (with certain exceptions, e.g. diagnosis and prevention of disease), even though the drug may also be used in more common diseases. The objective is to encourage clinical testing in the rare diseases. When a drug has been declared an orphan, a single company, not necessarily the original developer, can acquire rights to it and a degree of protection from competition. Japan defines an orphan drug as one intended for populations of up to 50 000.

orphan receptor   (Gr. *orphanos*, bereaved; L. *re*, again; *capere*, to take)
- **Receptor** identified from gene sequences (e.g., from close amino acid sequence **homology** with a known receptor) and for which an endogenous **ligand** has not yet been identified.

orphanin   (Gr. *orphanos*, bereaved)
- Provisional name ascribed to a newly identified endogenous ligand for what was previously referred to as an **orphan receptor**. Once an endogenous ligand has been identified, the receptor can be given a logical name (see **receptor classification/nomenclature/taxonomy**). *Orphanin* is not a useful term as all newly discovered endogenous ligands for orphan receptors qualify as orphanins.

OTC
- Over the counter (shop) – medicines sold directly to the public without a pre-

scription; also known as **home medicines**. OTC medicines may be *pharmacy only* or *general sale* (i.e. may be sold at any outlet).

otoxicity (Gr. *otos*, ear; *toxikon*, arrow poison, from *toxon*, arrow, and so, any poison)
- Drug-induced damage to the eighth cranial nerve, inner ear or vestibular apparatus (e.g. aminoglycoside antibiotics).

outcomes research
- This is a broad concept going beyond the ordinary strict concept of therapeutic **efficacy** examined in classic formal controlled therapeutic trials. It measures the overall impact of a treatment on the patient's life (*effectiveness*) as well as costs (*efficiency*). Such research is increasingly expected by health providers (managed care organizations, governments) seeking to allocate their limited/finite resources with fairness.
See **economics, quality of life, therapeutic trial**

outliers (Old Eng. *ut; licgan*)
- Observations that are highly inconsistent with the main body of data. They should not be excluded from the data analysis, but it is permissible to present analysis both with and without them. The term *rogue results* should not be used for outliers for it implies that there is something wrong with these observations, which may or may not be the case.
See **regression towards the mean**

outsourcing (Old Eng. *ut;* L. *surgere*, to rise)
- The practice of, for example, pharmaceutical companies, to employ independent specialised contract research organizations (CROs) to perform specific aspects of a drug development programme.

overall/overview analysis See **meta-analysis, systematic review**

overexpression of receptors (Old Eng. *ofer*, over, above; *expressus*, distinctly shown)
- A research technique in which **genetic engineering** is used to cause **receptors** to be synthesized (in vast numbers) and inserted into the membranes of convenient cell lines, so that the properties of the **receptors** and/or the **transduction** systems can be studied. See **clone**

Overton–Meyer hypothesis of anaesthesia
- The hypothesis that potency of a general anaesthetic is correlated with increasing lipid solubility (1901).

oxytocic (Gr. *oxy*, swift; *tokos*, childbirth)
- A drug that hastens childbirth, especially one that stimulates uterine muscle.

Q

p value   See **probability value**

pA_2/pA_x
- The negative $\log_{10}$ of the molar concentration of **antagonist**, which causes the ratio of equieffective concentrations (**concentration ratio** or *dose ratio*) of agonist in the presence and absence of antagonist to be *x*

$$pA_x = -\log[A]_x = \log(1/[A]_x)$$

where $[A]_x$ is the concentration of antagonist causing a rightward shift of *x*-fold in the agonist concentration–effect curve (i.e. a concentration ratio of *x*). For genuine **competitive antagonism** the pA_2 is the negative $\log_{10}$ of the **dissociation equilibrium constant** for the antagonist.

              See **Arunlakshana & Schild method**, **Schild equation/plot**

PAA
- **Partial agonist** activity.   See **ISA**

packaging and safety (of medicines)   (L. *pangere*, to fasten)
- Increasingly, *child-resistant packaging* (containers, closures) is used routinely for all medicines handled by patients; though it is also liable to cause difficulties for the elderly.
- Because of incidents of malicious (criminal) tampering (contamination) of medicines, special *security packaging* has been developed and applied especially to medicines on direct sale to the public; it is of two principal kinds: *tamper-evident* and *tamper-resistant*. In 1982 several people died in Chicago (USA) as a consequence of taking a proprietary brand of acetaminophen (paracetamol) that had been deliberately contaminated with cyanide.
- These (necessary) devices all add to the *cost* of medicines.
              See **original pack dispensing**

PACT
- Prescribing analyses and cost. A computerized procedure that allows prescribers individually to be kept informed of the cost of their prescribing (UK National Health Service). It allows prescribers to compare their costs with those of their peers. Such feedback has more impact than does general exhortation to prescribe economically. It also allows intervention by those authorities paying for prescriptions from public funds.
              See **indicative prescribing amount**

paediatric or **pediatric**   (Gr. *paidos*, of a child; *iatros*, physician)
- Considerations of age and development are relevant to pharmacology.
- The conventional periods of *childhood* are:
  - *Neonate*: birth to 1 month.
  - *Infant*: 1 month to 1 year.
  - *Early childhood*: 1 year through 5 years.
  - *Late childhood*: 6 years through 12 years.
  - *Adolescence*: 13 years through 17 years.

- The term 'child' has both general and specific connotations: paediatricians normally care for children from birth to 13 years of age. **See geriatric**

PAF–acether

- Platelet activating factor (PAF) is alkyl-acetyl-glyceryl-phosphorylcholine. Critically important portions of the molecule include the *acetyl* group and the *ether*-linked alkyl chain; hence PAF-acether. It is an important inflammatory **mediator**, as a potent activator of many inflammatory cells, e.g. neutrophils and eosinophils, as well as having effects on vascular smooth muscle. Much evidence also implicates the involvement of PAF in the aetiology of asthma.

PAGB

- Proprietary Association of Great Britain. The trade association representing companies that sell medicines directly to the public.

See OTC, home medicine

paired data   **See matched or paired data**

palliative care   (L. *pallium,* a cloak)

- To *palliate* is to relieve illness without curing. Drugs play a major role. The World Health Organisation defines palliative care as "the active total care of patients whose disease is not responsive to curative treatment. Control of pain, of other symptoms, and of psychological, social and spiritual problems, is paramount. The goal of palliative care is achievement of the best quality of life for patients and their families".

panacea   (Gr. *pan*, all; *akes*, remedy)

- An all-healing remedy (mythical).   **See specific, theriac**

paracrine   (Gr. *para*, alongside; *krinein*, separate)

- Non-nerve cells that release a chemical messenger (a local hormone) which produces effects on adjacent cells. The name is derived by analogy from **endocrine**.   **See autacoid, hormone**

paradigm   (Gr. *para*, alongside; *deiknumi*, to show)

- Example or pattern.
- A *paradigm* is a theory, a set of assumptions or a frame of reference that determines how we interpret the world.

paradoxical pain   (Gr. *para*, beside; *doxa*, opinion; L. *poena*, penalty)

- Rarely, a previously effective analgesic (opioid) may exacerbate pain. The mechanism is uncertain, but may involve competition for receptors between less efficacious metabolites and the parent drug.   **See opiate/opioid**

parallel group designs (in clinical trials)   (Gr. *para*; alongside; *allelos*, one another)

- Each treatment is given to a separate group of subjects, i.e. a non-cross-over study.   **See cross-over trial, therapeutic trial**

parallel importing (of drugs)   (Gr. *para*, alongside; *allelos*, one another;
                                           L. *in*, in; *portare*, carry)
- The importation of a drug from a country where the price is low to a country where the price charged is so much higher as to make the operation commercially profitable. Owing to the complexities of commerce and to government price-fixing, it can occur that a manufacturer finds its own exported product (re-)imported and underselling its home market. This annoys manufacturers. Parallel importing is open to abuse from badly manufactured and inappropriately labelled products and is therefore supervised by regulatory authorities.

parallel pharmacology   (Gr. *para*, alongside; *allelos*, one another;
                                   pharmakon, drug; *logy*, study)
- The properties of a drug other than that considered its main property. For example, chlorpheniramine is classified as an antihistamine, but it is also an antagonist at **muscarinic acetylcholine receptors**. While this causes the unwanted effect of a dry mouth, it can also be a useful effect in that it dries nasal secretions. When the potency of the drug for its parallel pharmacological properties is similar to the main pharmacodynamic action, the drug is of low **selectivity**. The term **side-effects** also describes this concept, but carries a pejorative connotation.   See **'dirty' drug, promiscuous drug**

Parallel Track Mechanism (regulatory term)
- A US Public Health Service policy that makes promising investigational drugs, e.g. for AIDS and other HIV-related diseases, more widely available while the formal therapeutic trials necessary for full licensing are being conducted. The objective is to allow availability to patients for whom there are no therapeutic alternatives and who cannot participate in the formal trials. The **EU** and other authorities have arrangements that have the same effect for rare (**orphan**) diseases.   See **regulation (official) of medicines**

parameter   (Gr. *para*, alongside; *metron*, measure)
- A measured variable characteristic, factor, aspect, feature or thing (a loose but common use).
- A measurement (derived from a set) constant in the case considered, but varying in different cases. For example, averages, standard deviations, regression coefficients.
- A **variable** that is kept constant to allow other variables to be investigated.
- A combination of physical quantities, usually more complicated than simple ratios. The term has been considerably diluted in common speech (after *DN Baron*).   See **metameter**

parametric and nonparametric statistics/test   (Gr. *para*, alongside;
                                                          metron, measure; L. *stare*, stand)
- *Parametric* tests, such as **Student's *t*-test** and the **analysis of variance (ANOVA)** are those based on an assumed form of distribution, usually the **normal distribution**, for the population from which the experimental samples are drawn.

– *Nonparametric*, or **distribution-free, tests** are those that, although they involve some assumptions, do not assume a particular distribution, e.g. **Wilcoxon signed ranks test**. A discussion of the relative 'advantages' of the tests is ludicrous. If the distribution is known (not assumed, but KNOWN), then use the appropriate parametric test. Otherwise do not.

parasuicide   (Gr. *para*, alongside; L. *sui*, oneself; *cidium*, kill)
– The term used for an apparent attempt at suicide that is so ineffectual (e.g. a low dose of a drug taken in circumstances in which it will be quickly discovered) that it may be doubted whether the individual was seriously intent on dying.

parasympatholytic   See **anticholinergic drug, antimuscarinic**

parasympathomimetic   (Gr. *para*, alongside; *sum*, with; *pathos*, suffering; *mimesis*, imitation)
– Definition as for **sympathomimetic** but applying to the parasympathetic (cholinergic) branch of the autonomic nervous system.

parenteral drug administration   (Gr. *para*, alongside; *enteron*, intestine)
– By a route other than the alimentary tract.

parsimony   (L. *parcere*, to spare, refrain)
– The principle (law) of parsimony states that the simplest explanation consistent with a data set should be chosen over more complex explanations. It is a guiding tenet in scientific study (*C-B Stewart*).   See **Occam's razor**

partial agonist   (L. *pars*, a part; *agon*, a struggle)
– A drug that combines with specific receptors but does not produce a response equal to the maximum that can be produced by other (full) agonists acting on the same receptors (i.e. the maximal possible response in that tissue), even when it occupies all the receptors.
– Because, like an **antagonist**, it competes with a **full agonist** for receptors, therefore reducing the response to (fuller) agonists, it is also known as *dualist* or *agonist–antagonist*.
– An agonist having low **intrinsic efficacy**. Note that this definition depends on the nature of the response that is measured. If a maximal response requires only, say, an **occupancy** of 5 per cent, an agonist may produce a maximum response, although it would obviously appear to be a partial agonist when a different response was measured, e.g. one that required 90 per cent occupancy for a maximal effect.
– A drug that is a partial agonist in one tissue may be a full agonist in another tissue, depending on the **receptor reserve** (and the drug's intrinsic efficacy).
                                        See **agonist**

partition coefficient   (L. *partire*, to divide; *co, com/cum, con*, with, together, in common, jointly, equally, reciprocally, mutually; *efficere*, to effect)
– The ratio of the concentrations of a substance in two different phases of a

system, e.g. of two immiscible liquids.   See **oil:water partition coefficient**
- *Hansch coefficient*: a numerical representation for the equilibrium.
- It gives an indication of the likelihood of a substance entering a cell.
See **hydophilic/-phobic, lipid solubility**

paste   (Gr. *pastos*, sprinkled)
See **ointment**

pastille   (L. *pastillus*, a small loaf, from *panis*, bread)
- A soft **lozenge**.

patch (skin)   See **transdermal drug delivery system**

patch clamp   (Middle Eng. *patche*, a piece of material used for mending;
klamp, brace, clasp or band)
- A research technique in which a hollow glass 'patch' pipette is made to form a tight (giga-ohm) seal with a cell membrane by applying suction. There are four variants of the technique:
  - *Cell-attached* patch, in which recordings are made through the pipette sucked on to the membrane of an intact cell.
  - *Whole cell* patch, in which extra suction is applied (to a *cell-attached* cell) and the piece of membrane across the tip of the patch pipette is disrupted, leaving the whole cell attached to the pipette, but with the cytoplasm of the cell continuous with the fluid inside the pipette.
  - *Inside-out* patch, made by pulling the pipette away from a *cell-attached* cell. This leaves a piece of membrane across the pipette tip with what was originally the intracellular surface of the membrane in the bathing fluid and the 'outside' of the patch in contact with the fluid in the pipette.
  - *Outside-out* patch, made from a *whole cell* patch by increasing the suction sufficiently for the cell to be drawn onto the pipette until the cell membrane opposite to the original puncture lies across the tip of the pipette. The pipette is then pulled away leaving a piece of membrane across the end of the pipette with its 'outer' surface in contact with the bathing fluid and its 'intracellular' surface in contact with the fluid in the pipette.
- Ionic currents can be recorded from the whole cell, or from one (or a small number of) channel(s) in an isolated patch. This technique has allowed major advances in our understanding of the properties of ion channels and of how their activity is altered by neurotransmitters/hormones/drugs/intracellular messengers.

patent for drugs   (L. *patere*, lie open)
See **generic drugs**

-pathy   (Gr. *pathos*, suffering)
- *As a suffix*: disease, e.g. neuro*pathy*, retino*pathy*, encephalo*pathy*. Useful when speaking of **adverse drug reactions**, e.g. isoniazid neuropathy.

patient med-packs   See **monitored dosage systems**

patient pack dispensing   See **original (patient) pack dispensing**

patient package insert (PPI)
- An information document for patients included by the manufacturer in a package of medicine designed to be given unopened to the individual patient.
                              See **original (patient) pack dispensing**

payments to research subjects and to investigators
- The tradition that healthy **volunteers** should act as research subjects for purely idealistic or educational motives has been lost. This is chiefly due to the large and increasing demands of drug developers preparing applications for regulatory authorities.
- Studies for this purpose (chiefly **pharmacokinetics**) are ordinarily tedious and prolonged and it is now usual to pay healthy volunteers.
- Payments should be enough to enable recruitment, but not so much as to induce subjects to volunteer against their better judgement or more frequently than is advisable for their own good. Payment should be for time and inconvenience, not for risk-taking. Student grants/costs and the national average wage may be taken as reference points for amount.
- Research **ethics committees** should review all payments of *any* kind, including gifts or travel.
- The view has been advanced that volunteering for research studies is a job like any other and rewards should be left to market forces. If people wish to make an occupation of such work, it is their own business and nobody else's. At present this is a minority view.
- Payments may be made to *patients* who undertake extra activities or clinic attendances which are therapeutically unnecessary on the same basis as those to healthy subjects.
- Payment to *investigators* and to *departments* (money, gifts, travel, etc.) have ethical implications and should also be subject to ethical review. "When it comes to the margin between what is acceptable and what is unacceptable, judgement may sometimes be difficult: a useful criterion of acceptability may be, 'Would you be willing to have these arrangements generally known?'" (*Royal College of Physicians of London*: this whole entry is based upon reports of the College).
- In *nonclinical (basic) research* also, employing institutions should know of any payments to investigators made by outside bodies.

PC
- *Pharmaceutical Codex* (previously *British PC*).

P2C2E
- Process too complicated to explain (*S Rushdie*).

PCP
- Pentachlorophenol, and also, by informal convention, phencyclidine.

PCR
- **Polymerase chain reaction.**

PDE
- Phosphodiesterase.   See **phosphodiesterase inhibitors**

PDGF
- Platelet-derived growth factor; one of the **cytokines**.

peer review or refereeing   (L. *par*, equal; *re-ferre*, to carry back)
- The practice of assessing scientific research proposals for support, and reports for publication, by putting them before suitably qualified individual referees or panels. Investigators' reputations are considerably enhanced if their work is published in major journals that are known routinely to use stringent peer review. Unfortunately, some referees have been suspected of holding up projects, of blocking innovatory as well as poor quality research, and even of stealing the ideas of investigators they deem to be professional rivals. There is increasing demand that peer review no longer be anonymous (as it usually still is), and that itself be subject to peer review and scientific evaluation.
- A peer-reviewed journal is one that has submitted most of its published articles for review by experts who are not part of the editorial staff (**International Committee of Medical Journal Editors**).
- Correspondence columns provide valuable *post hoc* peer review, (but many journals do not provide for correspondence). Prudent literature-searchers always check subsequent issues of the journal. But plainly it is not practicable for letters that may appear following publication of an article to be peer-reviewed, and the difficulty is overcome by allowing authors an opportunity to respond to major criticism. Critics should declare any interest.
                    See **impact factor (of a journal), interest (conflict of), Ingelfinger rule**

pegylation   (From **acronym** PEG for polyethylene glycol)
- The **half-life** of recombinant proteins can be increased by chemical modification techniques. One such technique is conjugation with polyethylene glycol (PEG). This technique has been successfully applied to, for example, recombinant (r) human (h) megakaryocyte growth and development factor (rhMGDF).

PEM
- **Prescription event monitoring.**

penetration (rate of)
- The **rate** of penetration (across a membrane) $= P \times S \times (C_1 - C_2)$, where P is permeability, S is surface area and $(C_1 - C_2)$ is the concentration difference (*Rowland & Tozer*, see Acknowledgements).

peptide
- Any substance derived from two or more natural **amino acids** by the combination of the amino group of one with the carboxyl group of the next. Peptides of three or more amino acids are *polypeptides*, e.g. insulin.

percentages   (L. *per centum*, out of every hundred)
- "Rates or proportions should not be given without any information on the total

numbers on which they are based. This is a fundamental rule, although constantly broken. The news media are great offenders in this respect. They will glibly report that influenza deaths, road-traffic accidents, or burglaries have risen fivefold in a week, but not whether the basic figures are 10 and 50 or 100 and 500. It is often stated that it is wrong to calculate a percentage when the number of observations is small, e.g. 50, *but so long as basic numbers are also given* it is difficult to see where the objection lies, and how such a presentation can be misleading – except to those who disregard the basic figures and who, therefore, in all probability will be misled by any presentation" (*A Bradford Hill, A short textbook of medical statistics*, 1977).

See **concentration, law of initial value**

percentile See **centile, decile, quantile**

perfusion (L. *per*, through; *fundere*, to pour)
– To pass a liquid through channels (e.g. vascular) in a tissue.

See **superfusion**

perilaunch (of a medicinal product) (Gr. *peri*, around; Anglo-Norman, *lancher*, to set in motion)
– The period between the issue of a marketing authorization (licence) for a drug and the act of marketing (launch).

perinatal pharmacology (Gr. *peri*, around; L. *nasci*, be born; G. *periodos*, circuit)
– For general clinical purposes, the period spanning a few days before and after birth. There is no agreed precise definition. Plainly this is a period of particular hazard for many reasons and presents special problems with regard to drug therapy for mother and child. Because the period is so important, official perinatal mortality figures are collected and for these there has to be a precise definition, i.e. from 28 weeks' pregnancy to 1 week postnatal.

permeability (of a membrane) (L. *per*, through; *meare*, to pass, go)
– Permeability (by passive **diffusion**) is the ease with which a drug can pass across a membrane. It is influenced by solubility (in lipid or water), molecular weight and membrane thickness.

See **lipid solubility, proportionality constant**

perturbation (L. *per*, through; *turbare*, to disturb)
– Disturbance of the normal function of a process.

pessary (Gr. *pessos*, plug)
– A solid formulation specially designed for insertion into an anatomic passage, particularly in the vagina. See **suppository**

PET
– Positron emission tomography.
– PET is an imaging technique which depends upon the detection of the two

photons of equal energy released simultaneously at 180° to one another in the process of mutual destruction which occurs when a positron emitted from certain isotopes meets an electron. Positron-emitting isotopes include ^{15}O, ^{18}F and ^{11}C. These isotopes can be incorporated into tracer molecules which are used in one of two main ways in imaging studies:

- Local blood flow can be constantly monitored with [^{15}O]-labelled water or [^{13}N]-labelled ammonia. Increased localised cellular activity (e.g., increased neuronal activity in the brain) results in increased blood flow and an increase in the PET signal in that region. Similarly, local cellular metabolism can be monitored with [^{15}F]-labelled deoxyglucose.
- Selective **ligands** labelled with positron-emitting isotopes can be used to visualise and estimate **receptor** occupancy in the brain (or other organs) of conscious subjects. The technique involves a two-stage process. In the first stage, the individual is injected with a known amount of a labelled standard ligand and the radioactivity is mapped. On a subsequent occasion, the subject is given a dose of the drug to be investigated, followed by the same dose of the labelled ligand. Reduction in the radioactive signal in a given location indicates that the receptors in that region are occupied by the test drug. Sophisticated procedures for calculating the level of receptor occupancy have been developed.
- PET imaging is invasive (in that it involves the injection of radioactively-labelled substance), has relatively low resolution (approximately 1 cm^3), and requires a sophisticated detection system, ready access to a cyclotron (positron-emitting isotopes have very short **half-lives**) and an organic chemistry laboratory to synthesise the labelled chemicals rapidly and to a high level of purity.

pH
- Negative logarithm to the base 10 of the molar hydrogen ion concentration. It is a measure of acidity (low pH, 1–7), and of alkalinity (high pH, 7–14): neutral = pH 7.0.　　　　　See **mole/molar/molal, pH partition hypothesis**

phaeochromocytoma　　　　　(Gr. *phaios*, dusky; *chroma*, colour; *kutos*, vessel, cell; *oma*, tumour)
- A tumour of the adrenal medulla having particular interest to pharmacologists because it secretes **adrenaline** and noradrenaline. It may be benign or malignant, single or multiple, and may appear in other chromaffin tissue sites. It characteristically causes paroxysmal arterial hypertension.

phagocytosis　　　　　(Gr. *phagein*, to eat; *kutos*, vessel, cell)
See **endocytosis**

pharma, pharmaco　　　　　(Gr. *pharmakon;* drug)
- A widely used prefix to indicate that the second part of the word relates to drugs: examples follow in the entries below.

pharmaceutical equivalence　　　　　(Gr. *pharmakeia*, making of drugs; L. *aequus*, equal; *valere*, to be strong)
- Products are pharmaceutical equivalents if they contain the same amount of

the same active substance(s) in the same dosage form that meet the same or comparable standards and are intended to be administered by the same route. Pharmaceutical equivalence does not necessarily imply **bioequivalence** as differences in the **excipients** and/or the manufacturing process can lead to differences in product performance (in **disintegration/dissolution** rate and/or **bioavailability**) **(WHO)**.

pharmaceutical product   (Gr. *pharmakeia*, making of drugs,
                                                                pro, forwards; *ducere*, to lead)
– Synonymous with dosage form.   See **formulation**

pharmaceutics   See **biopharmaceutics**

pharmacoanthropology   (Gr. *pharmakon*, drug; *anthropos*, human being;
                                                                          logy, study)
– The study of differences in **pharmacodynamics** and **pharmacokinetics** between genetically different populations.   See **ethnopharmacology**

pharmacodynamics   (Gr. *pharmakon*, drug; *dunamikos*, force)
– A term used for the biological effects, including mechanisms, of a drug, as opposed to its absorption, distribution and fate (**pharmacokinetics**).
– The study of the relationship(s) between dose of drug, time (from administration of drug) and response.   See **pharmacology**

pharmacoeconomics   See **economics**

pharmacoepidemiology   (Gr. *pharmakon*, drug; *epi*, around, following;
                                                                demos, the people)
– The study of the use and effects of drugs in large numbers of people.
– Epidemiology is the study of disease and its distribution in defined populations. It is concerned with both identifying individuals who have a disease, including drug-induced disease, and with enumerating those who do not. It allows the measurement of rates of occurrence and the characteristics of susceptible subjects. Epidemiological techniques involve the observation of subjects who are taking drugs in the ordinary way of medical care (and **controls**). They include **prescription event monitoring**, **case-control studies** and patient **record linkage** by computer.

pharmacogenetic polymorphism   (Gr. *pharmakon*, drug; *gignesthai*,
                                                to be born; *polus*, many; *morphe*, form)
– The existence in a population of two or more **alleles** (at the same locus), resulting in more than one **phenotype** with respect to the effect of a drug. *Pharmacogenetic polymorphism* usually takes the form of different drug metabolizing capacities, i.e. genetic differences in a single enzyme. Drug metabolic processes that display genetic polymorphism include the acetylation of drugs such as isoniazid, the aromatic hydroxylation of drugs such as dextromethorphan, and the hydrolysis of suxamethonium.

pharmacogenetics   (Gr. *pharmakon*, drug; *gignesthai*, to be born)
- Pharmacological responses and their modification by hereditary influences, including race.   See **idiosyncrasy**

pharmacogenomics
- The practice of designing drugs according to individual **genotypes** to enhance safety and/or **efficacy**; a form of drug **targeting**.

pharmacognosy   (Gr. *pharmakon*, drug; *gnosis*, knowledge)
- A term coined by Seydler (1815) to mean 'the knowledge of drugs'. This science is now subsumed in **pharmacology**.
- "A division of pharmacology which treats of simples or unprepared medicines" (1842).
- Study of the botanical, or other, sources and characteristics of crude drugs (this is the term's principal use).
- More recently the term **phytopharmacy** has been offered as preferable.

pharmacokinetic parameters: primary and secondary
- *Primary* pharmacokinetic parameters are dependent on physiological **variables**, including: absorption **rate constant**, hepatic **clearance**, renal clearance and **volume of distribution**.
- *Secondary* pharmacokinetic parameters are dependent on primary parameters, including: **half-life**, elimination rate constant, fraction excreted unchanged, **area under the curve**, steady state concentration, average plateau concentration (*after Rowland & Tozer*, see Acknowledgements).
- Most of the **parameters** listed here have individual entries in this book.

pharmacokinetics   (Gr. *pharmakon*, drug; *kinein*, to move)
- The **absorption, distribution, metabolism** and **elimination** of drugs and metabolites, including the variation with time of drug concentrations in tissues.
- *Pharmacokinetics* may be divided into:
    - *Macrokinetics* (Gr. *makros*, large): major factors that affect the total amount of drug in the body, e.g. hepatic metabolism, renal elimination.
    - *Microkinetics* (Gr. *mikros*, small): lesser factors that can influence responses and duration of action, e.g. diffusion across membranes, receptor binding.
- When writing of the kinetics of, e.g. propranolol, it is not (as at first sight it seems) a **tautology** to write 'the *pharmaco*kinetics of propranolol' because pharmacokinetics is concerned with metabolism and disposition in the body and not only with the kinetics of chemical reactions that might take place *in vitro*.
- *Population pharmacokinetics* is the use of data obtained from patients under treatment with a drug, using the (often sparse) data obtained in **therapeutic trials** or in **therapeutic drug monitoring** of routine therapy, as opposed to specially designed detailed study in limited numbers of subjects.
- Some symbols and abbreviations used in pharmacokinetics:

A	amount
A_{ss}	amount of drug in the body at steady state
AUC	area under the plasma concentration–time curve between zero time and infinity
C	concentration (amount/volume)
C_{max}	maximum concentration attained after a single dose
C_{ss}	concentration at a steady state
CL	clearance (volume/time)
D	dose, amount
F	total availability
k	first-order rate constant
K_m	Michaelis–Menten constant (amount/volume)
k_0	zero-order rate constant
k_p	equilibrium distribution ratio of a substance between tissue and blood, or partition coefficient
Q_H	hepatic blood flow
Q_R	renal blood flow
R	rate (amount/time)
t	time
t_{max}	time from administration of a dose (or start of a constant infusion) to when the concentration (in blood) reaches its peak
$t_{1/2}$	half-time (life)
$t_{1/2,z}$	half-life of the terminal exponential phase
V	volume of distribution
V_{max}	maximum rate of metabolism (enzyme).

(For more, see *M Rowland, G Tucker* Symbols in pharmacokinetics; *British Journal of Clinical Pharmacology* 1982;14:7–13.)   See **compartment**

pharmacology   (Gr. *pharmakon*, drug; *logy*, discourse, study)
- The study of drugs – what they are, how they work and what they do.
- The study of the manner in which the function of living tissues and organisms is modified by chemical substances.
- The study of the effect of chemical agents on living processes.
- The use of drugs to characterize biological systems and how to discover new drugs [medicines] using biologic systems (*TP Kenakin*).
- *Chronic pharmacology.* The consequences of prolonged drug administration as opposed to the effects of single or a few repeated doses (acute pharmacology).
- Pharmacology is commonly subdivided into **pharmacodynamics** (the biological effects of drugs) and **pharmacokinetics** (absorption, distribution, metabolism and elimination), also expressed as, respectively, *the effect of drugs on the body* and *the effect of the body on drugs.* It is also, for convenience, divided into *basic* and **clinical pharmacology**.
- "I believe that pharmacologists should be defined, like any other specialists, in terms of their primary interest and aims. Here is my credo. A pharmacologist starts with the phenomena of drug actions, as seen in physiological sys-

tems, and seeks to establish order, pattern and sequence among them. The ultimate aim is to determine the rules by which physiological 'information' can be coded into molecules so that, in the long term, the pharmacologists will be able to predict desirable as well as toxic consequences" (*JW Black*, Nobel Laureate 1988, writing in 1996).

– The purpose of, and the justification for, the practice of pharmacology (defined as the study of the effect of chemicals on living organisms, tissues or processes) is the hope of eventual benefit, of whatsoever sort, to humankind and to such other species as humankind chooses. The benefits may be direct (as in medicinal therapeutics) or indirect (as with pesticides). This applies whether or not individual scientists are consciously motivated by pure curiosity and/or by potential utility.
By its nature pharmacology raises inescapable ethical issues regarding respect for life (whether in isolated tissues or whole organisms) that are of concern to pharmacologists and also to society which, one way or another, pays for pharmacology. (The outcome of an informal survey conducted by *DR Laurence* published in *Trends in Pharmacological Sciences* 1997;18:153).

pharmacon　　　　　　　　　　　　　(Gr. *pharmakon*, active principle, drug)
– A substance having biological activity, whether healing or noxious; a term chiefly used in mainland Europe. The ancient Greeks used *pharmakeus* to mean both apothecary and poisoner.

pharmacophore　　　　　　　　　　(Gr. *pharmakon*, drug; *phoros*, a carrier)
– The specific part of a molecule that is responsible for the molecule's biological activity.

pharmacopoeia　　　　　　　　　　　(Gr. *pharmakon*, drug; *poiein*, to make)
– A book (especially one officially published) containing lists of drugs with standards of manufacture, purity, assay, etc., and directions for use.

pharmacovigilance　　　　　　(Gr. *pharmakon*, drug; L. *vigilare*, to keep awake)
– The process of identifying and responding to drug safety issues.
– Pharmacovigilance may be *passive* (the collection of spontaneous reports) or *active* (structured), where patients or prescribers are recruited and surveyed.
　　　　　　　　See **post-marketing surveillance, prescription event monitoring**

pharmacy/-ist　　　　　　　　　　　　(Gr. *pharmakeia*, making of drugs)
– Traditionally, the preparation (formulation) and supply of medicines/the one who undertakes this. Increasingly, pharmacists are undertaking activities in wider areas of drug use, patient information, etc.
– The place where community pharmacists practise; a dispensary.

pharmacy-only medicine　　(Gr. *pharmakeia*, making of drugs; L. *medere*, to heal)
– A medicine that may be sold directly to the public (without a prescription) but only from a pharmacy and under the supervision of a pharmacist.
　　　　　　　　　　　　　　　　　　See **supply of medicines**

pharmafood   See **nutraceutical**

pharming   (slang, from *farming*)
- The process of producing cheaply human protein/enzyme medicines from genetically engineered animals, e.g. goats, sheep.

See **transgenic animal bioreactors**

phases of clinical studies of new drugs
- These phases are divisions of convenience in what is a continuous extending process (which may be abridged where appropriate):
  - *Phase I – Clinical pharmacology (20–50 subjects):*
    - Healthy **volunteers** or patients, according to class of drug and its predicted safety.
    - **Pharmacokinetics** (absorption, distribution, metabolism, elimination).
    - **Pharmacodynamics** where practicable; acceptability; safety; efficacy.
  - *Phase II – Clinical investigation (50–300 subjects) (therapeutic exploration):*
    - Patients.
    - Pharmacokinetics; pharmacodynamics, dose-ranging in expanding, carefully controlled studies of efficacy and safety.
  - *Phase III – Formal therapeutic trials (randomized controlled trials; 250–1000+ subjects) (therapeutic confirmation):*
    - Efficacy on a substantial scale; safety; comparison with other drugs; studies are often multilocation.
  - *Phase IV – Post-marketing/licensing studies (2000–10 000+ subjects) (therapeutic use).*
    - *Surveillance* for safety and efficacy; and further *formal* **therapeutic trials**, including comparisons with other drugs. Post-marketing surveillance studies are sometimes designated *Phase V*.

See **post-marketing/licensing surveillance, therapeutic trial, women as subjects in early tests of new drugs**

phases of drug metabolism
- *Phase I reactions*: reactions in which a polar group (e.g. -OH, -COOH, -SH, -NH$_2$) is created or is introduced into a molecule by oxidation, reduction or hydrolysis. Oxidation is the commonest, and is generally accomplished by nonspecific enzymes (**cytochrome P450** isoenzymes) in the smooth endoplasmic reticulum of hepatic cells. The products of phase I reactions often retain a high degree of biological activity. Some drugs may be rendered sufficiently **polar** by phase I reactions to undergo elimination in the urine without further metabolism.
- *Phase II reactions*: or conjugation reactions, are those in which a drug already carrying a reactive group, or a metabolite from a phase I reaction, combines with an endogenous substrate (e.g. glucuronic acid, sulphate or glutathione). Phase II reactions almost invariably result in inactive products, which are highly polar and are readily excreted in the urine or in the bile.

See **lethal synthesis, prodrug**

phenazone   See **drugs as tools** (*Antipyrine*)

phenomenology   (Gr. *phainomenon*, appear; *logy*, discourse, study)
- That phase of science in which events and results are collected and studied – it usually occurs before theories and hypotheses are erected, and is an essential precursor of the numerate phase of scientific development.
- That branch of science concerned with **phenomenon**, rather with that of being (ontology/**ontogenesis**).

phenomenon (plural **phenomena**)   (Gr. *phainomenon*, appear)
- A thing that is perceived or observed.
- A highly exceptional fact or event.

phenotype   (Gr. *phainein*, seen, to appear; *tupos*, image, figure)
- The characteristics seen as a result of **expression** of the **genotype**.

PHI/PHM
- Peptide histidine isoleucine (mouse) and peptide histidine methionine (human). Vasoactive polypeptides with high **homology** with **VIP** and coded for by the same **gene**.

-philic   (Gr. *philos*, loving)
- Suffix meaning to have a preference for, e.g. **lipophilic**.

PHM   See **PHI/PHM**

-phobic   (Gr. *phobos*, fearing)
- Suffix meaning incompatible, to avoid, hate or fear, e.g. **hydrophobic**.

phocomelia   (Gr. *phoke*, a seal; *melos*, extremity)
- The characteristic effect of **thalidomide** taken in early pregnancy. The limbs fail to develop so that the hands or feet are attached close to the trunk, to that extent resembling the anatomy of the seal.

phorbol esters   See **drugs as tools**

phosphodiesterase inhibitors
- Drugs inhibiting phosphodiesterase, e.g. milrinone and the methylxanthines, have a range of effects on the heart, bronchi and nervous system, e.g. **caffeine**.   See **xanthines and methylxanthines**

photodynamic therapy   (Gr. *phos*, light; *dunamis,* power)
                                            See **photosensitivity**

photosensitivity   (Gr. *phos*, *phot-*, light; L. *sentire*, to feel)
- There are two forms of photosensitivity in which drugs are concerned:
  - *Phototoxicity*, in which skin burn occurs due to the presence of a substance that lowers the threshold to ultraviolet light (UVL);

- *Photoallergy*, in which a severe dermal reaction occurs with a small dose of UVL. In drug-induced cases a photochemical reaction occurs in which the drug combines with a tissue protein to form an **antigen**.
- *Photodynamic therapy* utilizes phototoxicity. It involves administering a photo-sensitizer and then activating it with, for example, UVL or laser. Used in the treatment of psoriasis and cancer, for example.

pH partition hypothesis   (L. *partire*, to divide; Gr. *hupothesis*, foundation)
- The rate of passage of a weakly basic or acidic drug through a membrane is dependent on the **pH** of the environment and the **dissociation equilibrium constant** (for ionization) of the drug (the pH at which half the molecules will be dissociated – into **anions** and **cations** – and half undissociated).
                    See **Henderson–Hasselbalch equation, ion trapping, lipid solubility, lipophilic, pK$_a$**

PhRMA
- Pharmaceutical Research and Manufacturers of America.

phylogenesis   (Gr. *phylos*, race, tribe; *genesis*, birth)
- Evolution of animal or plant species.   See **ontogenesis**

physiological antagonism   See **antagonism**

physiologically functional food   See **nutraceutical**

phytomedicines   (Gr. *phyton*, plant)
                    See **herbal medicines**

phytopharmacy/pharmacology (Gr. *phyton*, plant; *pharmakeia*, making of drugs)
- A term proposed to cover all aspects of the reciprocal relationships between plants and drugs, both plant-derived substances acting as drugs and drugs acting on plants.   See **pharmacognosy**

piggy-backing (slang regulatory term)
- An application for a product/marketing licence cross-referring to and relying on an existing licence as a basis to allow the applicant company to market the same product. The term is a corruption of *pick-a-back* where one object (or person) is carried on the back of a larger person.

PIL
- Patient (or product) information leaflet.

pill   (L. *pilula*, a little ball)
- A spherical or ovoid, solid, oral dose-form in which the active ingredients are evenly distributed throughout the vehicle. Normal diameter 3–8 mm. Super-seded by **tablets**. Also used in popular speech for any solid **formulation**.
- *'The Pill'* is universal (slang) as a synonym for oral contraceptive tablets.

pilot (clinical) trial   (Gr. *pedotes*, steersman, Old Fr. *trier*, to sort)
- A small study (generally) conducted to generate information that will assist the design and logistics of a definitive, formal, **pivotal clinical trial**, for the latter are very expensive investments (professional time, money etc.)

ping-pong bi-bi reaction
- A reaction in which an enzyme catalyses two reactions, separately or together. Each reaction separately is reversible, but where they occur together the outcome is irreversible. *Pratt & Taylor* (*Principles of drug action*, 1990) give as an example the enzyme *N*-acetyltransferase in relation to acetylcoenzyme A and to sulphanilamide. The study of such reactions is of medical interest in relation to the genetically determined slow and fast acetylation of drugs such as isoniazid and hydralazine.

pinocytosis   (Gr. *pineo*, to drink; *kutos*, hollow, vessel, and so *cyto*, cell; *osis*, condition)
See **endocytosis**

pivotal clinical trial   (*pivot*, etymology uncertain)
- A pivot is a centre on which something turns, and so the word is applied to a clinical trial that is of such high quality that decision-taking (clinical, regulatory) can 'turn' (rely) on it. A drug developer who achieves such a study of a product is a happy drug developer.   See **clinical trial, therapeutic trial**

pK_a
- The negative logarithm to the base 10 of the acid **dissociation equilibrium constant** (for ionisation). It is a measure of inherent acidity or alkalinity of the molecule: it is the pH at which the compound is 50 per cent ionized and 50 per cent unionized.
- Confusingly, various mathematical symbols are used to represent the (pharmacological) dissociation equilibrium constant of an **agonist**, for a **receptor**, including K_A, K_a, K_D and K_d – K_A is now preferred. Expressed in exponent form (i.e. as the negative $\log_{10}$), these become pK_A, pK_a, pK_D and pK_d. More confusingly, the *association* equilibrium constant (**affinity constant** – reciprocal of dissociation constant) of a drug for a receptor is also sometimes referred to K_A or K_a, and the corresponding exponent forms are thus pK_A or pK_a.

PL
- **Product licence** (regulatory term).

placebo   (L. *placere*, to please; *placebo*, I will please)
- Any component of *therapy* that is without specific (biological) activity for the condition being treated.
- A medicine given to benefit or please a patient not by any **pharmacodynamic** actions, but by psychological means. A placebo may be biologically inert (e.g. lactose) or may contain active substances (e.g. bitters, minerals, vitamins). All treatments, not only drugs, carry placebo effects. Placebos may cause adverse effects.

- As a **control** in the *scientific evaluation* of drugs (the term **dummy** is more appropriate). The chief functions are:
  - To distinguish pharmacodynamic effects from the psychological effects of the act of medication;
  - To distinguish drug effects from fluctuations of disease that occur with time;
  - To avoid false negative conclusions (e.g. if a comparison of two analgesics shows no difference, it may be that the technique used is incapable of distinguishing between active and inactive agents).
- Strictly, it is incorrect to use the term placebo for a **dummy** substance administered to an animal.

placebo-reactor/responder   (L. *placere*, to please; *re*, against; *agere*, to act, to do)
- A person who reports changes of physical or mental state after taking a pharmacologically inert substance. A person who reports adverse events is a *negative* placebo reactor, and if given with intent, the agent is a *nocebo* (L. I shall injure). Placebo response is not necessarily permanent. People may respond at different times, depending on circumstances. Prolonged use of an inert remedy alone leads to loss of effect or *placebo sag.*

placebo run-in
- The practice, in randomized controlled **therapeutic trials** in chronic diseases, of giving *all* potential entrants an initial period on **placebo** *before* random allocation to the protocol treatments (which may include placebo). The intention is to screen out non-compliers and placebo-responders and/or to obtain a baseline state. The procedure raises significant scientific and ethical issues.

plagiarism   (L. *plagiarus*, plunderer)
- The act of taking for one's own the thoughts, writings or inventions of another without permission or acknowledgement; sadly, an increasing form of fraud in science.
- "Plagiarism is the most serious of the known crimes against scholarship" (*Nature* 1992).
- Attempts are being made to identify plagiarism by computer scanning of word use in published texts.
- "To copy from one source is plagiarism, to copy from several is research" (*Anon*).   See **intellectual property, research misconduct**

plantibody   (Blend word of plant and antibody)
- Human **antibody** produced by transgenic plants (e.g. maize, soya bean, tobacco) that have been created by transplanting a human gene (and programmed with additional DNA that increases production of the foreign protein). Such plants may produce sufficient antibody for use in targeting drugs for therapeutic purposes, e.g. cancer.   See **targeting of drugs**

plasma concentration (drug) (interpretation of)   (Gr. *plassein*, moulded or formed)
- The clinical significance of a measurement requires consideration of a range

of information, including: history of drug administration (dose, formulation, route, times, compliance); time of sampling (relative to dose); previous plasma concentration (if known); clinical status of the patient (weight, gender, age, disease, etc.); renal and hepatic function; plasma protein binding; other drug therapy; active metabolites; assay method (after *Rowland & Tozer*, see Acknowledgements).

plasma concentration of drugs as a guide to therapy

- If the measurement is made occasionally, as is likely, then the timing of the sample in relation to administration is plainly important. Ideally the patient should have reached steady state, and a decision must be made whether 'peak' or 'trough' concentrations, or both (e.g. for an antibiotic with a short $t_{1/2}$), are required, taking the blood 1 or 2 hours after an oral dose for peak, and immediately before a dose for trough. In any case, the timing of the sample should be known if interpretation is not to be misleading.

See **half-life, therapeutic drug monitoring**

plasmid   (Gr. *plassein*, something moulded or formed)

- An independently replicating, ring-shaped DNA molecule separate from the bacterial chromosome and often transferable between bacteria. Genes mediating resistance to antibiotics are commonly carried on plasmids. This mechanism of spread of resistance may occur between (resistant) bacterial flora in food animals (given antibiotics on an enormous scale to promote growth as well as to treat and to prevent disease) and human bacterial flora.

plateau principle   (Gr. *platus*, flat; L. *principium*, beginning, basic tenet)

- With a constant rate of input of drug, a plasma plateau concentration is eventually reached, provided that the elimination of the drug follows **first-order kinetics**. The *principle* is that if the rate of input is increased or decreased, the half-time for the establishment of the new **steady state** plasma concentration is equal to the (elimination) **half-life** of the drug (i.e., one elimination half-life after the change in dosage, the plasma concentration will be half way to the new steady state concentration). The time course of such a shift is determined solely by the first-order **rate constant** of the output process (k_{out}). In practice, when a drug is given at a constant rate (continuous or intermittent) the *time to reach steady state* depends only on the $t_{1/2}$ and, for all practical purposes, it takes $5 \times t_{1/2}$ to reach the new steady state (i.e. for the plasma concentration to reach a plateau).

play-the-winner allocation (in clinical trials)   (Middle Dutch *pleien*, to dance; Old Eng. *winn*, strife, conflict; L. *designare*, to mark out)

- A type of **clinical trial** design in which the next patient is assigned the same treatment if this was successful in the previous patient, or is given the other treatment if it was unsuccessful in the previous patient.

See **adaptive allocation design, random**

pleiotropic response   (Gr. *pleion*, more; *tropos*, turning)

- A response to a drug that occurs by more than one mechanism.

plot (Old Eng., piece of land)
– To locate and mark a point, or points, on a **graph** by means of coordinates (horizontal/abscissa; vertical/ordinate).

PMS
– **Post-marketing surveillance.**

point/interval estimates See **estimate**

poison (L. *potio*, a drink)
– That which destroys or injures life by a small quantity and by means not obvious to the senses (*S Johnson*, 1755).
– A poison is a substance, the main, sole or most notable action of which is its harmful effect on man, animals or other specific living systems, e.g. a mitochondrial poison, a fish poison.
– A substance may cease to be regarded as a poison when a use is found for it. For example, curare – 'a South American arrow poison' – becomes a 'muscle relaxant' in anaesthesia.
– Traditionally **toxicology** is the study of poisons, their effects, dosage and, more recently, their mechanism of action. But modern toxicologists have also had to concern themselves with wider issues.
– "All things are poisonous and there is nothing that is harmless, the dose alone decides that something is no poison" (*Paracelsus*, 1493–1541, physician, Switzerland: *Alle Dinge sind Gift und nichts ist ohne Gift, allein die Dosis machts, dass ein Ding kein Gift sei*); arguably the most important statement ever made about drugs as medicines.

Poisson distribution
– The occurrence of a purely random distribution in a continuum of space or time, e.g. the number of cells visible per square of haemocytometer, or quanta of acetylcholine released at a nerve ending. The Poisson distribution is used as a criterion of the randomness of events of this sort (*SD Poisson*, 1781–1840, mathematician, France). See **random**

polar/nonpolar (L. *polus*, end of an axis, from Gr. *polos*, axis, pivot)
– A molecule that possesses two oppositely charged and spatially separated regions (dipole) in its structure is said to be *polar* (e.g. ethanol, CH_3CH_2OH); polar molecules are water soluble. A molecule in which the charge is distributed evenly is said to be *nonpolar* (e.g. carbon tetrachloride, CCl_4). Cell membranes are largely composed of nonpolar lipids. Nonpolar molecules are **lipid soluble** and so diffuse across cell membranes more readily than those that are polar and less lipid soluble. Water and alcohol mix so readily because they are both polar (fortunately for the drinker, ethanol has a molecule so small that it can cross membranes rapidly through water-filled pores). In general, drug-metabolizing enzymes convert nonpolar (lipid soluble) molecules to the readily excreted polar (water soluble) molecules.
See **chromatography, hydrophilic/-phobic, lipophilic/-phobic**

polarization   See **depolarization**

policies   (L. *politia*, administration)
- A plan of action pursued by an individual or an organization, e.g. government regulation of drug introduction, use or manufacture. In these areas, government may be regarded as a machine for devising and implementing policies for the benefit of society. "The implementation of every policy needs to be tested: and this is done not by looking for evidence that one's efforts are having the desired effects but by looking for evidence that they are not" (*B Magee*, in *Popper*, London, Fontana, 1982), e.g. whether regulation fails to prevent unacceptably hazardous drugs from being introduced and whether it stops the introduction of useful drugs (this latter is particularly hard to detect).
                                  See **bureaucracy, drug lag, government**

polymerase chain reaction (PCR)
- A technique for amplifying the DNA present in a sample. In an appropriate mixture the enzyme DNA polymerase produces copies of any strands of DNA added. In this way the amount of DNA present can be enormously increased (amplified) and the resulting molecules can be compared with known DNA sequences. The technique can also be used to amplify RNA. The DNA/RNA added is the 'template'; 'primers' to the sequences of interest are used in the reaction mixture. The polymerase chain reaction is the basis for genetic 'fingerprinting', used, for example, in forensic science to establish the origin of blood, semen, etc. It can also enable more rapid identification of microorganisms than can culturing. Uses of relevance to pharmacology include the identification of novel **receptor/G-protein/ion channel** nucleic acid sequences.

polymorphism   (Gr. *polus*, many; *morphe*, shape)
- Having many shapes. In biology, polymorphism was used originally with respect to morphology but is now applied to any biological characteristic.
                                  See **pharmacogenetic polymorphism**

polypeptide   See **peptide**

polypharmacy   (Gr. *polus*, many; *pharmakon*, drug)
- Treating a patient with several drugs simultaneously. Although this is often necessary, the term is generally used with a pejorative overtone, implying the uncritical use of an excessive number of drugs.

PoM or POM
- **Prescription-only medicine**   See **supply of medicines**

pool size   (Old Eng. *pol*, small body of standing water)
- The amount of substance present in the body (or a **compartment**). Used in connection with calculations of **turnover**.

pooled data/analysis   See **meta-analysis**

'pork barrel' research
- Slang term, 1916. Research grants supplied by the USA Federal Treasury to a locality, to the economic benefit of the local citizens and therefore, it is hoped, to the political advantage of the local legislator and to the central government. Such grants are commonly made without independent review and in an exaggerated belief that science and technology are the keys to regional economic development in the short term. Earmarked grants are known as 'pork' (*earmark*, mark on the ear of farm animals as sign of ownership).

posology   (Gr. *posos*, how much; *logy*, study)
- The science of dosage.

post hoc   (L., after this)
See **correlations between variables, data dredging,**
post hoc ergo propter hoc

post hoc ergo propter hoc   (L., after this, therefore on account of this)
- The fallacy of assuming that temporal succession is evidence of causal association.   See **science/scientific method**

post-marketing/licensing surveillance (PMS)   (Fr. *surveiller*, to watch;
L. *vigilare*, to be watchful)
- Any non-promotional measure to confirm the safety of new drugs after they have been licensed for marketing; usually **observational.**
- It is recognized that a drug must be released for general prescribing (licensed, registered, marketed) after it has had detailed study in only hundreds of, or perhaps a few thousand, patients. The assumption that the most dangerous stage of drug development was that passing from animals to man has now been replaced by recognition that risk is greatest when a drug passes from rigorously supervised therapeutic trial to the inevitably less supervised general therapeutic use, at a stage when there may still be much more to discover, especially the rarer effects, and effects in special groups of patients (the old, renal disease, pregnancy, etc.). New techniques are needed to obtain reliable data at this stage. Post-marketing surveillance is known as *phase IV* of new drug development.
- *USA* (**FDA**) *regulation*: Requirement that pharmaceutical companies report to the FDA **adverse events** (AE) of which they are aware for all marketed drugs. If the AE results in death, prolonged hospitalization, or permanent disability, the firm must report the incident within 15 days of their notification of the AE. All other AEs can be reported on an annual basis.
See **phases of clinical studies of new drugs,**
prescription event monitoring

postulate   (L. *postulare*, to demand)
- *Noun*: Something claimed or assumed as a basis for reasoning, discussion or belief.

– *Verb*: To put forward a theory or **hypothesis** for discussion, or to help support an argument.

potency (L. *potentia*, power)
– An expression of the activity of a drug, either in terms of the concentration or amount needed to produce a defined effect, or, less acceptably, with regard to the maximal effect attainable. An imprecise term that should always be further defined (**IUPHAR**, with permission; *Pharmacological Reviews* 1995;47: 255–266).
– The relationship between the amount of a drug and its effect. It is usually measured by assessing the dose or concentration (or more precisely the reciprocal of these) at which a drug causes a given, predefined response (often half the maximal response). Potency is a property of a drug. The equivalent property of the system upon which the drug acts is **sensitivity**.
See **EC_{50}, efficacy, E_{max}, homoeopathy, IC_{50}, potentiation**

potent (L. *potentia*, power)
– A term used to describe a drug that is effective at low dose/concentration, i.e. it has a high **potency**.

potentiation (L. *potentia*, power)
– To increase **potency**, i.e. when one drug, which itself has not the effect under consideration, causes an active drug to produce an effect at a lower than usual dose (or concentration), e.g. monoamine oxidase inhibitor potentiates amphetamine on the cardiovascular system. The maximal possible effect is unchanged. The term is often used indiscriminately to describe an increase in the size of a response to a fixed dose of drug. A better term in this circumstance would be **augmentation**. It is insufficient to claim that a drug has been potentiated if the response to a single dose is increased. Before a phenomenon can be described as potentiation, evidence must be provided of a shift to the left in the concentration–effect curve.
– Potentiation is measured in terms of **concentration ratio** (previously called *dose ratio*).
– The correct way to use the verb 'potentiate' is 'drug *x* potentiates drug *y*' (not 'drug *x* potentiates *the effect of* drug *y*' – the *effects* of a drug cannot be made more potent). See **additive responses, synergism**

povidone
– A mixture of synthetic polymers of vinylpyrrolidone (polyvinylpyrrolidone). Its viscosity can be varied. Versions can be used as blood plasma expanders, as suspending/dispersing agents and for binding and coating tablets. It is used as a carrier for iodine (see **iodophor**).

powder (L. *pulvis*, dust)
– A solid substance in a state of fine division.
– Powders for oral administration are almost obsolete. They are chiefly for topical application. They are graded using sieves of standard mesh, e.g. an *ultra-*

fine powder is one where the maximal diameter of 90 per cent of the particles is not greater than 5 μm and no particles exceed 50 μm diameter.

power in statistics   (L. *posse*, to be able)
- "Formally, the power of a significance test is a measure of how likely that test is to produce a statistically significant result for a population difference of any given magnitude. Practically, it indicates the ability to detect a true difference of clinical importance. The power may be calculated retrospectively to see how much chance a complete study has of detecting (as significant) a clinically relevant difference. More importantly, it may be used prospectively to calculate a suitable sample size" (*DG Altman*).
- The statistical probability of rejecting the null hypothesis when it is false. The probability of having a successful study (**FDA**).
                         See **confidence interval, statistical significance**

power spectrum   (L. *posse*, to be able; *specere*, to look at)
                                                      See **spectral density**

PPI
- **Patient package insert.**

PPRS
- Pharmaceutical price regulation scheme. A 'voluntary' (for the pharmaceutical industry) scheme devised by the government for limiting the profit margin of drugs sold to the UK National Health Service.

practolol   See **oculomucocutaneous syndrome**

pragmatic/-al/-ism/-ist   (Gr. *pragma*, act, from *prattein*, to do)
- A doctrine that evaluates any assertion solely by its practical consequences, i.e. a belief is true if it works.
- Dealing with matters according to their practical significance or immediate importance.

pre- and post-synaptic receptors   (L. *prae*, before; *post*, after;
                                  Gr. *sun*, with, together; *haptein*, to connect;
                                              L. *re*, again, back; *capere*, to take)
- At a nerve ending there are receptors specific for the released neurotransmitter on both the effector cell (postsynaptic) and on the nerve ending itself (presynaptic). The latter **modulate** the further release of transmitter (**feedback** mechanism).   See **autoreceptor, receptor**

precaution (prescribing)   (L. *prae*, before; *cavere*, beware)
                                                       See **contraindication**

precision   (L. *prae*, before; *caedere*, cut)
- The closeness of agreement of a series of measurements.   See **accuracy**

precompetitive research (L. *prae*, before, *co, com/cum, con*, with, together, in common, jointly, equally, reciprocally, mutually; *petere*, seek)
- A term introduced in 1984 in the then European Communities (now **EU**) meaning research that is far enough from the market to allow industrial companies to collaborate without giving away trade secrets and which the EC might therefore support. The term has outlived its usefulness, if indeed it ever had any.

precoupling (L. *prae*, before; *copulare*, to fasten together)
- When a substantial proportion of **receptors** is *precoupled* to the **G-protein** in the absence of agonist, the system is likely to show basal activity – **constitutive activity**. Antagonists that reduce this basal activity are known as **inverse agonists**.

predictive medicine (L. *praedicare*, to proclaim)
- Modern technology increasingly allows the *prediction* of disease in an individual with the accompanying possibility that preventive action may be taken (rather than to wait for the disease to manifest itself).

prescribing (L. *praescribere*, to write previously)
- The act of writing a **prescription**.
- More broadly, the process of choosing and using medicines. Prescribing should be *appropriate*, i.e. based on known therapeutic efficacy, on safety and on convenience relative to other drugs or treatments, etc. Unavoidably, cost can have an influential, and sometimes even an overriding role.
  See **evidence-based medicine, placebo**

prescribing cascade (L. *praescribere*, to write previously; *cadere*, to fall; Ital. *cascata*, a waterfall)
- The sequence when an adverse drug reaction is misinterpreted as a new medical condition for which a drug is prescribed that puts the patient at risk of an additional adverse effect for which another drug may be prescribed, and so on... (*PA Rochon, JH Gurwitz*).

prescription (L. *praescribere*, to write previously)
- A written order for a medicine with detailed instruction of what should be given to whom, how much, how often, by what route, for how long, by whom ordered.
- "Writing prescriptions is easy, understanding people is hard" (*Franz Kafka*, 1883–1924, novelist, Czechoslovakia).
  See **dispensing, indicative prescribing amount**

prescription event monitoring (PEM)
- Prescription event monitoring enables the study of large **cohorts** of patients who are identified by prescriptions written by general practitioners. Linkage is effected between general practice and hospital records, and the Office of

Population Census and Surveys (OPCS) which provides information from death certificates. PEM can be applied prospectively or retrospectively, and can both generate and test **hypotheses**. The initial target is the first 20 000 patients ever to receive a drug after its release for use in general practice (*WH Inman*). PEM is only practicable where prescriptions are easily accessible in a community health service (as they are in the UK, at pricing centres that arrange payment by the National Health Service to the community pharmacist who supplied the medicine).   See **post-marketing surveillance**

prescription-only medicine (PoM)
- Medicine that can be legally obtained only from a pharmacist upon presentation of a valid prescription (from a doctor, dentist or veterinarian).
- Criteria for classifying a medicine as *prescription only* include:
  - That the product is likely to present a risk to health even if used correctly, unless there be some professional supervision.
  - The product is known frequently to be used incorrectly.
  - The product is normally administered parenterally (by injection).

pre-systemic drug elimination
- Occurs when orally administered drugs are metabolized during their passage from the gut lumen to the systemic (general body) circulation (by the intestine and/or the liver).   See **hepatic first-pass metabolism, metabolism of drugs**

prevalence rate   (L. *prae*, before; *valere*, to be strong)
- The number of events, e.g. illnesses, *existing* at any instant or within a specified period (of time) and related to the average number of persons exposed to risk of the event during that period i.e.

$$\frac{number\ of\ persons\ with\ a\ disease}{total\ number\ in\ group/population}$$

- It is *not* the same as **incidence**.   See **cross-sectional study**

prevention of disease
- *Primary prevention*: measures are taken to avoid disease before the subject has experienced it, e.g. myocardial infarction.
- *Secondary prevention*: measures are taken after the subject has experienced a disease, to prevent further episodes, e.g. myocardial infarction.
- *Suppression* can be viewed as a variant of prevention. The causes of disease continue to operate, but clinical manifestations are avoided by a suppressive measure, e.g. malaria, hypertension.

primary agonist   (L. *primus*, first; Gr. *agon*, a struggle)
- Some **agonists** (e.g. glutamate) may only be effective in the presence of another **ligand** (the co-agonist – glycine in the case of glutamate) that binds to a different site on the **receptor** macromolecule. In the example above, glutamate is the *primary agonist* and glycine the *co-agonist* (after **IUPHAR**; *Pharmacological Reviews* 1995;47:255–266).
           See **allosteric interaction**

priming dose   See **dose**

principle   (L. *principium*, beginning, basic tenet)
- Fundamental truth or proposition, on which many others may depend.
- Fundamental assumption forming the basis of a chain of reasoning.
- Fundamental truth as a basis for reasoning.
- A general law or rule as a guide to action.

proadifen   See **drugs as tools**

probability   (L. *probabilis*, that may be proved)
- The condition of being probable, i.e. likely to happen (or to be) but not necessarily.
- The probability of an event is a number between *zero* (implying impossibility)
  and *one* (implying certainty).
- *Conditional probability*: The probability that one thing is true, given that we
  know some other thing to be true (*S Sutherland*).
- For practical purposes, probability can be regarded as *relative frequency*. For
  example, if *r* individuals out of *N* show some attribute, then the probability that
  a single individual, randomly selected from all *N*, will have the attribute is defined as *r/N*.
- "...the laws of probability, so true in general, so fallacious in particular" (*Edward Gibbon*, 1737–1794, historian, England).
     See **knowledge, laws (various)** (*Popper's*), **likelihood, science in phar-
  macology**

probability density (function)   (L. *probabilis*, that may be proved;
                                                        densus, thick)
- An extension of the idea of **probability** that is needed to deal with **continuous variables**, such as body weight. The probability of observing a weight of
  70 kg exactly (i.e. 70 000 g) is obviously infinitesimally small. Therefore we
  define a continuous function (curve), the *probability density function*, such
  that when it is plotted against the value of the variable (e.g. weight) the area
  under the curve between, say, 69 kg and 71 kg represents the probability of
  observing a weight in this range. The ordinates of all *distributions* of continuous variables are *probability density functions*.

probability distribution   (L. *probabilis*, that may be proved;
                                              dis, asunder; *tribuere*, to give)
- A function that gives the **probability** of observing each of the particular values that a **variable** may adopt. The probability (or, in the case of a continuous
  variable, the **probability density**) is plotted against the value of the variable.
  A **frequency distribution**, which is most commonly plotted as a **histogram**,
  describes the number of times (frequency) that a particular value, or range of
  values, of a variable is *observed* (ordinate) for each value of the variable (abscissa). For example, the number of people with weights between 69 and
  71 kg might be plotted as a vertical bar that extends from 69 kg to 71 kg on

the abscissa. The observations may, or may not, be well approximated by one of the following theoretical distributions: **binomial, chi-square, exponential, normal, Poisson.**   See **probability density**

probability scale
- A scale which can be used in graphical representations of normally-distributed data. The scale compensates for the non-linearity of the S-shaped cumulative normal curve by contracting the scale around the **median** and expanding it at low and high cumulative percentages.   See **probit**

probability (p) value
- The p value is the probability that, if two groups are random samples from populations equal in terms of the factor being studied, the group **(mean)** difference will differ by the amount observed or more (regardless of the direction of the difference for a two-sided test) by chance, due to sampling variation (*Gardner & Altman*).
- p is the probability of obtaining a result at least as unlikely as the observed one, if the **null hypothesis** of no effect is true. *The last part of this definition is essential*; to omit it leads to the common error of believing that p is also the probability so that we make the mistake by accepting the significant result as a real finding. This is just not so (*S Gore & D Altman*).
                    See **statistical significance**

probit   (L. *probare*, to prove, test, if not from *probus*, virtuous)
- Contraction of *probability unit*. A **transformation** devised to linearize quantal dose–response curves. The probit of the percentage responding will be linearly related to the dose (or a specified function, e.g. log of it) if the distribution of **individual effective dose** (or specified function of it) has a **normal distribution** in the population.   See **normal equivalent deviate, quantum/quantal**

proconvulsant   (Gr. *pro*, before; *convulsus*, tear up)
- A drug which, although not itself convulsant, lowers the threshold to convulsant stimuli, such as convulsant drugs.

prodrug   (Gr. *pro*, before; Old Fr. *drogue*, unknown origin)
- A biologically *inactive* substance which is metabolized to a biologically *active* substance, e.g. cortisone to hydrocortisone. It is incorrect to describe active substances having active metabolites as prodrugs.   See **lethal synthesis**

product liability (This entry is based on the **EC** Directive on Product Liability and official discussion documents.)
- Liability for injury due to defective products.
- Liability *without fault on the part of the producer* is the sole means of adequately solving the problem, peculiar to our age of increasing technicality, of a fair apportionment of the risks inherent in modern technological production.
- Protection of the consumer requires that all producers involved in the production process should be made liable, in so far as their finished product, component part or any raw material supplied by them was defective.

- The injured person shall be required to prove the damage, the defect and the causal relationship between the defect and the damage.
- A product is defective when it does not provide the safety that a person is entitled to expect, taking all circumstances into account, including:
  - The presentation of the product.
  - The use to which it could reasonably be expected that the product would be put.
  - The time when the product was put into circulation.
- A product shall not be considered defective for the sole reason that a better product is subsequently put into circulation.
- The producer shall not be liable as a result of this Directive if he proves (amongst other things):
  - That the damage is caused by the fault of the injured person;
  - That the state of scientific and technical knowledge at the time when he put the product into circulation was not such as to enable the existence of the defect to be discovered. (This defence is known as the '*development risk defence*' or, colloquially, as the '*state of the art defence*'.) The provision of 'state of the art defence' plainly leaves a substantial gap in protection of the consumer. But manufacturers have argued that it would be wrong in principle, and disastrous in practice, for businesses to be held liable for defects that they could not possibly have foreseen. They believe that the absence of this defence would raise insurance costs and inhibit innovation, especially in high-risk industries. Many useful new products, which might entail a development risk, would not be put on the market, and consumers as well as business would lose out. The UK Government has therefore accepted that this defence should be allowed; but some other countries have not. This discordance is allowed by the EC Directive.
- The above refers to what has curiously been termed (by lawyers) a *design* defect in a drug, i.e. when there is a 'flaw' inherent in the product, affecting all items. A *manufacturing* defect affects individual articles or batches of articles when the act of manufacturing has gone wrong, and in this case drugs are, in law, no different from other products.   See **liability**

product licence
- A licence issued by a regulatory authority, which allows the licence-holder to promote, supply and sell the medicine for clinical indications in accordance with the terms of the licence only.   See **regulation (official) of medicines**

progress
(L. *pro*, forward; *gradi*, to walk)
- Advance or development, especially to a better state, e.g. science progresses (after *Oxford English Dictionary*); e.g. *some* new drugs.
- "Progress is a noxious, culturally embedded, untestable, nonoperational, intractable idea that must be replaced if we wish to understand the patterns of history" (*Stephen Jay Gould*).

prokinetic
(Gr. *pro*, before; *kinesis*, motion)
- Enhancement of movement, contraction or emptying, especially applied to the stomach, e.g. the *gastroprokinetic* drug, metoclopramide.

promiscuous drug   (L. *pro*, before; *miscere*, to mix)
- A description applied to a drug that can interact with several types of **receptor**. If the drug's **potency** is similar at all these receptors, the drug has low **selectivity**: also known as a **'dirty' drug**.
- The term has also been applied to:
  - *Receptors*: receptors that can interact with several types of drug or, more usually, with several types of transducer molecule.
  - *Coupling*: one receptor type can interact with and activate several types of **transducer** molecule, or one type of transducer molecule can interact with several types of receptor. This can be achieved by experimental **overexpression** of receptors in unusual cell types.

                    See **parallel pharmacology, pleiotropic, side-effects**

promiscuous receptors   (L. *pro*, before; *miscere*, to mix)
- Receptors which share **effector couplers**, such as G-proteins.

promoter   (L. *promotum*, forward)
- The region of DNA at which **transcription** of a gene begins. It is the region where RNA polymerase binds to the DNA molecule.

                                                    See **tumour promoter**

promotion of medicines
- 'Promotion refers to all informational and persuasive activities' (**WHO**).

proof/prove   (L. *probare*, to test, demonstrate)
- Evidence that establishes the *truth* or validity of something.
- To establish the *quality* of; to subject to testing.
- Confusion between these two (above) meanings leads to the use of the popular maxim, 'The exception proves the rule', to mean, 'The exception establishes the truth of the rule', which is nonsense, instead of, 'The exception tests the validity of the rule' which is science, i.e. where an observation is incompatible with a rule (**hypothesis**) then the rule (hypothesis) is falsified and requires revision to accommodate the new observation. The alternative meaning sometimes offered, that the phrase demonstrates that there must be a rule, for without a rule there cannot be an exception, is so fatuous as not to deserve comment. *Fowler's Modern English Usage (1968)* stigmatizes the phrase as 'serious nonsense' and as 'constantly introduced into argument, so much more often with obscuring than with illuminating effect.' It is best avoided.
- "The great tragedy of science – the slaying of a beautiful hypothesis by an ugly fact" (*TH Huxley*, 1825–1895, biologist, UK).
- Legal standard of proof:
  - *Civil actions*: the balance of probabilities.
  - *Criminal actions*: beyond reasonable doubt.
- *Scientific standard of proof* is akin to (or surpasses) that of criminal law.

                                                    See **confirmation, true**

proof of concept
- A phrase sometimes used for the establishing in a small scale clinical study (phase II), whether a larger (phase III) study should be mounted.

See **phases of clinical studies of new drugs**

propellants (aerosol) (L. *pro*, forward; *pellere*, to drive; Gr. *aer*, air; *sol*, abbreviation of solution)
- Pressurized aerosol formulations usually employ **hydrofluoroalkanes** which are replacing **chlorofluorocarbons**, as gaseous propellants.

See **inhalation of drugs**

prophylaxis (L. *pro*, before; Gr. *phulaxis*, a guard)
- To prevent or protect from by prior treatment or advice.

See **prevention of disease**

proportion (L. *pro,* before; *portio*, a share)
- A fraction in which the numerator contains a subset of the items/individuals contained in the denominator.

proportional hazard regression model

See **Cox proportional hazards/regression model**

proportionality constant (L. *pro*, for; *portiare*, to share out; *cum*, with; *stare*, to stand)
- When two **variables** are related so that a graph of one plotted against the other results in a straight line with a positive slope, the two variables are said to be *directly proportional*. The slope of the line is the *proportionality constant*. For example, the rate at which a drug diffuses across a membrane is directly proportional to the concentration gradient across the membrane:

$$v = P_k(C_{out} - C_{in})$$

where v is the rate of diffusion, C_{out} and C_{in} are the concentrations of the drug outside and inside the cell respectively, and the proportionality constant, P_k, is the **permeability** *constant*.
- When the slope of the line is negative, the two variables are said to be *inversely proportional* (i.e. when one increases, the other decreases).

proposition 65 (California, USA) (L. *pro-positio*, a setting forth)
- Proposition 65 of the Safe Drinking Water and Toxic Enforcement Act (1986) requires that medicines containing, for example, preservatives will expose a person to no more than 1/1000th of an amount shown to have no adverse developmental effect in animal testing. "For the pharmaceutical industry there are sobering implications in having to modify nationally distributed drugs to satisfy any state's regulatory requirements" (*S A Furey* 1993). Although well-intentioned, such legislation needs to be national, or better, international, if the goal of *affordable* medicines is to be attained. See **Delaney clause**

proprietary name/product (L. *proprius*, one's own)
- A trade name given to a medicine by a pharmaceutical company; proprietary

names are always spelled with a leading capital letter, e.g. Inderal (propranolol). The proprietary name is the property of that company alone. Consequently, a medicine will have one approved or generic name but may have several proprietary names, one for each manufacturer.
- Any ready-prepared **medicinal product** placed on the market under a special name and in a special pack **(EU).** See **names of drugs**

prospective study (L. *pro*, before; *specere*, to look)
- Looking towards the future.
- A scientific study in which there is no knowledge of the outcome for any of the subjects at the time of entry into the study; a **cohort study.**
- A follow-up study. See **case-control study, random, control, retrospective study, therapeutic trial**

prostaglandins (prostanoids) (So named as they were initially believed to derive from the prostate gland)
- Twenty-carbon fatty acids (**eicosanoids**) formed in tissues from phospholipids via **arachidonic acid** in response to a wide variety of stimuli/injury, i.e. they are not found preformed, as are most **autacoids** or local hormones. They occur in virtually all tissues of the body and have a major role in, for example, inflammation. The biological community is so accustomed to the name that it does not feel uncomfortable about its obvious origin when speaking of, for example, the brain.

prosthetic group (Gr. *prosthesis*, an addition)
- A compound, other than an amino acid, which is coopted by an enzyme to provide extra reactive groups. Prosthetic groups are tightly bound to the enzyme and remain unchanged at the end of the catalytic reaction.

protagonist (Gr. *protos*, first; *agonistes*, actor)
- Principal character(s) in a play, debate or story. It is *not* an antonym of **antagonist**; the antonym for which is **agonist.**

protection (L. *pro*, before; *tegere*, to cover)
- When a system of **receptors** is exposed to a *reversible* binding agent (**agonist** or **antagonist**), the occupied receptors are protected from a subsequently-added *irreversible* agent (agonist or antagonist) which will have access only to unoccupied receptors. If exposure to the irreversible agent is transient (as in a brief attack with a chemical weapon), affected subjects will be at least partially protected from it. The principle was applied (inconclusively) against expected **nerve gas** attack during the Gulf War (1991).
See **competition, non-equilibrium antagonist**

protein binding (Gr. *proteios*, primary; Sanskrit *bindh*, bind)
- Plasma and other tissue proteins (macromolecules) have drug (small molecule, **ligand**, hormonal metabolite) binding sites that act as stores and do not mediate a biological effect. Free and bound drug are in equilibrium. Dis-

placement interactions occur; the bound drug is inactive. Protein binding is a transport mechanism for hydrophobic drugs (see **hydrophilic/-phobic**).

protocol   (Gr. *protos*, first; *kolla*, glue)
– The detailed written plan of an experiment or process.
– The rules that govern the way that different types of computers communicate with each other.

proton-pump inhibitor
– An agent that inhibits the enzyme H^+/K^+-**ATP**ase (proton pump) of the gastric parietal cell, providing dose-related inhibition (95 per cent or more) of gastric acid secretion, e.g. omeprazole.

proto-oncogene   See **oncogene**

pseudo-allergic reaction   (Gr. *pseudes*, false; *allos*, other;
                                      ergon, activity; L. *re*, again, back; *agere*, to act, do)
– An adverse reaction that mimics an allergic reaction but which has no immunological basis, e.g. an **anaphylactoid** reaction on first as well as on subsequent exposure to a dextran, caused by histamine release.

pseudo-hybrid   (Gr. *pseudes*, false)
                                                    See **hybrid drug**

psychedelic   (Gr. *psukhe*, soul; *delos*, visible)
– The property of 'heightening' or 'expanding' consciousness, perhaps merely by impairing attentiveness to immediate practically important detail/events.

psychodysleptic   (Gr. *psukhe*, soul; *dus*, abnormal; *lepsis*, a seizure)
– A substance that produces mental changes which resemble some psychotic states.   See **hallucinogen**

psychopharmacology   (Gr. *psukhe*, soul; *pharmakon*, drug;
                                                    logy, discourse, study)
– The study of drug effects on the mind, on behaviour, on thinking, on cognition.
– *Cosmetic psychopharmacology*: The use of drugs to alter personality traits that are within the normal range. It refers to drug actions that may induce people who are not ill (in any conventional sense) to feel 'better than well'; to alter personality traits, e.g. shyness, self-esteem. The term was introduced by P Kramer to describe **anecdotal** evidence that people who were not clinically depressed felt better when taking fluoxetine (Prozac), an **SSRI** antidepressant. The implications for society of such drug use, if it became widespread, could be enormous.

psychostimulant   (Gr. *psukhe*, soul; L. *stimulare*, to urge on)
– Drugs that increase the level of alertness (e.g. **caffeine**, amphetamine).

psychotomimetic   (Gr. *psukhe*, soul; *osis*, condition; *mimeisthai*, to imitate)
- Producing effects that mimic psychotic states (e.g. **LSD**).

psychotropic   (Gr. *psukhe*, soul; *tropos*, a turn)
- Affecting mental function.

publication   (L. *populus*, the people)
- To make generally known, e.g. by issuing printed copies.
- *Duplicate or redundant publication*: As the pressure to publish or perish increases, publication of the same scientific information in different journals increases. It is highly objectionable to editors (waste of editorial, refereeing and other resources, as well as exclusion of other articles) and to readers, by enlarging the literature. Journal editors, in flagrant cases, have published a notice that duplicate publication has occurred, naming the culprit(s). But duplication can sometimes be acceptable, e.g. where the original publication was in a minority language or in an obscure governmental report. However, editors expect to be consulted about this and are deeply antagonized when they are not. Duplicate publication may be *overt* (and so fairly readily detectable if detection is sought) or *covert* (where steps are taken to avoid detection, as by change of authors, of language, by adding extra data).
- *Salami publication*: Dividing a piece of research into *minimal publishable units* to generate multiple publications when it could appropriately have been published as a single item. The objective is commonly career advancement. However, the practice can be defended "in much the same way that salami is better served sliced than consumed whole, some readers may prefer to digest various key messages delivered separately in a short series of papers" (*MJ Bennie, CW Lim*). Salami (L. *sal*, salt) is an Italian sausage.
- *Publish or perish*: Professional careers, reputations, promotion and research grants are increasingly dependent on the number of publications – counting is easier than assessing quality. This leads to salami publication (above) and enhances references in the **Science Citation Index**. It also leads to excessive numbers of authors (see **authorship**) and to **research misconduct**.
  The first recorded instance of publish or perish is claimed to be the ancient Greek philosopher Socrates who was condemned to take poison (hemlock) in 399 BCE and who never published (we are grateful to Dr. L Lasagna for drawing this to our attention).
- *Publication bias*: Editors of scientific journals are naturally selective about what they publish. They want an attractive, interesting journal. To this end they are likely to give priority to publishing the positive, the interesting, the sensational contribution. Negative studies, e.g. that drugs A and X are similar, although they provide useful information, are, frankly, boring to read and therefore go unread. The suggestion that there should be a *Journal of Negative Results* has not been taken up by any publisher (though electronic storage/publication may remedy this). "But many completed therapeutic trials are not even offered for publication" (see **clinical trials, unreported**). Publication bias can have an important adverse effect on **meta-analysis**.

- *Delaying publication*: Commercial or government sponsors of research in universities sometimes wish to delay (or even prevent) publication of the results. This raises ethical issues. The matter should be addressed in the contract made before the research commences. The Committee of Vice Chancellors and Principals of the Universities of the United Kingdom has recommended that universities should allow sponsors the right to delay publication for a specified period, normally not more than 12 months. A longer delay of two years or, at the very most, three years may be appropriate in exceptional circumstances, but only if the sponsor presents a compelling case and this is agreed with the researchers concerned (1992).
- *Scientific papers for publication*: The **International Committee of Medical Journal Editors** has recommended uniform requirements for manuscripts submitted to biomedical journals. These are widely accepted by editors.
- *Ghost writing*: There are individuals and specialist companies who will prepare (review) articles to the satisfaction of commercial sponsors and then find a prominent/respected doctor/scientist to be 'guest' author (for an **honorarium**). The final version, when submitted to the journal, may contain no clues about its origins.
  - A widespread practice is for a potential author to be asked to collaborate in the preparation of an article which will be mainly written by a ghost writer, but with 'full' control by the 'author'. Many ghost-written reviews start life as an outline and list of references prepared by the 'author'. Several stages of drafts may be sent to the 'author' for correction and the final version will only be submitted to the journal when written approval has been provided by the 'author'. Ghost writers are sometimes acknowledged, but this usually only happens if the 'author' insists upon doing so.
  - In today's world, ghost writing is legitimate and even necessary, but it is open to abuse.   See **authorship**, **chauvinism in publication**, **interest (conflict of)**, **language of science**, **peer review**

purgative   (L. *purgare*, to purify)
- A medicine promoting the evacuation of the bowels and usually acting by increasing the water content of the colon. Synonymous, for practical purposes, with laxative, aperient and evacuant. 'Cathartic' is usually confined to the most violently effective substances. The notion that bowel evacuation 'purifies' no doubt has deep psychopathological roots.

purinergic
- Nerves having adenosine triphosphate (**ATP**) or a related nucleotide or nucleoside as a transmitter.   See **NANC**, **purinoceptor**

purinoceptors
- A family of receptors that is activated by purine nucleotides and nucleosides. P_1-purinoceptors are activated by adenosine and adenosine monophosphate; P_2-purinoceptors are activated by adenosine triphosphate. P_2-purinoceptors are further subdivided into those coupled to an integral ion channel (**ionotropic receptors**) and those coupled to a **G-protein** (**metabotropic recep-**

tors). Purines (e.g. **ATP**) are released from purinergic neurons in both the peripheral and central nervous systems.

purism   (L. *purus*, pure)
- A needless and irritating insistence on 'purity' and 'correctness' of speech or writing in the expression of which 'pride apes humility' (*Fowler's Modern English Usage*).

p-value   See **probability (p) value**

pyrexia, pyretic, pyrogen   (Gr. *puro*, fire)
- *Pyrexia* is fever/rise in body temperature. Agents that cause it are *pyretics* or *pyrogens*. Pyrogens (protein or saccharide substances) of microbial or fungal origin may contaminate water used for injectable formulations.

QALY
- **Quality-adjusted life year.**

quack   (Dutch *quacken*, to prattle)
- An ignorant pretender to skill; and the unevaluated medicines used by such persons.   See **nostrum**

qualitative data   (L. *qualis*, of what sort)
- These relate to distinctions of kind or of attributes; they are *non-numerical* and allow allocation only to groups.   See **quantitative**

qualitative methods in research   (L. *qualis*, of what kind)
- These derive from the social sciences; they do not primarily seek *quantitative* measurements; they develop concepts which help to provide understanding of social phenomena in natural rather than in experimental settings giving due emphasis to the meanings, experiences and views of participants; they are not inherently incompatible with rigorous quantitative studies (after *C Pope, N Mays*).

quality-adjusted life year (QALY) and quality of life (QoL)
(L. *qualis*, of what kind)
- QALY is a unit of health measurement that combines *quantity* (duration) of life with its *quality.*
- Use of QALYs in health delivery decisions remains controversial.
- QoL: The way people feel and how they function in day-to-day activities.
- Quality of life has four principal or general dimensions: psychological, social, physical, economic; and these embody four detailed dimensions: physical mobility, freedom from pain and distress, capacity for self-care and ability to engage in normal social intercourse (including work).
                                    See **economics, utility measurement**

quality assurance and control
- It is essential that *manufactured medicines* be of high and consistent quality.
  - *Quality control* means testing samples at the end of, and sometimes during, the manufacturing process.
  - *Quality assurance* means monitoring each stage of the manufacturing process.
- These are concepts of *good clinical practice* (**GCP**) in trials of **medicinal products** conducted to satisfy official regulatory agencies. Quality *control* comprises the operational techniques undertaken to ensure the fulfilment of quality assurance. Quality *assurance* comprises systems and processes established to ensure that the trial and the data generated are in compliance with GCP (*based on* **EC** *definitions*).

QUANGO   (L. *quasi*, as if; G. *autonomous*, living under one's own laws;
                      L. *non*, not; *gubernare*, to steer; *organum*, tool)
- Quasi-autonomous non-governmental organization.

- A semi-public administrative body outside the civil service but financed by the exchequer and having members appointed by the government (**OED**), e.g. the Committee on Safety of Medicines (UK).
- Quangos are useful, indeed necessary, accessories of good government. Members of quangos are sarcastically described, by people who are excluded, as 'the good and the great', and as members of 'the **establishment**'; an imagined, perhaps real, **CABAL** that exerts (hidden) power and influence.
- But quangos, though supposedly appointed to give independent advice, can be influenced, and governments know that by judicious selection of members they can minimize the frequency of being given advice that they would prefer not to hear.
- The **acronym** has attracted a derogatory connotation, and the abbreviation **NDGB** has been proffered as a substitute, but *quango* now has a secure place in the language.

quantile   (L. *quantus*, how much; *-ilis*, suffix denoting relationship)
- Quantiles are values used to divide a set of data into sections, each having the same number of observations. *Quartiles*, as the word suggests, divide the data into four equal parts, *quintile* into five parts and so on; the term refers to the cut-off points, not to the groups so obtained. A clever device to display a distribution (*Tukey* 1977) is set out thus:

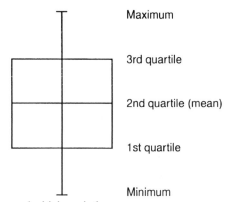

It is called a 'box and whisker plot'.

quantitative data   (L. *quantus*, how much; *data*, things given)
- Relating to amount or size; they are *numerical;* they may be *discrete* (whole numbers) or *continuous* (having fractional components).
- *Dishonest tricks* with quantitative data include suppressing the zero, inflating the scale, and extrapolation (*WM Castle, AF Ebbutt*). See **qualitative data**

quantum/quantal response   (L. *quantus*, how much; *re*, again; *spondere*, to promise)
- *General:* amount.
- *Of neurotransmitter:* in cases where the transmitter is released only in **integer**

multiples of a basic (more or less constant) amount, this basic amount is called a *quantum*.
- *Quantal response*: a discontinuously variable response, e.g. the number of individuals, out of a finite sample, showing a specified response, an **all-or-nothing** (present:absent) response as opposed to a **graded response**.

quartile   See **quantile**

quotation and permission to quote   (L. *quot*, how many; *per*, through; *mittere*, to send)
- Scientific and medical authors frequently need to quote from other authors for both scientific and educational reasons. Quotation involves consideration of the written (statutory) laws of **copyright** as well as the unwritten laws of courtesy.
- Scientists are in the business of disseminating their ideas and generally like to be quoted, but the question arises of when an author's permission is required and when it is not. Communication would be seriously impaired if permission had to be sought (from author and/or publisher) for even the smallest quotations from copyright texts.
- So various are the situations where quotations are used that the laws of copyright (e.g. USA, UK) understandably can give only general guidance.
- Permission to quote copyright material generally need not be sought where the quotation is *non-substantial* (in relation to the whole work is implied) or where it is made *for the purpose of criticism or review* (UK). The concept of *fair use* is also applied (USA), the relevant factors being, the *purpose and character* of the use, the *amount* in relation to the whole copyrighted work, and whether the quotation could affect the *market* for or *value* of the quoted work; the purpose of the quotation is also relevant, i.e. whether it is used for commercial or for non-profit educational purposes.
- Such general guidance, applied with common sense, should ordinarily be sufficient to tell us what quotations may be made without seeking the permission of authors or publishers. Plainly, where there is doubt, permission should be sought.
- The source of quotations of copyright material should always be acknowledged.
- **Plagiarism** is theft.   See **intellectual property**

racemate   (L. *racemus*, a bunch of grapes)
- One of the two or more **optical isomers** that make up a **racemic** mixture.
                                                              See **chirality**

racemic   (L. *racemus*, a bunch of grapes)
- An equimolecular mixture of two or more **streoisomers** (e.g. dextro, laevo) designated by the prefix *dl*, e.g. *dl*-propranolol. If the isomers are optically active, the mixture has no optical activity. Modern nomenclature for the configuration of stereoisomers is *R*, *S* (L. *rectus*, right; *sinister*, left).
                                                              See **chirality**

racemic therapeutic agents
- Fixed-ratio mixtures of **stereoisomers** ought to be regarded biologically as different compounds (*EJ Ariens*).   See **chirality**

radio-   (L. *radius*, ray)
- Prefix denoting a radioactive **isotope** of an element.

radioactive labelling/tagging   (L. *radius*, ray; *actus*, a doing, performance; Old Ger. *lappa*, a rag)
- By incorporating radioactive atoms into molecules of interest, e.g. drugs, the fate of these molecules can be followed by tracking the radioactivity. It is assumed that the molecule behaves in exactly the same way as the unlabelled molecules with which it is surrounded. The actual proportion of radioactive molecules in a dose (*specific activity*) is usually very small, partly because of the cost of incorporating a large proportion of labelled molecules, partly because of the technical difficulty of producing high specific activities, and partly because of the damage caused by high-intensity radiation, both to the surroundings (experimental tissue, animal or patient) and to the molecule itself (chemical breakdown caused by radiation – *autoradiolysis*). The most commonly employed **radioisotopes** in pharmacology are ^{3}H (tritium); ^{14}C, ^{32}P (β-emitters); and ^{131}I (γ-emitter).
- *In medical diagnosis*: a **radiopharmaceutical** in a dose just sufficient for it to be detected is called a *tracer*.
- *In research*: radioactive molecules (or atoms) are added to a biological system so that a biological process can be followed by keeping track of the radioactivity.   See **ligand-binding assay, PET**

radioactivity   (L. *radius*, ray; *actus*, a doing, performance)
- Emission of energy as particles or rays, e.g. electrons, X-rays, during spontaneous disintegration of **isotopes** of elements.

radioimmunoassay   (L. *radius*, a ray; *immunitas*, exemption; *exagium*, a trial of weight)
- An immunochemical procedure which requires the preparation of an **antibody** to the substance to be assayed (using it as a **hapten** according to standard immunological procedures) – the **antigen**. When this antibody is incubated

with a known concentration of radioactively-labelled antigen, the antibody will become radioactively labelled to an extent depending upon the concentration of the antigen and its affinity for the antibody. If the radioactively labelled antibody is incubated with a series of different concentrations of unlabelled antigen (the 'standard'), some of the radioactive antigen will be displaced. A 'standard curve' is prepared by plotting the ratio of bound to free radioactive antigen against the concentration of unlabelled antigen. When antibody that has been reacted with labelled antigen is incubated with the solution of antigen that is to be assayed (usually diluted to a known extent), some of the labelled antigen will be displaced. The bound:free ratio is measured and the concentration of the antigen can be determined by interpolation on the standard curve.

– Recently ways have been developed of making synthetic polymers with integral recognition sites. These can be used instead of biologically-raised antibodies.

– Radioimmunoassay is a form of **ligand-binding assay**.

radioisotope   (L. *radius*, ray; Gr. *isos*, equal; *topos*, place)
– An *unstable* **isotope** of an atom that spontaneously decays to a more *stable* isotope of the same, or more commonly a different, element by losing mass, either in the form of a particle (electron, positron, neutron, α-particle, etc.) or as a photon (γ-ray, X-ray). The emitted matter or photon can be detected, and the decay is characteristic for the particular isotope because of its unique energy profile.   See **radiopharmaceutical, radioactive labelling**

radioligand-binding assay   See **ligand-binding assay**

radionuclide   (L. *radius*, ray; *nucula*, nut, kernel)
– A nuclide (nucleus) of an atom that is radioactive. If it arises from the radioactive decay of another radionuclide, it is known as a daughter radionuclide, the parent **isotope** being the mother radionuclide.   See **radiopharmaceutical**

radiopharmaceutical   (L. *radius*, ray; Gr. *pharmakeia*, making of drugs)
– A preparation containing one or more **radionuclides**. Radioactive material in liquid, particulate or gaseous form (unsealed). Used in diagnosis and in therapy. (Sealed sources of radiation from which the radioactive substance cannot escape are not deemed radiopharmaceuticals.) Radiopharmaceuticals are used for research (to investigate physiology and pathology), diagnosis (scanning), treatment (radiotherapy), or new drug development (**pharmacokinetic** evaluation).   See **PET, radioactive labelling**

radiosensitizer   (L. *radius*, ray; *sentire*, to feel)
– An agent that renders cells more susceptible to ionizing radiation, when given before exposure.

random/-ization/ random sample/selection
                                  (Old Fr. *randir*, to gallop at great speed)
– Selection such that there is an equal (or predetermined) chance for each item, and selections are independent of each other.

- A random (or **stochastic**) process is characterized by the occurrence of events such that:
  - The probability of occurrence of an event in a time interval of a given length is always constant (no matter, for example, how long has elapsed since the last event occurred), and
  - The occurrence of an event in one time interval is independent of the occurrence of events in other (non-overlapping) time intervals.
- Random is not the same as **haphazard**. Randomization must be achieved by either physical means (throw of an unbiased coin or die), or by means of published tables of random numbers, or by a suitable computer program (these are strictly *pseudo*-random numbers because they have been generated according to a formula, as in gambling casinos; *Monte Carlo techniques*); randomization of the more complex designs (e.g. **Latin squares**) is not as obvious as it might at first seem (consult, for example, *RA Fisher & F Yates*, *Statistical tables*, 1963).
- The purpose of randomization is to minimize systematic **bias**.
- Any sort of statistical analysis (and any sort of intuitive analysis) of observations depends on properly-executed random selection and allocation.
- *Balanced* randomization ensures that numbers in each experimental group are equal at predetermined intervals.
- *Randomized consent in* **clinical trials**: see *Zelen randomization* in **therapeutic trial.**
- *Minimization* is a device for reducing to a minimum the imbalance (that may occur with simple randomization) between treatment groups where there are several factors known to affect prognosis, e.g. age, severity of disease.
- But it is not necessary to have equal numbers in each group, especially if the natural history of the disease is well known, when a 2:1 ratio can be used instead of the usual 1:1. Random number series can be adapted to provide unequal groups or allocation may be devised to change during the trial so that more patients are progressively allocated to the most successful treatment – **play-the-winner** allocation.
- Unsurprisingly, some, even many, patients (doubting the investigator's assertion that there is true **equipoise**) are unwilling to accept that the treatment they receive will be determined by chance (they are entitled to be told this); with resulting low recruitment and high drop-out rate. Trial designs are being developed in which *patient preferences* are taken into account for some or all patients, but they have less discrimination (*statistical power*) than truly randomized studies, for potential biases are uncontrolled, and therefore they require more subjects.
    See **power in statistics, convenience sample, therapeutic trial**

randomization test
- One on the most efficient types of non-parametric significance tests. The principle can be illustrated by observations on two treatments (of the type that **Student's *t*-test** would commonly be used for). If there were no real difference between the treatments (**null hypothesis**) then each individual would have shown the same response even if given the other treatment. Therefore

the observed difference between the treatments has arisen only because of the way the **random** numbers were distributed when the individuals were divided into two groups. The probability of this difference arising by chance can be assessed by writing all the observations down on cards, repeatedly dividing the cards randomly into two groups, and seeing how often the difference between the **means** of the groups exceed that observed (or simulation of this process on a computer). This procedure is simple, efficient, makes few assumptions but is rarely used.
- A statistical test to see whether the outcome of a putatively random selection does, in fact, contain systematic **bias**. See **parametric, probability (*p*) value**

randomized block design
- An experimental design in which each of two or more treatments is used once in random order in each subject (row). It is usual to arrange that the numbers allocated to each treatment are equal after every 'block' of patients has entered the study; for two treatments, the blocks are usually of four patients, two on treatment A and two on treatment B (balanced block); but unbalanced blocks (2:1, 3:1) are sometimes appropriate.   See **Latin square**

randomized controlled (therapeutic) trial (RCT)
- The classical method of evaluation/comparison of therapies.
                              See **control, prospective, random, therapeutic trial**

range   (Old Fr. *ranger*, to position)
- The lowest and highest values of a set of data.   See **centile**

rank/ing   (Old Fr. *ranc*)
- The arrangement of data in order from the smallest to the largest and their designation in numerical order, 1,2,3 and so on.   See **variables**

rankit
- Ranked normal deviate. For a standard **normal distribution** (i.e. a frequency distribution with a mean of 0 and a standard deviation of 1.0), rankits are the average scores obtained when *n* **variates** are sampled at random. These values are printed in tables. For example, if five items are chosen at random from a standard normal distribution, and the process repeated many times, once the items have been put into rank order, their average values (as given in tables of rankits) turn out to be −1.163 for the first item, −0.495 for the second, 0.0 for the third, 0.495 for the fourth and 1.163 for the last. Rankits are useful in testing for normality of distribution; when rankits are plotted against a ranked array of a normally distributed **variable** the points will lie on a straight line.   See **logistic regression analysis, probit**

rat race
- The relentless struggle to get ahead of one's rivals, particularly in professional and commercial occupations. *Rat* is used generally as a derogatory epithet (*Brewer's Dictionary of Phrase and Fable*).

rate (L. *ratus*, fixed)
- The frequency of occurrence of an event, e.g. death, disease; commonly expressed as the number of events per thousand or million of population per year.
- Amount ÷ time.

rate constant (L. *ratus*, fixed; *constans*, to stand firm)
- The **proportionality constant** for processes in which rate is proportional to concentration, electrical potential, etc.
- For a chemical reaction, see law of **mass action**.
- For any exponential process, see **time constant**.
                    See **elimination constant, dissociation equilibrium constant, exponential curve/equation/ function**

rate-limited kinetics
      See **Michaelis–Menten kinetics, saturation kinetics, zero-order kinetics**

rate theory See **receptors**

ratio (L. *ratio*, calculation)
- The quantitative relationship between two magnitudes determined by the number of times one contains the other integrally or fractionally.

rational drug therapy (L. *ratio*, reason, method)
- Use of an appropriate drug by a correct route in adequate doses over a sufficiently long or short time.   See **evidence-based medicine, prescribing**

raw data (regulatory term) (old Eng. *hreaw*)
- The original records (or certified copies) of clinical and laboratory findings.

RCT
- **Randomized controlled trial.**

reactivity (L. *re*, again; *agere*, to drive, do)
- The ability of a system to respond. It is often assessed in terms of the maximum response (e.g. of a blood vessel or airways). Sometimes the term is used interchangeably with **sensitivity**. This usage reduces the flexibility of the language for describing phenomena. However, the term is almost synonymous with **responsiveness**. The distinction is subtle, but reactivity suggests an undesirable or untoward response – as in **hyperreactivity**.
- Reactivity has also been defined in terms of both the maximal response (E_{max}) and the **sensitivity** of the tissue (**EC_{50}**) (*Hulbert et al.* 1985):

$$R = E_{max} / EC_{50}$$

rebound See **withdrawal syndrome**

recall bias   (L. *re,* again; Old Eng. *ceallian,* a herald; see **bias**)
- An assessment **bias** that occurs when individuals in one group are more likely to remember past effects than individuals in another of the study or control groups. Recall bias is especially likely when a **case-control study** involves serious disease and the characteristics under study are commonly occurring, subjectively remembered events (**FDA**).

receptor   (L. *re,* again; *capere,* to take)
- [Receptors are] cellular macromolecules that are concerned directly and specifically in chemical signalling between and within cells. Combination of a **hormone, neurotransmitter, drug** or intracellular messenger with its receptor(s) initiates a change in cell function. The regions of the receptor macromolecule to which endogenous **agonists** bind are referred to collectively as the *recognition site(s)* of the receptor (**IUPHAR**, with permission; *Pharmacological Reviews* 1995;47:255–266).
- A specific macromolecular (protein) binding site on or in a cell, to which structurally specific agonists (drugs, hormones, neurotransmitters, etc.) bind as the first step in evoking a response. It is supposed that **competitive antagonists** bind to the same site on the receptor as the agonist (i.e. **syntopic**), excluding the agonist, but evoking no response themselves.
- A cellular macromolecule with which drug/hormone/**autacoid** molecules of a specific class combine, the combination being essential for the production of their effect on the cell. It is useful to distinguish *active* receptors, whose function is expressed only when an agonist molecule is bound, and *passive* receptors (e.g. enzyme molecules, carrier molecules) whose normal function is inhibited by combination with a drug molecule.
- **Binding sites** that cannot mediate a biological effect (e.g. plasma albumin) are best not called receptors.
- *Characterization of receptors* (Gr. *kharacter,* distinctive nature) – Two problems have plagued a purely pharmacological definition of receptor subtypes. The first is the question of whether observed pharmacological differences represent different receptor molecules or simply cell-specific differences in the environment of a common receptor molecule...The second is the problem of knowing whether there is a pure receptor population in a given tissue, a problem that may generally have been underestimated...For the present, two ongoing systems of receptor definition, structural and pharmacological, appear to be necessary (IUPHAR, with permission; *Pharmacological Reviews* 1992;44:351–362).
- *Cloned receptors* – Receptors produced *in vitro* by inserting the gene for the receptor into a suitable *expression system* that does not normally express the receptor (e.g., Chinese hamster ovary cells). This allows the production of limitless identical copies of a receptor molecule for research. The expression system is usually such that the number of copies of the receptor (*level of expression*) can be controlled by the experimenter.
  - The technique has been used both to investigate the characteristics of a chosen receptor and its interactions with drugs and coupling systems (e.g., **G-proteins**) and to investigate whether a given gene is responsible for the expression of a receptor that has physiological significance. It may be that

it is possible to classify receptors on the basis of their amino acid sequence, although the significance of minor deviations in sequence and how these variants should be named is a matter of debate. It is also unclear how many changes and what type of changes in the sequence define a new receptor.

- Cloned receptors can be of naturally occurring receptors ('wild' type) or can be mutations (*recombinant*). Mutations can be either point deletions, where certain amino acids are missing completely from the sequence, or mutations in which one or more amino acids are replaced by other amino acids. If large segments of the sequence are replaced by sequences from other (but usually related) receptors, the product is usually known as a *hybrid receptor*. Hybrid receptors have been valuable for identifying the functions of different parts of receptor molecules. See **clone**
- *Endocytosis of receptors* (Gr. *endo*, within; *kutos*, vessel, cell) – Most G-protein-coupled receptors appear to undergo *cycling* in which they are constantly removed from the cell surface into *endosomes* from where they are either delivered to the cell surface again or are removed and degraded. The binding of a **ligand** to receptors increases the rate of *internalisation*, although the process continues at a basal rate in the absence of ligand. The process probably plays a part in **down-regulation** of receptors.
- *Families of receptors* – There are four main families of receptors:
    - **Ionotropic receptors** ('fast' receptors); in these the binding site is an integral part of an **ion channel** (**ionophore**).
    - **Metabotropic receptors** ('slow' receptors); these are linked to **G-proteins**.
    - *Tyrosine kinase-linked*; binding of the transmitter (usually a hormone or growth factor) stimulates the phosphorylation of a tyrosine residue on an intracellular protein, thereby setting in train a sequence of events leading to a (slow) response.
    - *Steroid (DNA-linked) receptors*; these are intracellular proteins that can bind both to transmitter (e.g. steroid or thyroid hormone) and to nuclear chromatin. Binding of the transmitter causes a conformational change which stimulates DNA **transcription** in the nucleus.
    See **superfamilies of receptors**
- *Heptahelical receptors* – Receptors belonging to a *superfamily* of related **G-protein**-linked receptors, the protein sequences of which contain seven highly lipophilic **domains** that span the cell membrane. Also known as 7TM [transmembrane] receptors, slow receptors, **metabotropic receptors**, serpentine receptors or heptaspan receptors.
- *Induction of receptors* – The stimulation of a cell to *express* a receptor that it does not normally express. Stimuli can be pathological (e.g., tissue injury) or physiological (e.g., angiogenesis). This results in the appearance of responses of which the cell was previously incapable.
- Models of receptor action:
    - *Classical* model: Drugs combine with receptors according to the law of **mass action**. If the drug is an agonist, the receptor is activated to an extent characterized by the drug's **intrinsic efficacy**.

- *Two-state* model: The receptor can exist in two forms or states, one of which leads to a tissue response, whereas the other does not. In general, drugs can combine with both forms, and relative affinity for the two forms will determine whether the drug is a **full agonist** (binds preferentially with the active conformation), an **inverse agonist** (binds preferentially with the inactive conformation) or a neutral **antagonist** (shows no preference for either conformation) – see **efficacy**.
- *Three-state* model: An extension of the two-state model to allow for *receptor promiscuity* and the finding that agonists can have different rank-orders of potency when interacting with the same receptor but where the receptor couples to different effectors. The model proposes that the receptor can exist in three conformational states and that interaction between the agonist and active conformations of the receptor therefore depends upon two **dissociation equilibrium constant**s rather than a single constant. See **promiscuous receptors**
- *Rate theory* model: The tissue response is considered to be determined by the number of new drug–receptor complexes formed in unit time, rather than by the number of complexes existing at a given time. There is no strong evidence for this theory and it is inconsistent with recent observations.
- *Operational* model: A model developed by **Black & Leff**, which describes responses to drugs in terms of the **hyperbolic** relationships between drug concentration and receptor occupancy, and between receptor occupancy and **stimulus**.
- *Modulatory site* – An **allosteric** site on a receptor macromolecule to which a ligand other than the agonist can bind as a result of which the action of an agonist is either increased or decreased.
- *Native (or wild type) receptors* – Receptors having the amino acid sequence that occurs in nature rather than an artificial sequence made in the laboratory.
- *Nomenclature* – The following are the recommendations of the IUPHAR Committee for Receptor Nomenclature and Drug Classification (**IUPHAR**, with permission; *Pharmacological Reviews* 1996;48:1–2):
  - Mammalian receptor systems are the basis of IUPHAR classifications. The nomenclature may extend to other vertebrates if useful, provided it does not compromise the mammalian classification. Evolutionary changes may be so great that invertebrate receptors are difficult to classify within mammalian-based nomenclature.
  - The receptor should be named after the endogenous agonist, or the appropriate collective term when a family of related substances may interact with a receptor.
  - The agonist abbreviation, followed by a numerical subscript, is to be preferred in naming new receptors. Further subdivision by subscript letters is allowed when there is a strong basis for grouping receptors together.
  - Species **homologues** should not be given separate names, but the species should be identified if necessary by a lower case prefix, i.e., $m5\text{-}HT_{2A}$ or $h5\text{-}HT_{2A}$ for the mouse and human receptor, respectively. [A list of spe-

cies abbreviations is given in the Table.] If necessary, further strain differences should be defined in the text [describing the receptor].

- Recombinant receptors without well-defined functional characteristics should be referred to by lower case letters, i.e. 5-ht$_6$, 5-ht$_{1f}$ or α_{1d}. When the recombinant receptor is shown to be of functional relevance in whole tissues and is fully characterized, upper case letters should then be used, e.g. 5-HT$_6$ or α_{1D}. When there is strong pharmacological evidence for a new receptor, but the amino acid sequence has not been defined, the receptor will be referred to in upper case italics, e.g. *H$_3$* histamine receptor.
- New *splice variants* [see below], if pharmacologically relevant, should be indicated by subscript letters in lower case, in parentheses, e.g., EP$_{3(a)}$, EP$_{3(b)}$, EP$_{3(c)}$, EP$_{3(d)}$ receptor.
- Greek letters and Roman numerals should be avoided in any new nomenclature. The name should not include 'R' or 'r' as an abbreviation for receptor. Where subscripts are used, there should never be subscripts to an existing subscript.
- Distinct names should be used for **G-protein**-linked receptors and ligand-gated **ion channel** receptors activated by the same agonist so that, in the future, the distinction does not depend solely on numerical subscripts as presently occurs for the 5-HT$_3$ receptor.

TABLE: Proposed list of species abbreviations to precede the receptor name, where further precision is required

Abbreviation	Species	Abbreviation	Species
b	bovine	h	human
ca	canine	mk	monkey
ch	chick	m	mouse
e	equine	p	porcine
f	feline	rb	rabbit
gp	guinea pig	r	rat

- *Orphan receptor* – A receptor for which a natural ligand has not been identified.
- *Recombinant receptors* – Receptors produced by **genetic engineering** in which one or more amino acids, or more often whole sequences of amino acids, are different from those in the natural or *wild* form of the receptor. Changes can be either *deletions* (in which one or more amino acids are omitted from the protein) or *mutations* (in which one or more amino acids are replaced with different amino acids).
- *Spare receptors* – The receptors surplus to the minimum number required to produce a maximum response in the presence of a full agonist.
  - It often happens that the capacity of a tissue to respond to an agonist reaches its maximum at an agonist concentration that is too low to occupy (and, *a fortiori* [L., with stronger reason], to activate) all the receptors. In such a case the maximum response will be seen at an agonist concentration that occupies, and activates, less than (sometimes much less than) 100 per cent of receptors at equilibrium. In such cases there are said to be

spare receptors (for the particular agonist, tissue and response under consideration). Note that this does not imply that there are two *kinds* of receptors, spare and otherwise. If a maximum response is produced by 1 per cent occupancy, all receptors eventually participate, each being activated for 1 per cent of the time, on average. Therefore the term 'spare receptors' is somewhat misleading – **receptor reserve** is preferred.

– *Species homologues* (Gr. *homos*, same; *logos*, word) – Receptors which subserve the same function and respond to the same endogenous transmitter(s) but which have minor differences in their amino acid sequence between different species.

– *Splice variants* – Within a species, a single gene can sometimes give rise to proteins with amino acid sequences that differ due to variations in assembly of sequences of polypeptides. These different forms are known as *splice variants*. Splice variants of the same receptor may have different pharmacological properties.

– *Up- and down-regulation* – The number (density) of receptors on cells can change in response to the concentration of the specific binding molecule (**ligand**). Prolonged high concentrations of agonist with high receptor **occupancy** cause reduction of the number of receptors (down-regulation) and prolonged occupation of receptors by inert molecules (**antagonists**) leads to an increase in the number of receptors (up-regulation).

See **chimeric receptor, receptor classification/nomenclature/taxonomy, regulatory subunit**

receptor classification/nomenclature/taxonomy

(L. *classis*, assembly; *nomen*, name; Gr. *tasso*, arrange)

– There are several ways of classifying and naming receptors.

– *By transmitter/hormone/mediator.* The first level of classifying receptors is to assign them to major groups, according to the transmitter/mediator/ hormone (i.e. endogenous **ligand**) that acts upon them, e.g. all *acetylcholine receptors* respond to the neurotransmitter **acetylcholine**; all **GABA**-receptors respond to the neurotransmitter GABA.

– *By selective agonists/antagonists*: The subdivisions of receptors within the major groups was originally achieved by studying the rank orders of potencies of related drugs, usually **agonists**. Because the development of selective **antagonists** has tended to follow the identification of receptor subtypes, the use of antagonists in the classification of receptors has usually been confirmatory, and has followed studies with agonists. Examples of this are **nicotinic** and **muscarinic acetylcholine receptors** (and the subdivision of muscarinic acetylcholine receptors into M_1, M_2, M_3 and M_4); $GABA_A$ and $GABA_B$ subtypes of GABA receptors. Such functional studies are now usually combined with **ligand-binding** studies, which allow direct measurement of **affinities** of drugs for particular receptors. Receptors of any one type will have a characteristic spectrum of affinities for a range of ligands. Classification according to affinity for standard drugs has been the chief tool of the receptor taxonomist for many years.

– *By transduction process*: It is often useful to group receptors according to how the response is brought about once a drug binds to the receptor. There are four main processes and, on this basis, receptors can be assigned to one of four 'families': ionotropic, metabotropic (G-protein-linked), tyrosine kinase-linked, DNA-linked (see **receptor** for a fuller account). Knowledge of **transduction** (*receptor–effector coupling*) mechanisms will usually provide important information relevant to the nature and structure of a given receptor type.

- *By structure*: **Molecular biology** now allows the molecular pharmacologist to determine the precise **amino acid** sequence and three-dimensional structure of receptors. The use of sequence **receptor probes** has also revealed the existence of gene sequences that code for receptors for which no functions are known (e.g. m5-muscarinic acetylcholine receptors). However, classification by total amino acid sequence can be complicated by the finding that receptors with different sequences can be indistinguishable as far as their sensitivities to drugs are concerned, although it is likely that such 'different' receptors have nearly identical sequences in their drug-binding **domains**.   See **receptor** (*Characterisation; Nomenclature*)

receptor-effector coupling   See **transduction**

receptor-mediated endocytosis
- The binding of some **ligands** to their cell-surface receptors can trigger **endocytosis**, in which both the ligand and the receptor are transferred across the cell membrane into the cytoplasm. The process is particularly common with peptide hormones, growth factors and antibodies, but also occurs for some transmitters. It probably forms part of the process known as *down-regulation*.
                                                                    See **receptor**

receptor probe   (L. *probare*, to test)
- A tool (a drug) designed to bind selectively to, and thereby identify, specific types of **receptors**.
- A characteristic sequence of known amino acids in a particular type of receptor can be used to make an **oligonucleotide** probe which can be used to screen DNA sequences in tissues to determine whether that receptor, or a closely related receptor, exists in a tissue.   See **reverse pharmacology**

receptor reserve
- In many tissues, an **agonist** can produce a maximal response when occupying only a small fraction of the receptors. This is a dynamic process; over a period of time all the receptors will be occupied briefly, but at any instant only some will be. This surplus of receptors is known as the *receptor reserve* and accounts for the fact that low doses of a **nonequilibrium antagonist**, which are known to inactivate a proportion of the receptors irreversibly, will often cause a rightward, parallel shift in the agonist log **dose–response curve** without reducing the maximum (i.e. a maximal response is possible when less than 100 per cent of the receptors are occupied by agonist). Similarly, a **partial agonist** will not induce a maximal response, even when it occupies all the

receptors. 'Receptor reserve' is synonymous with the term 'spare receptors' (see **receptor**), but is preferred because the latter term implies a static situation.

reciprocal plot   (L. *reciprocare*, moving backwards and forwards, alternating)
— A graphical device for converting a hyperbolic saturation curve (e.g. a curve relating reaction rate to a substrate concentration in an enzyme-catalysed reaction, or fractional occupancy to ligand concentration) to a linear form. A **hyperbola** is the locus of a point, the product of the coordinates (x,y) of which is constant (i.e. $x \times y = $ constant). The saturation curve has the general form:

$$y = \frac{ax}{(x+k)}$$

where x is the independent **variable**, y is the dependent variable and a and k are constants. Plotting y directly against x gives a curve such that y approaches a as x approaches infinity. The most commonly encountered reciprocal plots are:
— *Lineweaver Burk plot or double reciprocal plot:*

$1/y$ v. $1/x$
$(1/y) = (1/x) \times (k/a) + (1/a)$.

This is the equation for a straight line with a slope of k/a and an ordinal intercept of $1/a$. The abscissal intercept is $1/k$.
— *Scatchard plot:*

y/x v. y
$(y/x) = (-y/k) + (a/k)$.

With this plot the abscissal intercept measures a and the slope measures $-1/k$. In pharmacology the Scatchard plot is a useful graphical method for showing **ligand-binding** data. In this case $x/y = $ [bound ligand]/[free ligand]; $a = B_{max}$ and $k = K_d$. Before the wide availability of computers, Scatchard plots were widely used to analyze ligand-binding studies (*Scatchard analysis*), but this use has been (or should be) superseded by nonlinear curve-fitting techniques, for reasons given below.
— *Semireciprocal plot:*

x/y v. x
$(x/y) = (xa) + (ka)$.

With this plot the abscissal intercept is $-k$ and the ordinal intercept is k/a. The slope is $1/a$.
— Although these plots are still useful to provide a quick test of whether or not a set of experimental points conforms to a hyperbola, they are not very satisfactory as means of estimating the parameters a and k because of the unequal weighting that the **transformations** introduce. In particular, they should never be used in combination with linear **regression analysis** by the **least squares** method, which is rendered invalid by the highly uneven distribution of **variance**.

recognition (drug/receptor)   (L. *re*, again; *cognoscere*, to learn)
- When a drug molecule interacts with a **receptor**, the process, by definition, involves recognition by the receptor of the drug molecule. Drug molecules, or **ligands**, must have **selectivity**, must bind in a saturable manner, and, where appropriate, demonstrate **stereoselectivity** for the proposed receptor (**IUPHAR**, with permission; *Pharmacological Reviews* 1992; 44:351–362).
                    See **receptor, recognition subunit/-site**

recognition subunit/-site   (L. *re*, again; *cognosco*, learn; *sub*, below; *unus*, one)
- The part of a **receptor** molecule (or complex) that is structurally complementary to the **ligand** and at which the ligand interacts with the receptor. In **G-protein**-linked receptor systems, there are several subunits; the *recognition subunit*, the **regulatory subunit**, and the **catalytic subunit**. The recognition *site* is a small region on one of the transmembrane **domains** of the recognition *subunit*. In **ionotropic** receptors, the recognition site (or sites) resides on the extracellular surface of one (or more) of the subunits comprising the **ionophore**.

recombinant DNA   (L. *re*, again; *combinare*, join two together)
- DNA deliberately coupled from different sources.
- DNA into which new genetic material (e.g. from other species) has been introduced, or the rearrangement of genes in the chromosome (DNA) into an order different from that of either of its parents. It can be spontaneous or induced (**genetic engineering**). The technique is being used (among other things) to produce protein hormones, e.g. insulin and growth hormone, for use in therapeutics, and to produce large numbers of receptors which can then be inserted into simple test systems to investigate the properties of putative medicines.

record linkage   (L. *recordari*, remember; Old Ger. *gelenk*, joint, link)
- This entails collating medical information from separate sources on individual patients identified by name and date of birth to seek, for example, an association between a drug and a disease (*N Wald*).

recreational (use) drugs   (L. *re*, again; *creare*, to create, produce)
- The drug itself is not primarily recreational, rather the *mode of use* is. Recreational use (which is intermittent, to fit with an individual's social and recreational activities) may proceed to continual use and so to drug **dependence**. Examples of recreational-use drugs include: alcohol, tobacco, **caffeine**, amphetamines, cocaine, betel, khat, LSD and many more.
                    See **abuse and misuse of drugs, substance abuse**

reductionism   (L. *reducere*, to reduce)
- Analysis of complex entities into simple constituents as an aid to understanding. Its use depends on the view that the whole is the sum of its parts, which may not necessarily be so.

refereeing   See **peer review**

regimen/regime   (L. *regere*, to rule)
- A systematic course of treatment. The variant *regime* is acceptable, but more commonly employed of, for example, governments, as in *fascist regime* (fascist *regimen* would be considered odd).

regression analysis   (L. *re*, back; *gradi/gressum*, step;
                                                   Gr. *ana*, back; *lusis*, to loosen)
- Regression analysis describes mathematically the dependence of one linear **variable** on one or more other linear variables; it allows *prediction* of one variable from another.
- Where an outcome of treatment is nonlinear (i.e. an event scored as present or absent, failure or success), then linear regression calculations may predict improbable probabilities. To escape this, a logarithmic transformation is used, the **logit** transformation (logit (p)).
                              See **Cox proportional hazards/regression model**

regression curve   (L. *re*, back; *gradi/gressum*, step)
- Curve best fitting inexact **data**.

regression towards the mean   (L. *re*, back; *gradi/gressum*, step;
                                                   medius, middle)
- The tendency for initial *extreme* values to show change towards the **mean** (centre) on a second measurement rather than to become even more extreme; this can mislead (false positive effect) in **therapeutic trials**. The term is only meaningful where there *is* a mean towards which to regress.
- The idea or tendency, for it is not appropriate to call it a **law** (though this is sometimes done), does not represent some mysterious universal force, e.g. gravity; it is what empirical experience tells us; in its simplest, most powerful form, it simply points out that contrary to the imaginations of newspaper readers and editors everywhere, straight-line extrapolations of current trends, for example, do not continue forever; it is a statement of empirical experience across a wide variety of causally unrelated settings. In the case of the size of living things, first biology and eventually physics ensure that, for example, ants can never become as large as trucks. Its application to stock market prices, though interesting, is beyond the scope of this book (after *PL Bernstein*).

regret avoidance   (Old Norse *grata*, to weep; L. *vacare*, to be empty)
- Decision-makers have to deal with three kinds of uncertainties:
  - Of facts.
  - Of public reaction to facts.
  - Of the future consequences of their decisions.
- In respect of the last the decision-maker on behalf of the public (e.g. politician, civil servant), being human, is liable to favour the decision that dilutes responsibility and minimizes risk, and so also minimizes later regret (regret avoidance) if the outcome is unfavourable. Neither politicians nor civil servants like making enemies, and so their temptation to indulge in regret avoid-

ance is strong, with the result that much legislation is weakened by compromises that are not, in fact, in the public interest. No-one can object if cautious individuals allow risk avoidance and regret avoidance to dominate decisions in their own personal lives, but it is another matter when decisions are being made on behalf of other people (*Lord Ashby*, 1976, botanist and scientific policy-maker, UK). Regret avoidance is a substantial factor in **regulation (official) of medicines**.

regulation (official) of medicines
(L. *regulare,* to control)

- For definition of a *medicine* see **medicinal product**.
- Regulation, which is broadly similar worldwide, conforms to principles which are recognized as of general importance, but the details (with accompanying administrative **jargon**) on how each country or group of countries administers these generally accepted principles differ, and cause unnecessary difficulties to drug developers. Efforts are being made (the **International Conference on Harmonization**) to minimise the enormous waste of resources caused by the need for drug developers to adapt their research programmes to needlessly diverse national bureaucratic requirements (see **proposition 65**).
- The principles of official (statutory) medicines regulation are that:
  - No medicine shall be supplied without prior licensing by the **government**.
  - A licence shall be granted on the basis of scientific evaluation of:
    - *Quality*, i.e. purity, stability (**shelf-life**).
    - *Safety,* in relation to its use: evaluation at the point of marketing is provisional in the sense that it is followed in the community by a **pharmacovigilance** programme.
    - *Efficacy,* (now often including **quality of life** and **economics** studies).
    - *Supply,* i.e. whether the drug is suitable to be unrestrictedly available to the public or whether it should be confined to sales through pharmacies or on doctors' prescriptions; and what printed information should accompany its sale (**summary of product characteristics**).
- A licence shall specify the clinical indications that may be promoted and shall be for a limited period (5 years) which is renewable on application.
- A regulatory authority may order a drug to be taken off the market at any time for good cause.
  [*Note*: Some exceptions to the rigorous scientific evaluation are made in the case of some substances used in **complementary medicine** provided that suitably limited therapeutic claims for efficacy and safety are made; see *homoeopathic product* in **homoeopathy**.]
- The *dilemma of official regulation* is that the public wants a freewheeling deregulated society whilst also expecting to be protected from all risk (after *D Kessler*, 1997, ex-director of the US **FDA**).
- *Criteria of good regulation* (by the chairman of the **CSM**, UK):
  - Scientific integrity.
  - Fair appeals procedure.
  - Accountability.
  - Local **ADR** monitoring.
  - Confidentiality (commercial *only*).

- Minimal bureaucracy.
- Harmonization.
- Effective communication.
- Speed.
- Low-cost/self-funding.
- *Fast-tracking*: many countries have a flexible option for licensing a drug where there is urgent need, e.g. in the treatment of AIDS, on limited data; especially where patients may die before the full paraphernalia of developing and reviewing a **new active substance** is completed, and where patients knowingly accept the risks inherent in fast-tracking procedure, i.e. they will not expect compensation if they are injured (see **compassionate drug use, liability, Parallel Track Mechanism)**.
- *Some influential regulatory authorities:*
  - USA: The powerful Food and Drug Administration (FDA), decisions of which have worldwide repercussions, so big and important is the USA market. No multinational company can ignore FDA requirements (see **FDCA**).
  - European Community/Union: The European Medicines Evaluation Agency (EMEA), 15 countries in 1997 (see **subsidiarity**).
  - Japan: The Ministry of Health and Welfare (Koseisho) has a Pharmaceutical Affairs Bureau which acts using external assessors as a Central Pharmaceutical Affairs Council.
  - Other countries: Regulation by governments varies from high-quality, science-based, to virtually zero. The amount of duplication of complex review processes in the world is colossal and wasteful, and ought to be diminished (see **International Conference on Harmonization**). Most countries use external independent assessors in some way (see **QUANGO**).
- *Veterinary medicines* are regulated under laws similar to those for human medicines, making special provision for special uses such as growth promotion agents in animal feeds and manipulation of productivity, e.g. milk production.

[**Note**: Technical ('allowed') terms used by regulatory authorities worldwide are legion. A selection of terms used by major authorities and terms that particularly throw light on the bureaucratic process will be found throughout this book.] See **abridged application, drug lag, environmental impact assessment, need clause, well-established medicinal use, phases of clinical studies of new drugs, post-marketing surveillance, prescription-only medicine, toxicity tests, summary of product characteristics**

regulations (L. *regulare*, to control)
See **guidelines**

regulations to control inducements to prescribers
- In the UK there was sufficient concern in 1994 for the government to tighten controls as follows:
"Any attempt by drug companies to influence doctors' prescribing habits by

means of financial or other inducements is to be deplored. These regulations will bring breaches of hospitality norms within the scope of the Medicines Act and render offending companies or their sales representative liable to criminal prosecution.

"They will also make it a criminal offence for a doctor to solicit or accept expensive gifts" (Under-Secretary of State for Health: *Pharmaceutical Journal*).

regulatory creep (L. *regulare*, to control; Old Eng. *creopan*, to creep)
- The process by which restrictive official regulatory processes, introduced with promises of limited application, are gradually intensified and even spread to neighbouring activities for which they were not initially intended. For example: user **fees** to medicines regulatory authorities may be increased to support other activities, i.e. they become a tax.

regulatory subunit/site (receptor)
- That part of a **receptor**–effector complex that controls and regulates the activity of the **recognition** and/or **catalytic subunit**.   See **G-protein**

reify (L. *res*, thing)
- To treat an abstract concept as real (for the sake of argument): to mentally convert it into a thing.

relativism (L, *re*, back; *latus*, borne)
- The naïve belief that everyone's opinions are equally good, e.g. in **ethics.**

relaxation (L. *re*, return to a previous condition; *laxare*, to loosen)
- The time course of re-equilibration. If a system is perturbed (see **perturbation**) (for example by imposition of a sudden change of drug concentration or membrane potential), it will respond by changing, more or less gradually, until it reaches the equilibrium appropriate to the imposed condition. This temporal change is described as 'relaxation towards the new equilibrium'.
- The process by which a protein molecule (e.g. **enzyme, receptor**) changes conformation back to a thermodynamically favourable or 'resting' state after the dissociation of a **ligand** (e.g. substrate, drug).

replication studies See **science in pharmacology**

reporting bias (in clinical studies) (L. re, back; portare, to carry)
- An assessment **bias** that occurs when individuals in one group are more likely to report past events than individuals in another of the study or control groups **(FDA)**.

rescue treatment (L. *ex*, out; *cutere*, to shake; *trahere*, to pull; *mentum*, result)
- Therapeutic trials in serious disease or unpleasant symptoms are designed to provide for the introduction of known-to-be-effective alternative (rescue) therapy (where such exists) at an early stage should there be failure of a treatment under test.

- Use of a high (potentially fatal) dose of a drug to achieve an objective, followed by prompt reversal of its action to save vital tissues, e.g. folinic acid rescue in methotrexate treatment of acute lymphocytic leukaemia.

See **escape clause**

research (L. *re*, again; Old Fr. *cercher*, search)
- Careful search or enquiry, after, for or into.
- Endeavour to discover new, or collate old, facts.
- The scientific **verification** of a predicted but not proven relationship between **variables**.
- The definition of [clinical medical] research continues to present difficulties, particularly with regard to the distinction between innovative medical practice and medical research. The distinction rests on the *intent*. In medical practice the sole intention is to benefit the *individual* patient consulting the clinician, not to gain knowledge of general benefit, though such knowledge may incidentally emerge from the clinical experience gained. In medical research the *primary intention* is to advance knowledge so that patients in general may benefit; the individual patient may or may not benefit directly (*Royal College of Physicians of London*). The distinction is important in relation to the work of *research* **ethics committees**.
- *Pure versus applied research*: Politicians ask, "We support research. Why does not research support the national economy?" The complaint leads to the demand that research should be more 'relevant'. "Those who make it overlook, or have never understood, the huge gap there must be between discoveries about the natural world, which are the chief (but not exclusive) concern of the academic sector of the research community, and the development of innovations that can succeed on world markets" (*Nature*).
- The division of research into *pure* and *applied* has always been imprecise and intellectually unsatisfactory. But the general concept can be more than a distinction without a difference. In the UK a government advisory body has sought to divide research into 'mission-orientated' (applied) and 'curiosity-driven' (or 'strategic') (pure) with a view to differential financing which, if adopted, could render a range of long-term research activities more vulnerable to short-term political and economic pressures.
- "If *politics* is the art of the *possible* (*Otto von Bismarck*, 1867, Chancellor, Germany), *research* is surely the art of the *soluble*." [emphasis added] (*PB Medawar*, 1964, zoologist/immunologist, UK); it is commonly misquoted substituting *science* for *research*.
- It is better to have lived one day as a tiger than a thousand years as a sheep (ancient Tibetan proverb). See **animals in research, audit, clinical research, ethics committee, science/scientific method (observational study, experiment)**

research misconduct (See **research**; L. *minus*, less; *cum*, together; *ducere*, to lead)
- Competition in science is now so intense (for status, jobs, grants and personal wealth) that increasing numbers of scientists succumb to temptation "to simulate success and earn the rewards it brings" (*Nature*).

- The USA *Commission of Research Integrity* (set up by the US Department of Health and Human Services and by Congress) recommends the following *definition* (1996):

   Research misconduct is significant misbehaviour that improperly appropriates the intellectual property or contributions of others, that intentionally impedes the progress of research, or that risks corrupting the scientific record or compromising the integrity of scientific practices. Such behaviours are unethical and unacceptable in proposing, conducting, or reporting research, or in reviewing the proposals or research reports of others.

   Examples of research misconduct include but are not limited to the following:

   - *Misappropriation:* an investigator or reviewer shall not intentionally or recklessly

      (a) Plagiarise, which shall be understood to mean the presentation of the documented words or ideas of another as his or her own, without attribution appropriate for the medium of presentation; or

      (b) Make use of any information in breach of any duty on confidentiality associated with the review of any manuscripts or grant application.

   - *Interference:* an investigator or reviewer shall not intentionally and without authorization take or sequester or materially damage any research related property of another, including without limitation the apparatus, reagents, biological materials, writings, data, hardware, software, or any other substance or device used or produced in the conduct of research.

   - *Misrepresentation:* an investigator or reviewer shall not with intent to deceive, or in reckless disregard for the truth,

      (a) State or present a material of significant falsehood; or

      (b) Omit a fact so that what is stated or presented as a whole states or presents a material or significant falsehood.

- A major and regrettable aspect of this topic is that responsible bodies in many countries do not admit its substantial prevalence and so do not act. The pharmaceutical industry is very conscious of the risks of fraud in the clinical trials it sponsors and for which it pays large sums of money (that investigators might invent patients and invent data). Companies have also been known to suppress unfavourable data, which is also misconduct.

- Trading in pharmaceutical company shares by people who may have confidential information about the results of clinical trials (which can significantly influence share prices, e.g. in the treatment of AIDS) may breach insider dealing laws. Falsifying results to create a market may constitute deception that breaks laws against theft.

reserpine See **drugs as tools**

residence time See **mean residence time**

response to drugs See **all-or-none response, graded response**

responsiveness   (L. *respondere*, to return like for like)
- The ability to react to a given dose.
- The maximal response of which a system is capable, analogous to the term **intrinsic activity**, which is used to describe the maximal response that a drug can evoke.
- Often erroneously described as **sensitivity**; during an experiment *in vitro*, the properties of the tissue are likely to change with time. A reduction in the response to a given dose of drug can come about by either a change in *responsiveness* or by a change in *sensitivity*. Without knowledge of more than one point on the **dose–response curve**, these possibilities cannot be distinguished, but pharmacologists often (unthinkingly) ascribe alterations to changes in sensitivity.

resultant analysis   (L. *resultare*, to happen, to rebound;
                                                  Gr. *ana*, up, again, back; *luein*, to loosen)
- Method for distinguishing between true competitiveness at a common site on a receptor and **allosteric interaction**. The method involves measuring antagonism of the test antagonist in conjunction with that of a reference antagonist.   See **competition**

resume   See **curriculum vitae (CV)**

retro-   (L. *retro*, backwards)
- Prefix meaning backwards, as in **retrograde** (backward step).

retrograde messenger   (L. *retro*, backwards; *gradus*, step; *mittere*, to send)
- A transmitter (messenger) produced on the postsynaptic side (effector cell) of the synapse, which diffuses back across the synaptic cleft to act at a presynaptic **autoreceptor**.

retrospective study   (L. *retro*, behind, in time; *specere*, to look)
- Looking backwards in time; surveying the past.
- Describes a scientific study in which it is sought to distinguish (causal) relationships for an already observed event; a **case-control study**.
                                                  See **cohort study, prospective study**

'retrospectoscope' (use of)   (L. *retro*, behind, in time; Gr. *skopeion*,
                                                  to look at, examine)
- The only infallible scientific instrument; a whimsical version of *hindsight*, i.e. being wise after the event.

retrovirus   (L. *retro*, backwards; *virus*, slimy liquid, poison)
- A **virus** that inserts the DNA for its own synthesis into the DNA of the host.
                                                  See **reverse transcriptase/-ion**

revenge effect   (L. *re,* again, *vindicare*, to lay claim)
- The unintended, *ironic* results of mechanical, biological, chemical and

medical (supposed) improvements and ingenuity; examples include second cancers (but not loss of hair) due to cancer chemotherapy and drug-resistant microbes that are even harder to combat. E Tenner, who cleverly invented the term, offers a positive (optimistic) corollary "sometimes things can go right only by first going very wrong", e.g. in **regulation (official) of medicines**. See **laws, various**

reverse pharmacology (L. *revertere*, to turn back)

– The process whereby the knowledge of the pharmacology of a drug allows the discovery of a receptor and ligands or transmitters. For example, although the pharmacology of **cannabinoids** was quite well understood by the late 1980s, no **receptor** had been identified for them until **molecular biology** techniques revealed the presence of a receptor-like DNA sequence in the brain. When the properties of the receptor cloned from this DNA were examined, it turned out to be the missing cannabinoid receptor, for which (presumably) there is an endogenous ligand (the anandamines). A similar process employing more traditional technology enabled the isolation and characterization of the **endorphins**. The starting point for this search was the belief that opioid drugs *must* act via specific **receptors**. See **opiate/opioid**

reverse transcriptase/-ion (L. *revertere*, to turn again; *trans*, across; *scribere*, to write)

– The synthesis of DNA on an RNA template. Reverse **transcription** is the process by which a **retrovirus** incorporates its own DNA into the DNA of the host. It is accomplished by the enzyme *reverse transcriptase*.

review articles (L. *re*, again, back; *videre*, to see)

– The number of original scientific articles is, in many areas, overwhelming even to workers in those fields. Therefore review articles flourish – even up to 12 for every 100 articles published. Reviews are becoming the "cribs of the overworked scientist seeking a short cut". Do reviews (by casually chosen researchers) become the sole source of information? There are at least a dozen journals (in science generally) "devoted to a constant monthly issuance of reviews". "Is quality science and critical reading of the original literature best achieved through a rear-view mirror?" (*MJ Ignatius*, 1992). But high-quality, fully referenced reviews that are thorough, critically evaluate (not merely report) the claims of research reports, and offer syntheses and novel insights are to be treasured. *Pharmacological Reviews* is such a journal. See **publication** (*Ghost-writing*)**, systematic review**

Reye's syndrome (*RDK Reye*, pathologist, Australia)

– Fatty liver with encephalopathy seen in children under 15 years old. The cause (or causes) is unknown, but it is usually, although not always, associated with ingestion of **aspirin**. Although rare, it is serious (50 per cent mortality) and, in 1986, aspirin was labelled as **contraindicated** in children under 12 years old "unless specifically indicated", e.g. for juvenile rheumatoid arthritis (**BNF**). Although doubts have since been expressed, the association is generally accepted as being causal. Official medicines regulatory authorities are always in the dilemma – to warn *early, and* to be *right.*   See **regret avoidance**

rheology   (Gr. *rheos,* stream)
- The study of the deformation and flow of material; it includes blood flow and viscosity, flow of powders etc.

rhetoric of science   (Gr. *rhetoike,* the art of words)
- Rhetoric practices "Mere persuasion, in contrast to logic and scientific method that yield truth" (*Nature*).

right   (Old Eng. *riht*)
- A claim that should be recognized by **natural justice**, principles of morality and/or by law. A moral right is not necessarily protected by law. A legal right is protected by the legal system and may, or may not, have a moral basis. No moral right is absolute (for rights can conflict) and this is the reason rights are so contentious.   See **Declaration of Helsinki, law**

riot control or incapacitating agents   (Old Fr. *riote*; L. *in*, expresses negation; *capax*, hold)
- Also known as *harassing or disabling agents*; substances that are capable, when used in field conditions, of rapidly causing temporary disablement that lasts for little longer than the period of exposure (**WHO**). The **half-life** in the body is about 5 seconds; examples include CS (chlorobenzylidene malonitrile), a 'tear gas' (in fact disseminated as a solid **aerosol** or smoke), and CN (chloroacetophenone); CR (dibenzoxazepine) is stable in water and so can be used in 'water cannons'. Detailed pharmacological data are difficult to get as both users and producers are bashful about their business. Some particularly cause lachrymation (lachrymators; L. *lachrima*, tear) and others sneezing (sternutators; L. *sternutatio*). It is not clear that these substances are submitted to official (statutory) regulatory or licensing bodies that command general respect. **Formulations** are available for both group and individual use; the latter include pepper sprays.

risk   (L. *riscare*, to run into danger)
- The probability that a particular adverse outcome occurs during a given **quantum** of exposure to **hazard** (*Royal Society of London*). The concept also includes the *severity* of the adverse event, i.e. risk = probability × severity.
- *Calculated risk*: a risk deliberately taken (*not* a risk the exact magnitude of which can be determined). (L. *calculus*, small stone used in reckoning)
- *Acceptable risk*: the acceptable level is the level which is 'good enough', where 'good enough' means you think the advantages of increased safety are not worth the costs of reducing risk by restricting or otherwise altering the activity (*Fischoff et al.* 1978).
- *Attributable risk*: the difference between two **incidence** rates.
- *Objective and perceived risk*: the assessment based on statistical extrapolation and the assessment based on public perceptions. These can be very different.

– *Relative and absolute risk*: The results of therapeutic trials are commonly expressed as per cent reduction of an unfavourable (or % increase in a favourable) outcome, i.e. as *relative risk* (*risk ratio*) and this can be very impressive indeed until the figures are presented as the number of individuals actually benefited per 100 people treated, i.e. as *absolute risk*.

See **percentages**.

– Where a baseline risk is *low*, a statement of relative risk alone is particularly misleading (it implies big benefit where actual benefit is small); e.g., reduction of risk from 2% to 1% is 50% relative risk reduction, but it saves only one patient for every 100 patients treated. But where the baseline is high, say 40%, a 50% reduction in relative risk saves 20 patients for every 100 treated. This is expressed as the *absolute risk* or the **number needed to treat** (or the number of events prevented per 100 people treated).

– *Absolute risk* is the difference in the probabilities of an event in the control and treatment groups estimated as the corresponding difference in the event rates (*RJ Cook, DL Sackett*).

– *Relative risk* is the probability of an event in the active treatment group divided by the probability of an event in the control group. *Relative risk reduction* is derived by subtracting the relative risk from one; or by dividing absolute risk reduction by the probability of an event in the control arm (after *RJ Cook, DL Sackett*).

See **number needed to treat, odds ratio**

– *Floating absolute risk*: "The standard method of comparing the risk in each group with a baseline group is unsatisfactory because the standard errors and confidence limits relate to correlated parameters, all dependent on precision within the baseline group. We describe the construction of standard error for the parameters of all groups, without the need to select a baseline group. These standard errors can be regarded as relating to roughly independent parameters, so that groups can be compared efficiently without knowledge of the **covariances**. The method should assist in graphical presentation of relative risks and in the combination of results from published studies" (*DF Easton et al*. Floating absolute risk: an alternative to relative risk in survival and case-control analysis avoiding an arbitrary reference group. *Statistics in Medicine* 1991;10:1025).

– *Clinical research* **ethics committees** are now provided with **guidelines** from multiple sources, official and unofficial. In seeking to assist the committees in their assessment of risk, these guidelines commonly use qualifying terms that are not defined, and perhaps cannot be defined because interpretation is so **subjective**, and they have different implications for different people in different circumstances, e.g. according to whether the subject is healthy, or sick with minor or with major disease, or what expectation of personal benefit there may or may not be. Terms used to quantify (or qualify) risk include: acceptable, minimal, negligible, trivial, insignificant, unacceptable, substantial. Where guidelines and commentators do offer definitions, they are frequently obscure or contentious and differ from those of other guidelines. Research subjects, too, may take a view very different from that of a committee.

– *Phantom risk*: "Cause-and-effect relationships whose very existence is unproven and perhaps unprovable" (*KR Foster, DE Bernstein, PW Huber*, eds

Phantom Risk; Scientific Inference and the Law. MIT Press, 1993). For example, the assumption that all animal carcinogens lead to cancer risk in humans at all levels of exposure. The possibility that a substance may cause an undetectably small increase in, for example, the rate of cancer or birth defects, cannot be ruled out by science. Proof that something does not occur is logically impossible. It is in these situations that precise knowledge of causative mechanisms can come to the rescue; which is an argument for increased research (and funding).

- *Risk rating scale*: Despite the lack of consensus we offer a risk rating scale (UK Department of Health, 1996)

High	–	>1:100
Moderate	–	1:100–1:1 000
Low	–	1:1 000–1:10 000
Very low	–	1:10 000–1:100 000
Minimal	–	1:100 000–1:1 000 000
Negligible	–	<1:1 000 000

See **benefit/risk evaluation, odds ratio**

risk tolerance   (L. *riscare*, to run into danger; L. *tolerare*, to endure)
- The preparedness to accept a certain level of **risk** in order to enjoy a given level of benefit: "...tolerability does not mean acceptability. It refers to the willingness to live with a risk to secure certain benefits and in the confidence that it is being properly controlled. To tolerate a risk means that we do not regard it as negligible or something that we might ignore, but rather as something we need to keep under review and to reduce still further if and as we can" (from *F Layfield*, Sizewell B [nuclear power station] public enquiry: Summary of considerations and recommendations. London, HM Stationery Office, 1987). This also applies to drugs.

robust   (L. *robustus*, firm, from *robus*, oak tree)
- A statistical procedure is robust if its assumptions can be violated without substantial effects on its conclusions **(FDA)**.

routes of administration of drugs   (Old Fr. *rute*)
- Virtually every route that ingenuity can devise and technology can allow has been used, e.g. intravascular (intravenous, intra-arterial), intramuscular, subcutaneous, inhalation, topical (local, e.g. skin, eye), intradermal, transdermal, intranasal, intrapleural, per rectum, intrathecal. The terms are generally self-evident and a comprehensive list would be wearisome. But see **inhalation (of drugs)**

run-in period   (Old Eng. *rinnan*; *in*; Gr. *peri*, around; *odos*, way)
- Preparing a research subject to meet the formal entry requirements in a clinical experiment/**therapeutic trial**, e.g. adjusting pre-existing treatment.

safety (L. *salvus*, safety)
- Not involving danger.
- In the case of drugs, safety is a *relative* concept, relative to other drugs for the same purpose and to importance of the disease (e.g. cancer or insomnia).
- Safety refers to the freedom from harm or damage resulting from **adverse drug reactions** or physical, or behavioural abnormalities that occur as a result of drug or non-drug use (after **FDA**).
- Safety of **medicinal products** is judged in relation to the purpose for which they are proposed to be administered (Medicines Act, UK).

Salvarsan (L. *salvare*, save + arsenic = the arsenical substance that saves)
- Proprietary name for arsphenamine, Ehrlich's 'compound 606' (the 606th synthetic compound tested). Prepared in 1907, but at first thought to be inactive against syphilis, it entered human trials in 1910. Ehrlich announced the successful treatment of syphilis with Salvarsan in April of that year. It went on the market at the end of 1910, and it and its close **analogues**, e.g. *Neosalvarsan*, remained the standard treatment for syphilis until the introduction of penicillin in 1945. This was the breakthrough compound for which Ehrlich had searched, and to which he had given the name 'magic bullet' (*Paul Ehrlich*, 1854–1915, German scientist). See **chemotherapy**

same drug/different drug
- The USA **FDA** has proposed the following to determine whether two drugs are the 'same drugs' or 'different drugs' for the purpose of granting market exclusivity. The agency proposes that two drugs would be considered the same if their principal, but not necessarily all their structural features were the same, unless the subsequent drug were shown to be clinically superior. Thus, for macromolecules, two protein drugs would be considered the same if the only difference in structure were minor differences in amino acid sequence. This would protect the first approved drug product against a second sponsor's attempt to defeat exclusivity by introducing minor and biologically insignificant molecular changes. See **generic drugs**

sample/sampling (Old Fr. *essample*)
- A representative subset of a group or population.
- In biological and medical science it is often desired to know what are the characteristics of large populations. Since it is impractical to study each member of a large population, it is necessary to study a small population and to draw conclusions that will be accurate when applied to the large population. This is done by *sampling*. Samples should be drawn by a strictly **random** process to minimize the chance of **bias** (sampling error); but sometimes **convenience sampling** is unavoidable.
- *Sample size*: The number of items/elements/subjects in a sample. The size of a sample is determined by the needed accuracy of the final estimate/outcome. It depends on the variability of the collected data, the magnitude of the effect to be detected and the acceptability of **error** in relation to certainty. See **power in statistics**

sample size in therapeutic trials
– "If the smallest difference of clinical relevance can be specified we can calculate the sample size necessary to have a high probability of obtaining a statistically significant result – that is, high power – if that is the true difference" (*DG Altman*).   See **power in statistics, convenience sample**

SAR
– **Structure–activity relationship.**

sarafotoxin   See **drugs as tools**

saralasin   See **drugs as tools**

saturation kinetics, dose-dependent kinetics(L. *satus*, enough; Gr. *kineo*, move)
– *Saturation*: stage at which no more can be achieved.
– In *drug elimination*, if the plasma concentration of a drug is high enough, enzymatic elimination mechanisms may become saturated, so that further increases in concentration are accompanied by *proportionately* smaller increases in elimination rate than at lower concentrations, i.e. the elimination process is no longer **first-order**. At saturation the elimination rate becomes constant, and independent of drug concentration (i.e. **zero-order**) and not first-order, and therefore cannot be characterized by a **half-life**. At saturation, increases in dosage cause the plasma concentration to rise without coming to **steady state**. Saturation kinetics are sometimes misleadingly termed 'non-linear kinetics'. Another term is **Michaelis–Menten** kinetics.
                    See **exponential curve/equation/function, exponential kinetics**

saxitoxin   See **drugs as tools**

Scatchard plot   See **reciprocal plot**

scatter diagram/plot   (Old Eng. var. of *shatter*,
                                               Gr. *dia*, through, between; *grapho*, write)
– A **plot** of observations (e.g. death rate) against an independent variable (e.g. time, temperature) or, more commonly, against another observation (e.g. body weight). Useful in the preliminary evaluation of numerical data: it reveals to the observant eye the likely presence (or absence) of a relationship between two characteristics, and broadly the nature of any relationship, e.g. whether it is a straight line or not.

scedasticity   (Gr. *skedasis*, a scattering)
                                          See **heteroscedasticity, transformation**

scepticism   (Gr. *scepsis*, enquiry, doubt)
– An attitude of mind that questions facts, truth, soundness of inference.

Schild equation/plot
– *Gaddum–Schild equation*:
    – An equation that describes, under a wide range of assumptions, the effect

(as measured by the **concentration ratio** or *dose ratio*) of a competitive antagonist at equilibrium, as a function of the antagonist concentration:

Concentration ratio $= 1 + B / K_B$

where B is the concentration of antagonist and K_B is the **dissociation equilibrium constant** for binding of the antagonist to the agonist binding site (**receptor**).
- *Schild equation*:
  - If the Gaddum–Schild equation is expressed in logarithmic form, it becomes the equation for a straight line:

Log(concentration ratio-1) $= \log B - \log K_B$.

- *Schild plot*:
  - A graphical method for measuring the **potency** of **competitive antagonists**. For a fuller account see **Arunlakshana & Schild method**.
  See **Cheng & Prussoff equation, pA_2/pA_x**

science/scientific method (in pharmacology)   (L. *scientia* knowledge; Gr. *meta*, with; *hodos*, way)
- The persistent effort of men and women to purify, extend and organize the knowledge of the world in which they live (*A Flexner*, American physician and educator, b 1866).
- The body of knowledge obtained by scientific method.
- Ordered knowledge of natural phenomena and of the relations between them.
- Systematic, organized, formulated knowledge.
- The unity of all science consists in its method alone, not in its material.
- Science is merely common sense writ large. It is a part of common sense to be critical. It is part of common sense to submit our common-sense views to criticism, and science is, simply, the result of this criticism.
- A theory belongs to **empirical** science if we can say what kind of event we should accept as a refutation. Or, in other words, a theory belongs to science if it is, in principle, refutable. A theory that cannot clash with any possible or conceivable event is, according to this view, outside science (e.g. religions, Freudianism).
- We cannot identify science with truth, for we think that both Newton's and Einstein's theories belong to science, but they cannot both be true, and they may well both be false. But they are both testable, which means that if they do not stand up to tests they are refuted. "Thus I take testability, or refutability, as a criterion of scientific character" (*K Popper*).
- Thus the general picture of science is: we choose some interesting problem. We propose a theory as a tentative solution. We try our best to criticise the theory, and this means we try to refute it. If we succeed in our refutation, then we try to produce a new theory, which we shall again criticise, and so on...The whole procedure can be summed up by the words: bold conjectures controlled by severe criticism which includes severe tests. And criticism, and tests, are attempted refutations...Observation and experiment are essentially

- At any one time the overwhelming majority of scientists are not trying to refute prevailing orthodoxy, but are working happily within it...what they are doing is putting accepted theories to work.
  (The above items are largely from Karl Popper (1902–1994), professor of Logic and Scientific Method, London School of Economics and Political Science, UK.)
- Hermann Bondi (b. 1919, mathematician, UK) has stated simply: "there is no more to science than its method, and there is no more to its method than Popper has said".
- *Replication studies* are a cornerstone of science in general and of pharmacology and clinical science in particular. Replication studies do not necessarily have to copy *precisely* the original study, for then they would repeat any defect of design.
- There are two principal kinds of scientific method:
  - **Observational study** or **survey**, in which there is no active intervention or interaction by the investigator and which provides *correlations*, e.g. **case-control studies**, but which alone gives little information on causation, and
  - **Experiment**, in which the investigator creates a situation as wished, to test a hypothesis; information on causation may be gained through appropriately designed experiments (see *Magee* above and ***post hoc ergo propter hoc***).
- *To decide whether an observed association (correlation) is causal*, several criteria, no one of which alone is sufficient, must be satisfied. These include:
  - *Consistency* of association: diverse methods of approach should give the same answer.
  - *Specificity* and *strength* of association: specificity means the precision with which the presence of, say, chronic bronchitis or lung cancer, can be used to predict that the victim smokes and vice versa – also that the size of effect should be sufficient not to be obscured by any associated but noncausal factors, e.g. alcohol consumption; and a correlation of effect (disease) with dose (amount smoked) is also important. See **confounding**.
  - *Temporal* association: the supposed cause (e.g. smoking), must operate before any evidence of the disease appears.
  - *Coherence* of association: the associated event should fit in with all known facts of the natural history of the disease.
  - To these may be added: biological gradient; biological plausibility; experiment; analogy.
- "There is not one science of chemistry, another of electricity, another of medicine and so on; there are not even distinct sciences of peace and war. There is only one natural world and only one knowledge of it" (*W Bragg*, 1941, physicist, UK).
- "Science is the topography of ignorance" (*OW Holmes*, 1809–1894, author, US).
- "Science is nothing but perception" (*Plato*, ?427–347 BCE, philosopher, Greece).
- "The great tragedy of science – the slaying of a beautiful **hypothesis** by an ugly fact" (*TH Huxley*, 1825–1895, biologist, UK).

- "There are no such things as applied science, only applications of science" (*L Pasteur*, 1822–1895, chemist, France).
- "The whole of science is nothing more than a refinement of everyday thinking" (*A Einstein*, 1879–1955, physicist–mathematician, US).
- "Vacuum-cleaner science": the idea/practice that the mindless accumulation of observations is sufficient to constitute scientific activity.
- Science is the search for generalization.
- Science has *two main aspects*; the systematic recording of observations and the construction of rigorous theories to explain them (*Nature*).
- Scientific discovery is made when both the technology is available and the concepts are in place.
- The practice of science – "construct a refutable hypothesis: test: publish" (*JH Baron*).
- Science is a self-correcting institution striving to find truth based on published data.
- The scientific method is a device to compel objectivity and restrain the natural urge of experimenters to believe in their own ideas (*N Wade*).
- "For the great majority of people, believing in the truths of science is unavoidably an act of faith. Most of us neither witness the successful experiments nor would we be able to understand them if we did. So we put an extraordinary amount of trust in things we know virtually nothing about (very few people interrogate their anaesthetists)" (*A Phillips*).
  See **deduction, hypothesis, induction, knowledge, law, true/truth**

science and technology   (L. *scientia*, knowledge; Gr. *tekhne*, art)
- Science creates *understanding* of the world. Technology applies science in order to *manipulate* the world, particularly to achieve practical useful ends.

Science Citation Index   (L. *citare*, to set moving; *in*, within; *dic*, point out)
- "A citation index is a directory of cited references where each reference is accompanied by a list of source documents which cite it." "The user begins a search with a specific known paper (target reference). From this starting point one is brought *forwards* in time to subsequent papers related to the earlier paper" (*Institute for Scientific Information Inc., USA*). An enquirer can thus follow up work on a subject *subsequent* to a publication. The *Index* is enormous and therefore expensive, and it expands rapidly. Consequently it is available only in large science libraries. Up to 50 per cent of scientific publications are never cited.   See **impact factor**

science (neutrality of)
- This concept makes the claim that science is not the source of social/moral problems. These arise from the misuse of science. Science is neutral if it is uncontaminated by values. The concept is advanced to protect scientists from social, governmental and economic values. But science serves three masters, the cause of **truth**, the moral values current in society, and the often utilitarian requirements of those who pay. In medical pharmacological research the concept arouses little debate – values and utility reign.

scientific evidence in courts of law
- Issues involving drugs, particularly adverse reactions, increasingly reach the courts of law. "The question of what constitutes valid scientific data, suitable for admission as evidence in court has plagued judges for decades." "Judges have a legal duty of deciding what may or may not be presented to a jury." The US Supreme Court has clarified the rules on the use of scientific evidence, making judges responsible for ensuring that "any and all scientific testimony or evidence admitted is not only relevant, but reliable". The Supreme Court says the test should be *whether the methods used to reach conclusions are sound*. That means that US judges must now sift reliable from ill-founded science by considering *whether the claim is testable, whether it has been empirically tested and whether testing has been carried out according to a scientific methodology* (*Nature* 1993).

scientific imperialism   (L. *imperium*, command, authority, empire)
- Imperialism is the extension of one state's rule or influence over another whether in general government or in particular areas, e.g. economics, science. So enormously financially powerful are multinational companies that they now have what is the equivalent of the power of a state in relation to developing countries. A sum of money that is enough to transform an individual's life is trivial to such companies, seeking to obtain advantage.
- A manifestation of scientific imperialism is the conduct of clinical drug development in developing societies or countries where people are unlikely to benefit from their role as research subjects because most of the population is too poor to buy effective treatment in the future, including that which has benefited them in the clinical trial in which they have participated.
- Reasons for such studies include lower research costs and risk of litigation, less stringent ethical review, the availability of populations prepared to give unquestioning consent, anticipated under-reporting of adverse reactions due to lower consumer awareness, and the desire for personal advancement (in both investigators and patients) (after *P Wilmshurst*).
- For discussion of this under-discussed area by a range of informed and concerned people, see *British Medical Journal* 1997;314:840 & 887–891.

scientific misconduct   See **research misconduct**

scientific papers for publication
See **authorship, clinical trials (unreported),
IMRAD, International Committee of Medical Journal Editors, publication**

scientism
- The belief that science/scientific method *alone* can provide **knowledge**. Denial of any validity to non-scientific approaches, e.g. moral reasoning, the literary arts, religious experience.

scientist   (L. *scientia*, knowledge)
- "We need very much a name to describe a cultivator of science in general. I

should incline to call him a *scientist*" (*W Whewell*, 1794–1866, mathematician, geologist, etc. UK; in 1840 he also coined the words *anode* and *cathode*).

scintillation proximity assay (L. *scintillare*, to sparkle; *proximare*, to approach; *exigere*, to examine or test; hence *exagium*, a weighing)
- Technique developed for *high throughput* **screens** in which microspheres containing a scintillant are structurally modified so that they will selectively bind biologically active molecules. When radioactively-labelled molecules bind to the microspheres, light will be emitted and this can be used as a signal that binding has occurred. The technique depends critically on the choice of isotope – the decay must result in the emission of a particle that has a very short path-length in the medium, so that it will reach and excite only the scintillant in microspheres in close proximity (ideally the microsphere to which the molecule is bound), but will not reach other microspheres in the medium.

sciolism (L. *sciolus*, someone with a smattering of knowledge, from *scire*, to know)
- The practice of giving opinions on matters of which one has only superficial knowledge.

sclerosing agents (Gr. *skleros*, to harden)
- Highly irritant substance used to cause inflammation with subsequent fibrosis (e.g. sodium morrhuate to obliterate varicose veins).

screen/-ing (Old Fr. *escren*, to examine for the presence of something)
- The **empirical** process of submitting compounds to a biological test or tests to detect an effect of particular interest ('goal-directed' screen), or simply the hope that something interesting will turn up ('blind' or 'open' screen).

SDA
- Serotonin–dopamine antagonist.

second gas effect
- The second gas effect occurs during induction of general anaesthesia when a mixture of two gaseous agents is inhaled. If one of them (e.g. nitrous oxide) being at high (75%) concentration enters the blood very rapidly (as much as one litre per minute) then "fresh gases are literally sucked into the lung" (*SK Kennedy, DE Longnecker*) with the result that the alveolar concentration of a concomitantly administered agent (e.g. enflurane at 1%) is increased.

See **diffusion hypoxia**

second messenger See **first messenger**

second-order kinetics See **first-order kinetics**

secretagogue (L. *secretum*, apart; *agoge*, a drawing forth)
- A drug that stimulates **exocrine** glandular secretion, e.g. pilocarpine.

316

sedative   (L. *sedatus*, assuaged)
- A drug (or dose of a drug) that calms or soothes without inducing sleep, although it may cause sleepiness. A small dose of a **hypnotic** or **anxiolytic** often suffices for sedation.

seeding trials   (Old Eng. *saed*; Old Fr. *trier*, to sift)
- Some company-sponsored trials of approved drugs appear to serve little or no scientific purpose. Because they are, in fact, thinly veiled attempts to entice doctors to prescribe a new drug being marketed by the company, they are often referred to as 'seeding trials.' Features that distinguish such trials from scientifically rigorous studies include the use of a design that does not support the stated research goals, the recruitment of investigators not because they are experts or leading researchers but because they are frequent prescribers of competing products in the same therapeutic class, disproportionately high payments given to 'investigators' for their work (although the only work may be to write prescriptions for the drugs), sponsorship of the studies by the company's sales and marketing division rather than its research department, minimal requirements for data, and the collection of data that are of little or no value to the company. Typically, these trials involve introducing a new drug in a crowded therapeutic class. The success of such a new product may depend on undoing physicians' comfortable habits of prescribing a competing, more established product (*DA Kessler*, ex-director US **FDA** and others, *New England Journal of Medicine* 1994;331:1350).

selective/-ity   (L. *se*, apart; *legere*, to choose)
- *General*: characterized by careful choice.
- *Pharmacology*: the capacity of a given concentration of substance to affect a single biological function, leaving others unaffected. Selectivity is fundamental to pharmacology, toxicology and therapeutics.
- Can be expressed as ratios of median effective doses or concentrations for different tissues (ED_{50} or EC_{50}), but more conveniently as ratios of potencies at the different tissues.
- The property of drugs to distinguish between receptors is often improperly called **specificity**. 'Selectivity' is almost always to be preferred.

selection bias (in clinical studies)   (L. *se*, apart; *legere*, to choose)
- A **bias** in assignment that occurs when the study and control groups differ from each other by one or more factors that affect the outcome of the study [but which are not the subject of the study] (**FDA**).
- Anything that produces systematic error (bias) in a study threatens its validity. In particular, studies conducted in hospital may give different (worse) results from those conducted in a primary care (general practice) setting because the severity of disease and prognosis of the patients is very different. This is known as *Berkson's paradox.*
- Great care must be taken in forming treatment groups in **therapeutic trials** and the comparability of the groups for relevant factors should be demonstrated in the report.

self-medication
- Use of a medicine "Intended for use without the intervention of a medical practitioner, with the advice of a pharmacist, if necessary" (**EC**).
See **supply of medicines**

self-poisoning   (Old Eng. *seolf*, distinct identity; L. *potio*, a drink)
- This may be accidental or deliberate, and medicines are the principal vehicle in communities where they are easy to obtain. If deliberate, it may be genuine attempted suicide or a gesture not intended seriously to endanger life (**para-suicide**). This latter occurs particularly in young women. The delinquent behaviour of young men is as troublesome, but commonly takes different forms (e.g. violence). The social causes are complex.

semantic   (Gr. *semantikos*, having a significance)
- Relating to the meaning of words.

semilogarithmic transformation   (Etymol., see **logarithm, transformation**)
- When one variable (usually the dependent **variable**) has a distribution which is **skewed, homoscedasticity** can often be achieved by plotting the *logarithm* of this variable against the untransformed variable. This is the case for dose– or concentration–response data (but note that the independent variable – dose or concentration – has the skewed distribution). Hence pharmacologists' predilection for log-concentration–response curves.
See **logarithmic transformation, normal distribution**

sensitivity   (L. *sentire*, to feel)
- *Of a test*: the percentage of subjects reliably classified for a property by use of the test, e.g. patients having a disease.
- A measure of the capacity of a tissue to recognize (react to) the presence of drug molecules: measured as the **dilution** at which a given effect is produced. It is the tissue-related equivalent of **potency**. Although EC_{50} is generally thought of as a property of a drug, it is also a convenient way of expressing the sensitivity of a tissue numerically. The relative sensitivities of different tissues can be expressed as the ratios of the EC_{50}s of a single drug when measured in each tissue.
- Sometimes used to mean the extent of **reactivity** to an external stimulus. This can be misleading as a large response can arise from either high sensitivity or from high **responsiveness**. Unless the dose(concentration)–response curve can be shown to be located at low doses (concentrations), i.e. the EC_{50}/ED_{50} is small, then it is dangerous to claim a high sensitivity.
See **hypersensitivity, responsiveness, sensitize, supersensitivity**

sensitivity analysis
- A technique used to test how **robust** a **model** is, especially in (pharmaco)-**economic** studies; the model is run several times with the assumed values of important **variables** changed systematically.

sensitize   (L. *sentire*, to feel)
- To increase the **sensitivity** (of a responding system). The correct way to use

the verb 'sensitize' is 'drug *x* sensitized the tissue to drug *y*' (not 'drug *x* sensitized the tissue to *the effect of* drug *y*' – effects are not measured in the same units as **sensitivity**).

sequential analysis   (L. *sequi*, to follow; Gr. *analusis*, a dissolving into parts)
– In a study (often a therapeutic trial) employing sequential analysis, the observations are examined as they become available, and the total number of subjects entering the study is not predetermined, but depends on the accumulating results. This approach has an appeal in clinical research since all the subjects of a proposed trial are rarely available at the outset. It also has ethical value, since it minimizes the use of inferior treatment by allowing the trial to cease as soon as the predetermined level of statistical significance has been reached. In this it is distinguished from the **fixed-sample trial**, where numbers to enter are predetermined. But sequential analysis is unsuitable for studies where a difference is, in the event, not found, for it is then liable to involve enormous numbers of subjects. Various modifications have been developed, e.g. **interim analysis**, to avoid the disadvantages while retaining the advantages of sequential analysis, i.e. *modified sequential designs*.

serendipity
– The faculty of making fortunate discoveries by accident or by general sagacity. A term coined by Horace Walpole (1678–1757) from a fairy tale of three princes of Serendip (Ceylon, Sri Lanka) who possessed this happy capacity.
– The serendipity berry (*Dioscoreophyllum cumminsii*) contains a protein called monellin which is 100 000 times as sweet as sucrose and has been used as a low calorie food sweetener; but it is heat labile.

serenic agent   (L. *serenus*, calm weather)
– A drug producing (the illusion of) serenity.
– A drug that induces a dose-dependent inhibition of aggression in animals (and, it is hoped, in man), without causing sedation, motor impairment, sensory incapacity or reduced social interaction. The term is little used.
                                                           See **tranquillizer**

serotonin: 5-hydroxytryptamine: 5-HT   (L. *serum*, whey; Gr. *tonos*, tension)
– An **autacoid** and neurotransmitter that stimulates most smooth muscle. It is present in blood platelets, enterochromaffin cells (e.g. in the gastrointestinal tract) and brain. It acquired its name because serum from clotted blood has a vasoconstrictor effect, although some vessels, e.g. those in the skin, are dilated.   See **argentaffin/-oma**

serpentine receptors   See **receptor** (*Heptahelical*)

shelf-life   (Old Eng. *scylfe*, partition; *lif*, life)
– The time for which a drug formulation can be stored (under stated conditions, e.g. of temperature) without significant (specified) deterioration. Five years is generally deemed appropriate for medicines, where it can be achieved. The

expiry date, i.e. the date at which the production batch reaches the end of its shelf-life, should be stated on the container.

'shelf shaking'
– In the search for new drugs, chemical entities that have been synthesized and **screened** for one type of activity are not thrown away when they seem to have no interesting action. They are stored in a 'chemical library'. At some later date, when a new type of drug is being sought, the storage shelves may be 'shaken' and these old chemicals screened for the new activity. A number of successful medicines have been found in this way, for example the benzodiazepines. Many potentially useful (and profitable) drugs are probably still sitting on shelves that have not been shaken.

'shot-gun' preparation
(Old Norse *skot*, shot; Icelandic *Gunnhildr*, a notable fierce woman)
– A formulation containing a large number of ingredients in the hope of benefiting any disease or deficiencies the patient has or may have (e.g. vitamins, minerals, folic acid mixtures as haematinics and as **tonics** for the ageing).

sialorrhoea/-agogue
(Gr. *sialon*, saliva; *rhein*, to flow; *agoge*, drawing forth)
– Increased flow of saliva, e.g. as caused by **parasympathomimetic** drugs (e.g. **muscarinic acetylcholine receptor** agonists).

side-effect
(Old Eng. *side*; L. *efficere*, to accomplish)
– An unwanted effect of a drug that is a predictable, dose-related action, occurring at ordinary therapeutic doses. It may be best to confine this term to minor effects and not to use it as synonymous with adverse reaction, but both terms are often used loosely to include trivial and serious effects.
– The effects of a drug other than those by which the drug is normally classified. The effects may be useful or adverse.　　　See **adverse drug reaction, parallel pharmacology, promiscuous drug, selectivity, unwanted effects**

SIF cells
– Small intensely-fluorescent cells.　　　　　　　　　See **APUD cells**

sigmoid
(Gr. *sigmoeides*, sigma-shaped)
– S-shaped.

Simpson's paradox
(Gr. *para*, beside, beyond; *doxa*, opinion)
– Where the association between two variables is confounded by a strong association with a third variable, it can happen that analysis including this third variable reverses the first observed effect. This can have clinical importance. See *EH Simpson*, The interpretation of interaction in contingency tables. *Journal of the Royal Statistical Society*, 1951;13(2):236.　　　See **confounding**

single-blind study
(L. *singulus*, individual; Old Eng. *blind*; L. *studere*, to be diligent)

– Where the patient, or the observer, but not both, is ignorant of what is being given. **See double-blind**

single-patient clinical (therapeutic) trial: *n* = 1 trial

– It is part of ordinary medical practice in patients having chronic stable disease that several treatments may be used serially on an informal trial-and-error basis to select that most suitable for the individual. Efforts to put this clinical practice on a firmer basis, and even to begin to allow extrapolation to other patients, employ the paraphernalia of the formal **therapeutic trial** in these single patients, random order of treatments, placebo, double-blind, etc., and these studies have been dignified by the term *n=1 trial*. Where the outcomes of several n=1 trials are put together and *appropriately* analysed statistically they provide a (small) **within-patient, cross-over trial**, though it generally has the disadvantage that each patient has been managed by a different investigator at a different place. Nevertheless useful information may be obtainable in chronic or rare diseases.

SI units (Système International d'Unités; International System of Units)

(L. *unus*, one)

– SI is the culmination of over 100 years of international effort to develop a universally acceptable system of units of measurement. It is essentially an expanded version of the metric system. It comprises units of three types: *base* units, *derived* units and *supplementary* units, and also includes a series of prefixes by means of which decimal multiples and submultiples of units can be formed. The base units are defined and redefined by the *Bureau International des Poids et Mesures* (BIPM), which meets every 4 years.

See tables displayed on pp. 322–323

skewed

(Old Fr. *eschuer*, to shun, avoid)

– Distorted or biased (in a non-technical sense) see **bias.**
– Of a **probability density function**: not symmetric (so, for example, **mean** and **median** differ). The **normal distribution** is symmetrical (not skewed); the **exponential distribution** is highly skewed.

SKF–525A

– A commercial code number of Smith Kline and French for *proadifen* (see under **drugs as tools**).

skin patch

See transdermal drug delivery system

SLAPP

– Strategic lawsuit against public participation. A device whereby "legal actions are used to harass citizens who speak out in a way threatening to developers, government bodies and other vested interests", e.g by alleging defamation (*B Martin*).

slip

(Middle Low Ger., *slippen*)

– Biochemical processes such as ion pumps are not always completely cou-

- Strategic lawsuit against public participation. A device whereby "legal actions are used to harass citizens who speak out in a way threatening to developers, government bodies and other vested interests", e.g. by alleging defamation (*B Martin*).

slip (Middle Low Ger., *slippen*)
- Biochemical processes such as ion pumps are not always completely coupled. This lack of coupling, or 'slip', is advantageous to the function of biochemical transport mechanisms, because it balances the accumulated high-energy intermediate formed during certain energy flow steps and hence prevents over-energization of membranes. Some **ATP**ases exhibit slip.

slow receptors
- **Jargon** name for **receptors** that are linked via a **G-protein** either to an enzyme that produces an intracellular **second messenger** or to an **ion channel**. These receptors belong to a **superfamily of receptors** all of which consist of a single, continuous, polypeptide chain with seven membrane-spanning regions (**domains**) (see Figure).
   See **fast receptors, metabotropic receptors, receptors** (*Heptahelical*)

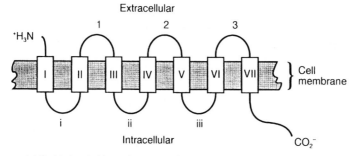

I–VII: Hydrophobic regions embedded in cell membrane
1–3: Hydrophilic extracellular loops
i–iii: Hydrophilic intracellular loops

See SI units, tables displayed on pp. 322–323

— *NAMES AND SYMBOLS FOR **SI** BASE UNITS (see p. 320):*

Physical quantity	Unit	Symbol
length	metre	m
mass	kilogram*	kg
time	second	s
electric current	ampere	A
thermodynamic temperature	kelvin	K**
luminous intensity	candela	cd
amount of substance	mole	mol

*For historical reasons one of the SI units, the kilogram, *incorporates a prefix [k]*. The symbol (kg), when unmodified, should be regarded as an entity. However, decimal multiples and fractions of the kilogram are formed by attaching the appropriate prefix to the symbol g (*not* to kg) despite the fact that *the gram is not a base unit for SI*. Thus 10^{-6} kg is written mg (*not* μkg). It follows that 10^{-3} kg is written g (*not* mkg), so *the appearance of gram or g is valid when the context requires it (DN Baron).*

** The thermodynamic temperature scale is based on the relationship between heat and mechanical work, but the kelvin is defined in terms of a measurable *thermometric point*, the triple point of water. Zero on the Celsius scale is now *defined* as 0.01 K below the triple point of water (i.e. the triple point of water is 273.16 K, and 0°C = 273.15 K). Temperature *differences* may be expressed in either degrees Celsius or in kelvins; for this purpose °C and K are interchangeable. It should be noted that the unit of measurement is the 'kelvin', not 'degree kelvin', and that its symbol is K, not °K (**WHO**, *DN Baron*).

*** Symbols for units do not change in the plural. Example: five kilometres is written 5 km , not 5 kms.

Symbols for units are never followed by a full stop (period), unless they occur at the end of a sentence. Examples: 5 g (not 5 g.); 10 ml (not 10 ml.).

In writing numbers, either a comma or a dot on the line may be used as the decimal marker in English text, but a dot on the line should not be used as the decimal marker in any text in which this symbol is used to indicate multiplication. (In languages other than English, only the comma is used.) Most international bodies have indicated a preference for the use of the comma. A raised dot (for example, 5·2) should never be used (the raised dot is reserved as a symbol to indicate multiplication). (The SI for the Health Professions: **WHO**). The implications for international travellers are evident.

****Use of the *solidus* (stroke). No more than one solidus should ever be used in the symbol for a unit, e.g. mg/kg/day, unless ambiguity is removed by the use of parentheses, e.g. (mg/kg)/day is intended, not mg/(kg/day).

— *NAMES AND SYMBOLS FOR SUPPLEMENTARY UNITS:*

Physical quantity	Unit	Symbol
plane angle	radian	rad
solid angle	steradian	sr

— *PREFIXES*: the following prefixes should be used for decimal fractions and multiples of SI units, rather than 10^{x} or 10^{-x}

Factor	Prefix	Symbol	Factor	Prefix	Symbol
10^{-1}	deci	d	10^{1}	deca/deka	da
10^{-2}	centi	c	10^{2}	hecto	h
10^{-3}	milli	m	10^{3}	kilo	k
10^{-6}	micro	μ	10^{6}	mega	M
10^{-9}	nano	n	10^{9}	giga	G
10^{-12}	pico	p	10^{12}	tera	T
10^{-15}	femto	f	10^{15}	peta	P
10^{-18}	atta	a	10^{18}	exa	E

(Some more extreme prefixes have been named: zepto, yocto, xenno, vendeko).

– *SOME SI DERIVED UNITS:*
(i.e. units formed by multiplying a base unit by itself or by combining two or more base units by multiplication or division).

Quantity	Name of derived unit	Symbol
area	square metre	m^2
volume	cubic metre	m^3
speed	metre per second	m/s
acceleration	metre per second squared	m/s^2
substance concentration	mole per cubic metre	mol/m^3

– *SOME SI DERIVED UNITS WITH SPECIAL NAMES:*

Name	Symbol	Physical quantity
becquerel	Bq	Activity (radionuclide)
coulomb	C	Electric charge
degree Celsius	°C	Celsius temperature
farad	F	Capacitance
gray	Gy	Absorbed dose (radiation)
hertz	Hz	Frequency
joule	J	Energy/work/quantity of heat
newton	N	Force
ohm	Ω	Electric resistance
pascal	Pa	Pressure
siemens	S	Electric conductance
sievert	Sv	Dose equivalent (radiation)
volt	V	Electric potential
watt	W	Power

– *NON-SI UNITS ACCEPTED FOR GENERAL USE:*

Physical quantity	Name of unit	Symbol
time	minute	min
time	hour	h
time	day	d
plane angle	degree	°
plane angle	minute	'
plane angle	second	"
volume	litre	l, L
mass	tonne	t

– For extensive treatment of SI units and related topics, see *DN Baron* (ed.); *Units, symbols, and abbreviations: a guide for medical and scientific editors and authors*, Royal Society of Medicine Press, London, W1M 8AE, UK; also international reports obtainable from national standardization institutes (current editions).

slush fund   (*Slush*, origin unknown – possibly Old Eng., onomatopoeic)
- A fund accumulated to buy extra luxuries for seamen by selling waste fat from a ship's galley after a voyage (in the days of long sailing voyages).
- A secret fund for financing political corruption.
- The term used informally in business and in academia for funds that may be spent for purposes that are not formally approved, e.g. entertainment, gifts, travel. Corruption is not an essential feature, although secret, unaudited spending inevitably leads to suspicion.   See **discretionary fund**

SMART
- Submission Management and Review Tracking (**FDA** regulatory term).

'smart' drugs
- A vulgar term for **nootropic** drugs. The USA regulatory authority (**FDA**) has warned that it may intervene over the promotion, as smart drugs, of vitamins, minerals, amino acids and prescription drugs.

smoking as a route of drug administration   (Old Eng. *smeocan*, emit smoke)
- A variety of drugs may be smoked (inhaled) for local pulmonary or systemic effect, e.g. stramonium for asthma (obsolete), marihuana, cocaine.
- In 1995 the **FDA** designated *cigarettes* (tobacco) as *drug delivery systems*, and as such liable to official drug regulation. The tobacco industry signified its opposition to this decision.   See **inhalation of drugs**

SMON   See **clioquinol**

SNRI
- Serotonin noradrenaline/norepinephrine reuptake inhibitor.

societal drug   (L. *socius*, companion)
- A drug, the use of which has impact beyond the patient for whom it is prescribed, e.g. **antimicrobial drugs** and the spread of drug-resistant organisms, some **psychotropic** drugs.

SOD
- **S**uper**o**xide **d**ismutase.   See **free radical scavenger**

'soft' drug   See **'hard' drug**

solid-dose imprinting
- It is self-evident that solid-dose forms (e.g. **tablets**, **capsules**) should be easily identifiable. Increasingly, regulatory authorities are requiring that **formulations** must bear a mark that, in conjunction with the product's shape, size and colour, permits identification of the active ingredients, dose, and manufacturer or distributor. The imprinted code may consist of numbers and/or letters, company name, and symbol, or a combination of these (after **FDA** regulations). With the smaller items, technical problems are considerable.

solidus (L. *solidus*, a gold coin)
- A short, oblique stroke used in written texts to separate items, alternative words, or numerator and denominator in fractions, e.g. mg/m^2/day. Avoid more than one solidus in any expression unless ambiguity is removed by the use of parentheses, thus (mg/m^2)/day. The tiresome solidus may be replaced by raising the function to the power −1. Thus mg/ml becomes mg ml^{-1}, and (mg/m^2)/day becomes mg m^{-2} day^{-1}. See **SI units**

solubility (L. *solvere*, to dissolve, release)
- The extent to which one substance will dissolve (i.e. be dispersed) in another:

Very soluble	1 in less than 1
Freely soluble	1 in less than 10
Soluble	1 in 10 to 1 in 30
Sparingly soluble	1 in 30 to 1 in 100
Slightly soluble	1 in 100 to 1 in 1000
Very slightly soluble	1 in 1000 to 1 in 10 000
Practically insoluble	1 in more than 10 000

(*British Pharmacopoeia*)

soluble tablet (L. *solvere*, to dissolve)
- The **tablet disintegrates** within 3 minutes when placed in water, and the active agent dissolves, although the solution may be opalescent due to added insoluble substances (**excipients**) used in the manufacture of the tablet.
See **dispersible tablet**

soma (Sanskrit *haoma*, juice)
- An intoxicating plant juice used in Vedic rituals. (The Vedas are ancient sacred Hindu writings.)
- L Lewin (*Phantastica*, 1927) regarded soma (or homa) as a strong alcoholic drink obtained by fermentation of a plant, and worshipped like the plant itself. He stated that none of the plants named as a source are able directly to induce the effects described, which are similar to those of alcohol.
- In 1932 Aldous Huxley in his novel *Brave New World* used the term to describe an imagined social drug that could be taken to provide holidays from reality but which had no adverse effects.

SOP
- **Standard operating procedure(s).**

sophisticated (Gr. *sophizesthai*, to act craftily; *sophistes*, a wise man)
- *Of a person*: having cultivated and refined tastes and habits.
- *Of methods, apparatus or machines*: complex and technically refined.
- The word and variations of it have long carried a pejorative (L. *pejorare*, to make worse) implication, but this no longer applies to the second use above.
See **state-of-the-art**

SPA See **scintillation proximity assay**

spare receptors   (Old Eng. *spaer*, sparing, frugal)
See **receptor**, **receptor reserve**

spasm   (Gr. *spasmos*, pull)
– A state of maintained muscle contraction.

spasmolytic   (Gr. *spasmos*, pull; *lusis*, loosen)
– Drug that relieves **spasm**. Usually applied to drugs that relieve intestinal colic
– usually **antagonists** at **muscarinic acetylcholine receptors**.

SPC (SmPC)
– **Summary of Product Characteristics**: in **EU** it replaces **data sheet**.
– Supplementary Protection Certificate. Certificate confirming the extension of a
pharmaceutical patent beyond its original term.

'special K'
– Street name for the drug ketamine used illicitly.
See **dissociative anaesthesia**

specialization   (L. *specere*, to look)
– "Knowledge is one. Its division into subjects is a [necessary] concession to
human weakness" (*HJ Mackinder*, 1861–1947, geographer, UK).

species   (L. *specere*, to look, and so, appearance, kind)
– Class of individuals/things having common qualities and/or characteristics.
– Kind, sort.

specific   (L. *specere*, to look and so, appearance, kind)
– *Noun*: An archaic concept. The name for a drug that is the perfect and only
cure for a condition. The *specific* was to the physician what the philosophers'
stone was to the alchemist.
– *Adjective*: Having only one effect. No drug is truly specific, although some are
highly **selective**.
– *Structurally specific*: Drugs that act by virtue of their precise three-
dimensional molecular structure, in contrast to those (structurally nonspecific) that act by virtue of their general physicochemical properties. Structurally specific drugs usually act via a **receptor**, which has complementary
structural features.   See **specificity**, **theriac**

specificity   (L. *specere*, to look and so, appearance, kind)
– A unique one-to-one relationship between an agent and that which is acted
upon, or an agent and the effect it produces. The **paradigm** of all specific relationships in biology is that which holds between **antigen** and **antibody**. It
commonly depends on the relative molecular configurations of the interacting
agents. In pharmacology the paradigm is drug and **receptor**, but at best a
drug is highly **selective** rather than (totally) specific.

- *Of a test*: the percentage of subjects reliably classified as having or not having a property by use of the test, e.g. healthy people as not having a disease.
See **selectivity, sensitivity, specific**

spectral density   (L. *spectare*, to observe; *densus*, thick)
- The spectral density function is a function of frequency that is used for analysis of electrical **noise**. It represents the amount of noise at each frequency; more precisely the area under the curve between two frequencies (compare **probability density**). The current through a piece of membrane containing ion channels that are randomly opening and shutting shows fluctuations (noise), described by a particular spectral density function called a *Lorenzian* (*LV Lorenz*, 1829–1895, physicist, Denmark), which can be regarded as the equivalent, in terms of noise, of an **exponential curve**. Spectral analysis of noise can give estimates of the properties of single channels when it is not possible to estimate the characteristics of a single ion channel directly (e.g. by **patch-clamp** analysis).

spectrophotometry   (L. *spectare*, to observe; Gr. *photos*, light; *metron*, measure)
- A technique for measuring the quantity of a substance on the basis of how much light of a particular wavelength it absorbs. Pure light of a single wavelength, usually in the visible or near-visible (i.e. including infrared and ultraviolet) spectrum, is shone through a solution of the substance under test. The absorption of light is proportional to the amount of substance in the light path, hence the concentration of the substance can be calculated from a separately-prepared calibration curve ('standard curve') of concentration v. absorption.

splicing
- The process by which **introns** are removed and **exons** joined together in RNA.

sponsor (regulatory term)   (L. *spondere*, to promise solemnly)
- An individual or an organization which takes responsibility for the initiation, management and/or financing of a clinical trial [or other research]. When an investigator independently initiates and takes full responsibility for a trial which may subsequently become a part of an application for a marketing authorization, the investigator then assumes the role of the sponsor as well (**EC/EU**).
- Investigators who negotiate contracts with sponsors should ensure that their freedom, in areas of ethics especially, is not restricted, e.g. by according the sponsor rights to prevent publication of results that the sponsor does not like.
- The proceedings of industrially sponsored promotional symposia sometimes achieve publication as supplements to reputable journals without effective **peer review**.

spreadsheet   (Old Eng. *spraeden*, to spread; *skeat*, cloth)
- A computer application, designed for analysis and prediction in economics

but useful in data collection and processing. A spreadsheet comprises an array of 'cells', each of which can contain a 'label' (a string of characters), a number, or an arithmetic expression that includes **variables**. The variables in the latter can be the numeric contents of other cells, which may themselves be arithmetic expressions. Changing the value contained in any one cell causes the contents of all the other cells which refer to this cell (directly or indirectly) to change, so that the values of all the expressions are simultaneously correct.

SR
– **Sustained-release (formulation).**

SRS-A
– Slow-reacting substance of **anaphylaxis**: now known to be a mixture of **leukotrienes**.

SSRI
– Selective **serotonin** reuptake inhibitor.

stability of medicinal products   (L. *stabilis, stare;* stand)
– Stability relates to the resistance of a product to change by chemical, physical and microbial reactions during transport, storage and use. Stability is expressed quantitatively as **shelf-life**; it is determined by long-term storage tests, 'field' (real-life) tests and by 'accelerated' tests (in which stresses, temperature, humidity, light, are exaggerated).   See **cold chain**

standard deviation   (L. *extendere,* to stretch out; *de,* from; *via,* road)
– Of a *sample*: A measure of the scatter, or dispersion, of the values in the sample. If the sample consists of n values of a variable y, i.e. $y_1, y_2, \ldots y_n$ the sample standard deviation (s) of y is:

$$s(y) = \sqrt{\frac{\sum (y_i - \bar{y})^2}{(n-1)}}$$

where $\bar{y}$ is the sample mean and $i = 1$ to n.
– Of a *population*: The true value, $\sigma(y)$, of which $s(y)$ provides an unbiased estimate.
– Of a *function*: If some quantity, such as a **mean** or slope of a line, is calculated from a sample of observations, we may wish to know its standard deviation as a measure of how precise it is. If only one experiment is done then we have only one mean (or slope) so the usual formula above cannot be used. However, it is possible to estimate theoretically the scatter that would be expected in repeated experiments. For example, the standard deviation of the mean of n values, $s(\bar{y})$ can be estimated as:

$$s(\bar{y}) = s(y) \div \sqrt{n}$$

This quantity is often called the **standard error of the mean (SEM)**.

standard deviation of the mean (L. *extendere*, to stretch out; *de*, from; *via*, road)
- A measure of **dispersion** or *scatter* of the sample means about the population **mean**; obtained by extracting the square root of the mean of the squared deviations of the observed values from their mean in a frequency distribution. It is synonymous with *sample* **standard error of the mean**.

standard error (SE) (L. *extendere*, to stretch out; *errare*, to err)
- Another term for **standard deviation**. Usually applied to an estimate of the standard deviation of some quantity (such as the **mean** of the slope of a line) calculated from a single sample of observations. See **estimate**

standard error of the mean (SEM)
- The distribution of the means of samples taken from a population with a **normal distribution** are themselves normally distributed about the population **mean**, but with a smaller standard deviation. This **standard deviation of the means** about the population mean is the *standard error of the mean* and is a statistic of *precision*, rather than of *dispersion*. It can be estimated from a sample standard deviation but, unlike the standard deviation of the sample, it is dependent upon the size of the sample. Consequently it is meaningless as a statistic unless the size of the sample ('n') is also quoted. It is popular among pharmacologists because it gives a rough estimate of the 95 per cent confidence interval for any mean, but being smaller than the **confidence interval** it looks tidier on graphs (95 per cent confidence interval = SEM × t, where t is **Student's t** for $n-1$ **degrees of freedom** and probability = 0.05).

standard gamble (Old Eng. *gamen*, game)
- "The standard gamble is the classical method of measuring cardinal preferences, being based directly on the fundamental axioms of utility theory. In order to measure preferences for chronic states preferred to death the subject is offered two alternatives; either the gamble, a treatment with two possible outcomes (death or return to normal health for the remainder of his life); or the certain outcome of remaining in the chronic state for the rest of his life. The probability of a successful outcome to the gamble is varied until the respondent is indifferent between the gamble and the certainty. This probability can then be used to calculate the preference value for the health state" (*MF Drummond*). See **time trade-off, utility measurement**

standard operating procedures (SOPs)
- Sponsor's standard, detailed, written instructions for the management of **clinical trials** (EC).
- Standard, detailed, written instructions describing the approved way of executing any task in academia or business. SOPs minimize arguments over trivia, and when well devised they facilitate tasks and establish a high standard. When poorly conceived, SOPs give cause for petty grievances and create bad will because the intelligent worker can see that there are better ways of doing things. See **GCP, GLP, GMP**

standardization   See **biological standardization**

starch blocker
- The trivial name for α-glucosidase inhibitors, e.g. acarbose, that reduce the digestion of dietary polysaccharides and sucrose to monosaccharides, and may be used as **adjuvant** therapy in diabetes mellitus.

state-of-the-art
- Used of a technically advanced and up-to-date device or process; high performance, efficiency and reliability are implied but not assured.
- *State-of-the-art defence*: see **product liability**

-static/-asis   (L. *stare*, to stand)
- Suffix meaning to prevent further growth, development, etc., as in *bacteristatic*.

statistical moment   (L. *stare*, to stand; *momentum*, moving power)
- The product of two **variables**. See, for example, **first moment**.

statistical regression   (L. *stare*, to stand; *re*, back; *gradus*, step)
- The tendency of extreme measures to move closer to the mean when they are repeated (*F Galton*, 1885, statistician etc., UK), e.g. individuals who score high (or low) in tests tend to do worse (or better) in repeat tests. It is a random phenomenon. In practical terms it means that baseline measures before an intervention should always be multiple, not single.
                                    See **law of initial value, regression to the mean**

statistical significance   (L. *stare*, to stand; *signum*, mark, token)
- The *probability* that an observed difference is the result of chance rather than of causal influences in an experiment. More precisely, the probability that the difference between an observed value of a **variable** and some specific (or hypothetical) value of the variable would be as observed or greater, as a result of **random** errors (factors), if the true (or population) value of the difference were zero. Calculations of such probabilities are commonly optimistic because
  - A number of untested assumptions is made.
  - The calculation takes no account of systematic (nonrandom) errors.
- A difference may be real (and therefore usually statistically significant at the conventional level) but nevertheless be too small in magnitude to be of any practical importance (a very precise experiment can detect very small differences).
- 'Not statistically significant' is compatible with there being no difference between treatments (**null hypothesis**), but does not *prove* this; the study may lack **power**.
- *Levels of statistical significance*: values that differ from their mean by more than twice the **standard deviation** as a result of random factors are relatively rare. Therefore differences of twice the standard deviation or more are conveniently adopted as 'significant', i.e. unlikely to be due to chance. In fact

such differences would occur 5 times in 100 tests (p=0.05) (repeated to an identical design). If this is thought too lenient, the level may be raised to 2.5 or 3 times the standard deviation, when differences would occur by chance approximately once in 80 or 370 tests ('highly significant', conventionally $p \leq 0.01$). The problem is always one of **probability** and workers are free to adopt any level they wish, so long as they make this clear. For this reason it is better to say in reporting results that the observed difference is *x* times the standard deviation rather than to say it is 'significant', or 'highly significant' (*A Bradford Hill*; A short textbook of medical statistics, 1977).

See **probability (p) value**

- In assessing the *meaning* of statistical significance in a comparative study account *must* be taken of **confidence intervals**. See **clinical significance**

statistician
(L. *stare*, to stand)
- One who practises statistics; an important discipline in modern societies.
- *Unjustly*: A tedious fellow.
- *Less unjustly*: "A person who can draw a mathematically precise line from an unwarranted assumption to a foregone conclusion" (*Anon*).
- Manipulation of data by statisticians caused Mark Twain (1835–1910, author, US) to write: "There are three kinds of lies – lies, damned lies and statistics."

statistics/statistic
(L. *stare*, to stand)
- The collection and arrangement of numerical facts or data, especially for large quantities or numbers.
- A body of methods for making wise decisions in the face of uncertainty. Statistics cannot provide proof or certainty; it provides **probabilities**.
- A *statistic* is a numerical entity (e.g. **mean, standard deviation, equilibrium constant**, slope of a line, etc.) calculated according to a specified method with the intention that it should provide a better (in some sense) estimate, from experimental data, of a **parameter**.
- The main function of that section of statistics that deals with tests of significance is to prevent people making fools of themselves (*DC Colquhoun*).
- *Use of statistics*: When criticized for using mathematical manipulations without understanding how they worked, O. Heaviside (physicist, UK, 1850–1925) replied: "Should I refuse a good dinner because I do not understand the process of digestion?" (The *Heaviside–Kennelly layer* is a region of the ionosphere.)
- *Statistics and statisticians* seem particularly to incur the odium of non-scientists.
- Thou shall not lie with statisticians,
  Nor commit a social science.
  (attributed to *WH Auden* 1907–1973, English poet).
- Statisticians are like alienists [psychiatrists] – they will testify for either side (*Fiorello H La Guardia*, Mayor of New York, US, 1933). See **statistician**

statistics and general clinical impressions
- One of the first heavyweights in the field was Francis Galton (UK:1822–1911) who in 1879 wrote:

"In our general impressions far too great weight is attached to what is mar-vellous...Experience warns us against it, and the scientific man takes care to base his conclusions upon actual numbers. The human mind is...a most imperfect apparatus for the elaboration of general ideas...General impres-sions are never to be trusted. Unfortunately when they are of long standing they become fixed rules of life, and assume a prescriptive right not to be questioned. Consequently, those who are not accustomed to original en-quiry entertain a hatred and a horror of statistics. They cannot endure the idea of submitting their sacred impressions to cold-blooded verification. But it is the triumph of scientific men to rise superior to such superstitions, to devise tests by which the value of beliefs may be ascertained, and to feel sufficiently masters of themselves to discard contemptuously whatever may be found untrue...the frequent incorrectness of notions derived from general impressions may be assumed..." *(Proceedings of the Royal Insti-tution, 1879).*

steady state   (O. Eng. *stede*; L. *stare*, to stand)
- The state in which the value of a specified variable (e.g. concentration) does not vary with time. A state of minimum (but not necessarily zero) **entropy** production.
- The state achieved when the rate of drug intake equals the rate of drug elimi-nation (hence steady state concentration, C_{SS}).   See **plateau principle**

stereoisomer   (Gr. *stereos*, solid; *iso*, same; *meros*, shape)
- Chemical in which structural groups can be arranged in different three-dimensional ways. In general, this does not change the chemical properties of the compound, but biological properties can be altered dramatically. Stereo-isomers can be **optical isomers** or conformational isomers (e.g. *cis-/trans-isomerism*).
- Where a drug is a **racemate** the British Pharmacological Society recom-mends that the prefix rac- should be used (e.g. rac-propranolol). It also rec-ommends that the absolute configuration should be indicated where possible (e.g. (S)-warfarin), and that geometrical isomers should be indicated by the prefixes Z/E or cis/trans.   See **chirality**

stereoselectivity   (Gr. *stereos*, solid; L. *legere*, to choose)
- Where a drug can exist as two or more **stereoisomers**, the structure of the **receptor** with which it interacts may be such that **recognition** of one isomer is preferred. That isomer will then be more **potent** than the other(s). If the other isomer(s) has (or have) no measurable effect, then it is allowable to use the term *stereospecific*. This is seldom, if ever, the case.   See **selectivity**

stereotype/-y   (Gr. *stereos*, solid; *typos*, image)
- Having all the classical characteristics of a particular class of thing, i.e. exem-plary of its type.
- Invariant, repetitive behaviour, e.g. that induced by amphetamine in experi-mental animals.

– The term probably arises from an obsolete printing technique. A stereotype was made by taking a mould from already set type-face (*forme*), filling this mould with molten metal and printing from this casting without having to re-compose the forme.

steric exclusion   (Gr. *stereos*, solid; L. *excludere*, to shut out)
– The process by which a drug, or a structurally important part of a drug (**phar-macophore**), is prevented from exerting its effect because it is physically prevented from reaching its target site (e.g. a **receptor** or a critically important part of a receptor) by the presence of a structural group on another drug which does not itself bind with the target site. *Steric* exclusion differs from other types of interference because the precise geometric arrangement of the interfering group is important; the same chemical group attached to a similar molecule, but having a different steric relationship to the rest of the molecule, will not exclude an active phamacophore.   See **competition**

sterilization   (L. *sterilis*, unfruitful)
– The killing of all forms of microorganisms, including bacterial spores and vi-ruses: liquid chemicals cannot be relied on to sterilize: heat, under carefully controlled conditions, is required.
– Removal or rendering nonfunctional the reproductive organs of either sex.
                    See **Tyndallization**

steroid
– *Chemical*: Complex lipids (17-carbon nucleus) including sterols, some hor-mones (sex, adrenocortical), glycosides (digoxin), vitamin D.
– *Clinical* **jargon**: "Is the patient on steroids?" means: "Is the patient being treated with an adrenocortical steroid?"

stilbestrol (stilboestrol, diethylstilbestrol)
– Stilbestrol, the first synthetic oestrogen in general clinical use, caused vaginal adenosis and cancer in the postpubertal offspring of mothers who took it dur-ing pregnancy in the hope of preventing miscarriage (an example of a *sec-ond-generation adverse effect*). Stilbestrol was used for this purpose for dec-ades after its introduction in the 1940s, on purely theoretical grounds (see **theoretician**). Controlled therapeutic trials were not done and there is no valid evidence of therapeutic efficacy. Male fetuses developed nonmalignant genital abnormalities. Claims for (increased) compensation still reverberate in the 1990s.   See **liability** (*Market-share liability*)

stimulus   (L. *stimulus*, goad)
– Incentive.
– An agent or influence that causes cells or tissues to respond.
– In 1956 RP Stephenson drew attention to the fact that response was seldom directly proportional to receptor **occupancy**. He concluded that different drugs have different capacities to initiate responses when bound to **recep-tors**. He called this property **efficacy** (*e*) and it is the **proportionality con-**

stant that relates receptor occupancy to the *stimulus*, *S*. The response, he proposed, is some (simple) function of *S*:

$$\frac{E}{E_{max}} = f(S) = f\left(\frac{e[DR]}{[R_T]}\right)$$

where *E* represents the effect, E_{max} represents the maximal effect that can be induced in the tissue, *f* denotes some function, [DR] represents the concentration of occupied receptors and R_T represents the total receptor concentration (free + occupied).

stochastic process   (Gr. *stokhos*, aim; L. *pro*, before; *cedere*, go)
- **Random** process: processes that involve probability theory because of their inherently random characteristics. The term is ordinarily used for processes that vary randomly in time, e.g. length of queues, the size and composition of populations (births, deaths, epidemics), the binding and dissociation of a drug molecule, or opening and closing of an ion channel (see **exponential distribution**).
- In the *17th century* stochastic meant an *educated guess* (e.g. "He was no prophet, yet he excelled in the stochastick art") which is the opposite of the above.

stoichiometry   (Gr. *stoikheion*, element; *metron*, measure)
- The branch of chemistry concerned with the proportions in which compounds react together (e.g. study of the binding of drugs/small **ligands**, to protein); relative proportions of substances in a reaction.

strain (genetic)   (L. *struere*, to construct)
- A population of the same stock descended from a common ancestor or derived from a single source.

stratification   (L. *stratus*, something strewn or spread)
- Division of a population or group of subjects into subgroups, layers or *strata*.
- In **therapeutic trials** stratification is used to enhance precision by grouping patients with similar characteristics, e.g. age, sex, duration or severity of disease, where it is believed that these characteristics are likely to affect the outcome. Stratification may be **prospective** (with balanced **randomization**) or **retrospective**. The former is preferred because it is not open to bias in choosing the criteria for the strata by knowledge of the outcomes.

Straub phenomenon
- The characteristic S-shaped erection of the tail of the mouse, associated with anal spasm, caused by opioid **agonists** and used as a test for opioid activity (*W Straub*, pharmacologist, active in the early 20th century, Germany).

See **opiate/opioid**

'street drugs'
- Drugs of any kind illicitly sold in places where the public gather, in streets, bars, cafés, etc.

streptozotocin   See **drugs as tools**

stress   (L. *strictus*, strict)
                                                              See **hysteresis**

strong/weak
- Commonly used adjectives applied to drugs or their effects. They are seem-ingly convenient terms, but are vague and cannot be expressed numerically. Usually employed instead of **potent/impotent**, but sometimes in place of **se-lective**/*nonselective* or *efficacious/inefficacious*. The more precise terms are always better (see **efficacy**).
- There may be a useful place for these words in describing the **intrinsic effi-cacy** of drugs. A drug with high intrinsic efficacy could be described as a strong agonist, in contrast to a drug with an intermediate intrinsic efficacy, which could be a weak agonist or **partial agonist**. However, there is still room for misunderstanding in this usage, as a partial agonist may have high **affin-ity** (i.e. bind 'strongly') and yet have low ('weak') intrinsic efficacy, whereas a full agonist could have low affinity (bind 'weakly') but high ('strong') intrinsic efficacy.

structure–activity relationship (SAR)   (L. *struere*, build; *agere*, go;
                                                              relatio, carry back)
- The relationship between chemical structure and biological activity.

Student's *t*-distribution
- If observations follow a **normal distribution**, then this (normal) distribution may be used to conduct statistical tests on the observations, but only if the **scatter** (standard deviation) of the observations is *known*. However, when the sample is small, not only is the **mean** subject to uncertainty (variability from sample to sample) but so also is the **standard deviation**. The correct way to allow for uncertainty about the standard deviation was given by WS Gossett in 1908. Gossett was Head Brewer for the Guinness brewery in Dublin (Ire-land), where he encountered small-sample problems. He derived his '*t* distri-bution' during a visit to University College London, UK, and published it under the pseudonym 'Student'. Although valid for small samples, it still assumes that observations follow a **normal distribution**.   See **Student's *t*-test**

Student's *t*-test
- A test of significance used for small samples of observations that follow a **normal distribution**, based on **Student's *t*-distribution**. Commonly used to test the reality of the difference between two **means**. If the two means are calculated from two entirely independent samples of observations, the test is described as *unpaired*. If both treatments are tested (random order) on each individual (cell, animal, patient, etc.), then it is reasonable, in order to maxi-mize precision, to look at the *difference* between the pairs of responses on each individual, a *paired test*.

styptic   (Gr. *stupho*, contract)
                                                              See **astringent**

subjective   (L. *sub*, beneath; *jacere*, to throw)
- Belonging or related to the mind or feelings of an observer or thinker rather than to the actual nature of the object being considered.
- Affected by emotion or personal **bias**; value-laden.
                                                     See **double-blind, objective**

sublingual drug administration   (L. *sub*, beneath; *lingua*, tongue)
- Sucking below the tongue instead of swallowing a solid dose form may permit absorption from the lingual or buccal membranes. Onset of effect by this route is rapid, and drug absorption can be terminated by spitting out the **formulation. First-pass** elimination in the gut wall or liver is avoided, e.g. of glyceryl trinitrate.
                          See **buccal drug administration, hepatic first-pass metabolism**

subsidiarity   (L. *sub*, down; *sedere*, to sit)
- A 'Eurospeak' term (invented by the European Community) for delegation, devolution or decentralization. What *can* be done at a lower level *should not* be done at a higher, thus, in Eurospeak, "...the Community shall take action, in accordance with the principle of subsidiarity, only if and in so far as the objectives of the proposed action cannot be sufficiently achieved by the member-States and can therefore, by reason of the scale or effects of the proposed action, be better achieved by the Community." Applied to official medicines regulation, the issue is the extent of the powers that should be accorded to the *European Medicines Evaluation Agency* (EMEA), and what powers should remain with member states (recognizing that there are significant national differences in the practice of medicinal therapeutics).
                                            See **regulation (official) of medicines**

substance abuse   (L. *sub*, beneath; *stare*, to stand)
- This imprecise but convenient term was introduced for social/recreational abuse of 'non-drug' substance, e.g. solvents of glues, cleaning fluids, hair sprays, butane gas, petrol (gasoline), shoe polish (vaporized), generally by inhalation. Its scope is sometimes broadened to include tobacco, alcohol and medicinal products such as anti-parkinson drugs, benzodiazepines.
                              See **abuse and misuse of drugs, recreational (use) drugs**

substance P
- A polypeptide **neurotransmitter** (CNS and **NANC** nerves) and local hormone (or **autacoid**) (gastrointestinal tract). It may be involved in pain transmission and many other functions.
- One of the **tachykinins**.
- There are various explanations for how it came by its name. The official version is that the discoverers were able to dry it to a **p**owder. It is also said that the original discoverers gave it this name because they first extracted it from urine.

'substantial evidence' (of efficacy)
- The US Food, Drug and Cosmetic Act requires 'substantial evidence' of effi-

cacy if a drug is to receive regulatory approval. Substantial evidence "is not what experts believe or conjecture, but empirical evidence adduced in clinical investigations that is of such quality and character that it would allow a representative, fair-minded, impartial, disinterested, and appropriately qualified expert to conclude reasonably from that evidence alone that the drug product in question will have the effect claimed" (*P Leber*).

See **evidence-based medicine**

substitute or alternative formulation   (L. *sub*, beneath; *statuere*, to set up; *alter*, other; *-ate*, function)
- The following distinction is sometimes made:
  - A *substitute* differs from another formulation in no significant way. Its introduction would not, for example, alter a pre-existing pharmacokinetic **steady state**.
  - An *alternative* formulation provides clinical efficacy, but differs sufficiently from another formulation so that it is not a *precise* replacement/substitute.
- These matters arise particularly in commercial competition between generic and proprietary formulations of the same drug.

  See **bioequivalence, generic substitution, names of drugs, equivalence trial, therapeutic equivalence**

substrate   (L. *sub*, beneath; *stratum*, something spread or laid down)
- Substance upon which an enzyme acts.
- Medium upon which microbes are grown (cultured). Usually implies a solid.

suicide   See **self-poisoning**

suicide (enzyme) inhibitor or suicide substrate   (L. *sui*, of oneself; *caedere*, to kill; *sub*, beneath; *stratum*, something spread or laid down)
- Where an enzyme, by its action on an inactive substrate (a **prodrug**), generates an irreversible inhibitor of itself, the enzyme can be said to commit suicide. For example, vigabatrin (γ-vinyl GABA) (antiepileptic) is inert, but is converted by GABA-aminotransferase into an active form that irreversibly inhibits GABA-aminotransferase.   See **clavulanic acid, GABA**

Summary of Product Characteristics (SPC, SmPC)
- A regulatory term (**EU**) for the summary document that accompanies an application for a marketing licence. When a licence is granted the approved SPC controls the therapeutic claims that may be made, the prescribing information and advertising. It can only be changed with regulatory approval.
- The SPC (EU) comprises:
  - Name of medicinal product
  - Composition of product
  - Pharmaceutical (dosage) form
  - Clinical particulars
    - indications
    - dose

- contraindications
- special warnings and precautions, including effect on ability to drive and use machines
- pregnancy and lactation
- unwanted effects
- overdose
- Pharmacology: pharmacodynamics and pharmacokinetics
- Preclinical safety data
- Pharmaceutical data: excipients, incompatibilities, shelf-life, storage, form of container, instructions for handling, name and address of the licence (market authorization) holder.

summation   (L. *summa*, main part, highest)
- In pharmacology, summation occurs when the combined effects of the application of equieffective doses of two drugs is the same as that produced by a double dose of either of the drugs given alone.   See **synergism**

sunscreen   (Old Eng. *sunne*; *escran*, barrier)
- A substance that, applied to the skin, absorbs or reflects (scatters) ultraviolet radiation. The performance of a sunscreen is expressed as a *sun protective factor (SPF)*, but techniques, at present, are inadequately standardized.

superfamilies of genes   (L. *super*, above; *familia*, household; Gr. *genos*, birth)
- Closely related genes that control the synthesis of proteins with very similar amino acid sequences, i.e. with high homologies.
                          See **homology, superfamilies of receptors**

superfamilies of receptors
- **Receptors** with close structural and operational similarities, the syntheses of which are controlled by genes within the same *gene superfamily*. For example, all receptors linked to **G-proteins** have very high **homologies** and all contain seven hydrophobic α-helical **domains** which span the plasma membrane. Superfamilies of receptors are numerous.
                                        See **superfamilies of genes**

superfusion   (L. *super*, above, over; *fundere*, to pour)
- To pass a liquid over the surface of an organ or tissue.   See **perfusion**

supergene family   (L. *super*, above, over; Gr. *genos*, birth)
                                        See **superfamilies of genes**

supersensitivity   (L. *super*, above, beyond; *sentire*, to feel)
- An enhanced **sensitivity** to a drug, i.e. the system responds to lower doses/concentrations than expected, e.g. *denervation supersensitivity* (which is largely due to an increase in receptor numbers on the target cell).

supply of medicines
- Medicines may be supplied:

- On prescription by an authorized health professional: prescription-only medicine (PoM).
- From a pharmacy only (P).
- By general sale (GS): any sales outlet.

suppository   (L. *sub*, below; *ponere*, to place)
- A solid dose form for convenient insertion into a body orifice other than the mouth to medicate locally or for systemic absorption.   See **pessary**

suprabioavailability   (L. *supra*, on top of; see **bioavailability**)
- The term is used in official regulatory practice where an otherwise **essentially similar** product provides higher blood concentrations (at the same dose intervals) than does the comparator product. See **bioavailability, bioequivalence**

suprainfection/superinfection   (L. *super, supra*, on top of; *in*, in; *facere*, to make)
- A fresh infection in addition to one already present, often as a result of the use of an antimicrobial drug that alters existing flora, reducing biological competition so that resistant organisms flourish (e.g. *Candida* infection following the use of broad-spectrum antibiotics).   See **opportunistic infection**

suramin   See **drugs as tools**

surfactant   (Blend or portmanteau word from *surface-active agent*)
- A substance that increases the spreading or wetting properties of a liquid by lowering surface tension: a cleansing agent, a **detergent**.
- A compound that can reduce the interfacial tension between two immiscible phases; they may be anionic or nonionic.

surmountable and nonsurmountable antagonism   (L. *sur*, above; *mons*, mountain; Gr. *anti*, against; *agon*, struggle, contest)
- Where a maximal response to an **agonist** can be restored in the presence of an **antagonist** by increasing the concentration of agonist, the **antagonism** is said to be *surmountable*, i.e. it can be overcome. This can create confusion because the antagonism is still there, as is evident from the increased concentration of agonist needed to restore the maximal response. Surmountable antagonism is an operational description of what happens and does not imply any particular mechanism. Where the maximal response is no longer achievable, the antagonism is *nonsurmountable*.   See **competition**

surrogate endpoint or marker   (L. *surrogare*, to substitute)
- A clinical measurement known to be statistically associated with and believed to be pathophysiologically related to a clinical outcome (*P Rolan*).
- Where a short-term drug effect can be correlated *reliably* with long-term therapeutic benefit, then demonstration of the short-term (surrogate) effect becomes acceptable as evidence to allow a regulatory authority to approve a therapeutic claim, which would otherwise require clinical studies sometimes lasting many years. Examples include, for their principal actions: hypolipi-

340

daemic, antihypertensive and antidiabetic drugs. Rejection of surrogate end-points could, it is widely agreed, diminish the incentive to develop new drugs for chronic diseases.

survey/surveillance　　　　　　　　(L. *super*, above; *vigilare*, to keep watch)
- Close and generally continuing observation.
- An observational study, not involving intervention.
- Surveillance studies of drugs for safety and efficacy, being less rigorous than the controlled **therapeutic trial**, can be conducted on a much larger scale; they are particularly useful for detecting rare events.
　　　　　　　　See **case-control study, cohort study,post-marketing surveillance, prescription event monitoring**

sustained-release formulation　　　　　See **modified-release formulations**

switch campaigns/switching
- Efforts by companies (manufacturers, mail-order providers) to encourage the switching (changing) of patients from their original prescriptions to **'me-too'** drugs. The outcome may benefit the patient (equal efficacy at lower cost), but it may not, because there is not always evidence of equal efficacy.

SWOT analysis
- A marketing technique that involves examining the **s**trengths of a product, its **w**eaknesses, **o**pportunities for its use (or sales) and **t**hreats to its market.

sympatholytic agent　　　　　　　(Gr. *sun*, with; *pathos*, feeling; *lusis*, loosen)
- A substance, the effect of which is to reduce the consequences of sympa-thetic nerve stimulation or activity. The term is sometimes used to include **an-tagonism** of injected **catecholamines**.　　　　　See **adrenolytic**

sympathomimetic agent　　　　(Gr. *sun*, with; *pathos*, feeling; *mimesis*, imitation)
- "...compounds which...simulate the effects of sympathetic nerves not only with varying intensity but with varying precision...a term...seems needed to indi-cate the type of action common to these bases. We propose to call it 'sym-pathomimetic', a term which indicates the relation of the action to innervation by the sympathetic system, without involving any theoretical preconception as to the meaning of that relation or the precise mechanism of the action" (*G Barger*, chemist & *HH Dale*, physiologist/pharmacologist, 1910, UK).

sympathoplegic　　(Gr. *sun*, with; *pathos*, feeling; *plege*, stroke, and so paralysis)
- A drug that paralyses the sympathetic nervous system.

symposium　　　　　　　　　　(Gr. *sun*, with, together; *potes*, drinker)
- Drinking party (ancient Greece) with conversation.
- Friendly discussion at which various points of view are put at a meeting or in a journal or book.
- "Doctors should be suspicious of symposiums that are sponsored by single

pharmaceutical companies" (*British Medical Journal* 1992) as a special issue or as a special section of a regular issue of a medical journal. Such symposiums often bypass **peer-review** processes. Symposiums on a *single* drug, but with a *general* title, e.g. *Advances in treatment of anxiety*, are particularly likely to be commercial promotion rather than education.

See **promotion of medicines**

synaptic cleft/gap   (Gr. *synapsis*, connection, junction)
- The region between two neurons, or a neuron and effector organ (e.g. muscle cell), across which **neurotransmitter** diffuses when the *presynaptic* neuron terminal is activated.

synaptosome   (Gr. *synapsis*, connection, junction; *soma*, body)
- Artificial vesicies made by gently homogenizing brain tissue. Synaptosomes are pinched-off, resealed nerve endings, containing all the normal apparatus of nerve endings. They can be prepared in high concentrations and are useful for examining drug effects on transmitter synthesis, storage, release, reuptake and inactivation *in vitro*.

syndrome   (Gr. *sun*, together; *dromos*, running)
- A group of symptoms and/or signs of disorder that forms a recognized entity. The cause may be unknown or there may be multiple causes. Where a single specific cause is known, then the *syndrome* is promoted to being a *disease* entity.

synergism   (Gr. *sun*, together; *ergos*, work)
- Combined effects of drugs having the same actions; sometimes confined to where the effect is more than the sum of the parts, e.g. $2 + 2 = 5$.

See **additive responses, potentiation, summation**

synonymous   (Gr. *sun*, similar, alike; *onuma*, name)
- Words having the same, or nearly the same meaning are synonyms (synonymous), e.g. *scatter* and *dispersion*.

synthetic, semisynthetic   (Gr. *sun*, together; *tithemi*, put; *hemi*, half)
- *Synthetic*: making a compound in the laboratory or in the body from its elements or from much simpler compounds.
- *Semisynthetic*: making a compound in the laboratory using a naturally occurring complex substance as the starting material, thus bypassing some tedious (and expensive) stages of synthesis, e.g. plant steroids are used in the manufacture of adrenocortical steroids.

syntopic   (Gr. *sun*, together; *topos*, place)
- Acting at the same molecular site. Thus, in syntopic **antagonism** the **agonist** and **antagonist** interact with precisely the same target or site.
- "Syntopic antagonists are the best tools that pharmacologists possess" (*JW Black*).   See **allotopic**

syrup (Arabic, *sharab*)
− A concentrated aqueous solution of sugar or other sweetening agent.

systematic (Gr. *sun*, with; *histemi*, set up)
− Consistent, methodical (not **random,** or casual, or unintentional).

systematic review/overview (Gr. *sun*, with; *histemi*, set up;
L. *re*, again; *videre*, to see)
− A **review article** containing a 'methods' section describing in detail how it was prepared.
− All **meta-analyses** of controlled **therapeutic trials** are systematic reviews, but not all systematic reviews are meta-analyses.

See **Cochrane Collaboration**

systemic (Gr. *sun*, with; *histemi*, set up)
− Affecting or involving the entire body, as in systemic administration of a drug, meaning it enters the general or systemic circulation.

systemic availability See **bioavailability,**
hepatic first-pass metabolism, pre-systemic drug elimination

$t_{\frac{1}{2}}$

See **half-life**

tablet

(L. *tabula*, table)

- Solid single dose-form made by compaction from granular (powdered) ingredients. Tablets may be **coated** or *uncoated,* **soluble, dispersible, effervescent, gastroresistant,** *or* **modified-release.**

tachykinins

(Gr. *takhus*, swift; *kinesis*, motion)

- The name given by V Erspamer to a group of small polypeptide transmitters or mediators that produce rapid responses, in contrast to **bradykinin** which produces slow responses. All have the terminal amino acid sequence –Phe–X–Gly–Leu–Met–NH$_2$, the so-called 'canonical sequence'. The three known mammalian tachykinins are **substance P,** neurokinin A and neurokinin B. Eledoisin comes from a Mediterranean octopus and physalaemin from a toad. Receptors for tachykinins belong to the **G-protein**-linked **superfamily.**

tachyphylaxis

(Gr. *takhus*, swift; *phulaxis*, guarding)

- Progressive diminution of response to *frequently* repeated doses; distinct from **tolerance**. In tachyphylaxis the maximal response is reduced, whereas in **tolerance** there is reduced **sensitivity** of the end/target organ.
- If music be the food of love, play on;/Give me excess of it, that surfeiting,/The appetite may sicken, and so die (*W Shakespeare*, 1564–1616, *Twelfth night* I.i).   See **desensitization, hyposensitization**

TAME

- N-α-p-tosyl-L-arginine methyl ester (as in the allergic mediator TAME-esterase).

tamper-resistant packaging

(L. *temperare*, mingle)
See **packaging and safety**

tardive dyskinesia   (L. *tardus*, late coming; Gr. *dus*, bad; *kinesis*, motion)

- An abnormality of movement, especially of face, jaws, tongue and limbs, characteristic of *long-continued* therapy with **neuroleptic** drugs that are dopamine antagonists (e.g. phenothiazines).   See **extrapyramidal reaction**

targeting of drugs   (Several old European languages *targe* or *targa*, a shield)

- A tissue may be highly **selective** for a drug of appropriate molecular structure, i.e. it is the target for the drug. Where structural selectivity is poor, tissue selectivity may be gained by special delivery techniques, varying from simple **topical** application or local regional arterial infusion, to attaching the drug to an **antibody** that is selective for the desired site of action, e.g. cancer cells, also **liposomes** and virus **vectors**. 'Targeting' generally means these latter techniques.

tautologous/-y

(Gr. *tauto*, the same; *logos*, word)

- Saying the same thing twice over in different words.

- Statement that is necessarily true.
- *Examples*: the reason for this is because; new innovation; gastric stomach; 8 a.m. in the morning; therapeutic treatment; human volunteer; absolutely unique, past history.

taxonomy   (Gr. *tasso*, arrange; *nomia*, distribution)
- Principles or science of classification.

TD$_{50}$
- Abbreviation of toxic dose 50 per cent. The **median** toxic dose, i.e. the dose that produces a toxic effect in 50 per cent of a population.   See **LD$_{50}$**

TDM
- **Therapeutic drug monitoring.**

tea   (Chinese Amoy dialect *t'e*; Mandarin dialect *ch'a*; Eng. slang *cha*)
- Fermented and dried leaves or buds of the plant *Camellia thea*. Contains **caffeine** (2–3%) and theophylline.   See **xanthines & methylxanthines**

TEA   See **drugs as tools** (*Tetraethylammonium*)

technique or technic   (Gr. *teknikos*, a skill, art, craft)
- A practical way of doing something.   See **technology**

technobabble   (Gr. *teknikos*, a skill, art, craft; L. *babulus*, fool)
- Composite word from *techno*logy and *babble*.   See **jargon**

'technological turkeys' (slang)
- New products or procedures whose danger and expense might have been minimised by proper study (*R Wyden*, Congressman, USA).
                                                                           See **state-of-the-art**

technology   See **science and technology**

teleology   (Gr. *teleos*, end; *logos*, word, subject of study)
- The study of the evidence for design or purpose in nature.
- The belief that natural phenomena have a predetermined purpose and are not determined by, for example, chance or natural selection.
- PB Medawar illustrates the philosophical dangers of too supine a dependence on the notion, from a 10-year-old schoolgirl's essay on a cow (quoted by Gowers in *The complete plain words*):
    "The cow is a mammal...At the back it has a tail on which hangs a brush. With this it sends the flies away so that they do not fall into the milk. The head is for the purpose of growing horns, and so that the mouth can be somewhere. The horns are to butt with, and the mouth is to moo with. Under the cow hangs the milk. It is arranged for milking. When people milk the milk comes and there is never an end to the supply. How the cow does it I have not yet realized, but it makes more and more. The cow has a fine

sense of smell: one can smell it far away. This is the reason for the fresh air in the country...the cow does not eat much, but what it eats it eats twice so that it gets enough. When it is hungry it moos, and when it says nothing it is because its inside is full up with grass."

teratothanasia (Gr. *teras*, monster; *thanatos*, death)
- The term is applied where an agent diminishes the rate of birth defects by selectively inducing abortion of affected conceptuses. The term is preferred (etymologically) over *terathanasia* (*Lancet* 1997;350:1712).

teratogen (Gr. *teras*, monster; *genesis*, be produced)
- An agent which causes physical or developmental abnormalities in the embryo or fetus.

terminal care
- The care of the dying; usually the final few weeks of life.
See **euthanasia, palliative care**

ternary complex (L. *ternarius*, of three)
- The complex between **agonist** molecule, **receptor** and **effector coupler** (e.g., **G-protein**) which must form before a response to the agonist can develop. It is assumed that ternary complexes do not form with antagonist molecules. See **inverse agonist**

tetraethylammonium (TEA) See **drugs as tools** (*Tetraethylammonium*)

tetrodotoxin See **drugs as tools** (*Tetrodotoxin*), **fugu**

textbook (L. *textus*, tissue, literary style; Old Engl. *boc*)
- "A supposedly objective compendium of established knowledge. It is this intent that causes their well deserved reputation for insipidity engendered by a style that blots out all vigour of prose and personal belief" (*Stephen Jay Gould*).

TGF
- Tumour growth factor. One of the **cytokines**.

thalidomide
- Ph**thal**imi**do**glutari**mide**. The most famous drug of this century, perhaps, after penicillin: thalidomide for the harm (**teratogenesis**) it caused, and penicillin for the good it does. The thalidomide disaster took place in 1960–1961, beginning in Germany, where thalidomide (a hypnotic) was on general sale to the public. It has provided the principal impetus to rigorous governmental drug regulation. At the time this entry was compiled, demands for further compensation (for the UK survivors) were still being raised in the courts. Thalidomide has found a limited role as an immunosuppressive, e.g. in leprosy, but its history renders its availability controversial.
See **accidents, phocomelia, regulation (official) of medicines**

theoretician (Gr. *theorein*, to gaze upon)
- The task of the theoretician is to predict what will happen and then to explain why the opposite occurred (*W Gratzer*).

theory (Gr. *theorein*, to gaze upon)
See **hypothesis**

theraccine
- **Thera**peutic va**ccine.**

therapeutic/-s (Gr. *therapeuein*, cure)
- Curative healing.
- Branch of medicine concerned with the treatment of disease/symptoms. Therapeutics may be:
  - *Curative*, e.g. bacterial infections.
  - *Suppressive* of disease or symptoms, e.g. diabetes, hypertension, pain.
  - *Prophylactic* (preventive), e.g. malaria, **antiplatelet drugs.**

therapeutic drug monitoring (TDM)
- Evaluation of therapeutic effect by clinical observation and particularly by measurement of drug or metabolite concentrations in blood or other fluids (e.g. saliva) or tissues as a guide to achieving *therapeutic* **efficacy,** avoiding **toxicity** and treating overdose. Drug concentrations are particularly useful where clinical assessments do not speedily provide evidence of effect, e.g. epilepsy, intermittent cardiac dysrhythmia; or of safety, e.g. avoidance of aminoglycoside toxicity.
- *Therapeutic range of plasma (or other tissue) concentration*: the range of concentrations in which therapeutic effect is expected. The upper limit is determined by the occurrence of adverse reactions (in 5–10 per cent of patients) and the lower by loss of therapeutic effect. It is usual to aim at the centre of the range. See **plasma concentration of drugs as a guide to therapy, therapeutic window**

therapeutic equivalence (L. *aequalis*, equal; *valere*, to be worth)
- Drugs, e.g. members of a series, that provide similar benefits with similar risks, i.e. they are essentially interchangeable as far as outcome is concerned.
- The concept also applies to generic versions of proprietary medicines.
- Lack of **bioequivalence** may be a cause of two formulations of the *same* drug lacking therapeutic equivalence. See **generic drugs, names of drugs, substitute or alternative formulation, therapeutic substitution**

therapeutic index/ratio (margin of safety) (Gr. *therapeuein*, cure; L. *index*, forefinger, informer, sign; *ratio*, reckoning)
- The concept was devised by Paul Ehrlich (1854–1915, scientist, Germany) as the ratio between maximal tolerated dose and minimal curative dose. A high number implies a safe drug, and *vice versa*. It is seldom calculated as above

because, in general, it does not truly represent reality, and because data, especially on 'curative' dose, are seldom available in a suitable form. However, the concept embodies a valuable way of thinking about safety of drugs. Consider, for example, penicillin (very high index) and lithium (very low index). In animal laboratories a ratio of **LD$_{50}$** and **ED$_{50}$** is sometimes offered as the therapeutic index.

therapeutic substitution: therapeutic alternative (drug): therapeutic interchange
- The practice whereby pharmacists may substitute medicines they deem (on reliable evidence) to be therapeutically equivalent to the medicines prescribed by the doctor. The practice may produce economic benefits and may be convenient, but it may also introduce risk since the pharmacist (inevitably) lacks access to full knowledge of the patient.
- "A cost-containing initiative which involves the dispensing of a drug *different in chemical structure* from the one prescribed. The substitute or therapeutic alternative is selected from the same therapeutic class and is deemed to have similar pharmacodynamic and pharmacokinetic properties, and similar therapeutic benefits, when administered in therapeutically equivalent doses" (*American College of Physicians,* 1990).   See **generic substitution, therapeutic equivalence, substitute or alternative formulation**

therapeutic trial   (Gr. *therapeuein*, cure; Old Fr. *trier*, to sift)
- The determination of comparative therapeutic efficacy.
- The classic randomized controlled trial (RCT)
     "is a carefully, and ethically, designed experiment with the aim of answering some precisely framed question. In its most rigorous form it demands *equivalent groups of patients concurrently treated in different ways* [emphasis added]. These groups are constructed by the random allocation of patients to one or other treatment; such an allocation may sometimes preferably be made within more but smaller homogeneous subgroups composing the total groups. Sometimes carefully matched pairs of patients may provide the contrast. In some instances patients may form their own controls, different treatments being applied to them in random order and the effects compared. In principle the method is applicable with any disease and any treatment. It should be designed to promote rather than hinder the traditional method in medicine of acute observation of disease by the clinician at the bedside."
     "In short, in the controlled clinical trial our endeavour is to measure the relative value of a defined treatment (or treatments) by the comparison of a group of patients treated in one way with a similar group not so treated. Everything turns upon the validity of that final deduction from the results of the trial. And, in turn, it is this that dictates the rules for the specific trial – whether it be double-blind, whether we use a placebo, whether there be constraints upon the variability of the patients admitted. There is no hard-and-fast 'cookbook' recipe to fit every trial. The trial itself promotes the choice of rules." (*A Bradford Hill, A short textbook of medical statistics,* 1977; the author was the 'father' of the modern therapeutic trial.)

- *Patient preference trial*: "Patients may be placed in one of three groups according to preference and willingness to be randomised: (a) patients who have no strong preference and therefore consent to randomisation; (b) patients with a preference who still consent to randomisation; (c) patients who refuse randomisation and opt for a treatment of choice" (*DJ Torgerson, B Sibbald*). Accommodating patient preferences complicates the analysis of a trial, but has advantages in respect of **compliance** and **ethics**.
- *Zelen randomization*: In a conventional randomized controlled trial, the consent of patients is invited to accept treatments (one of two) chosen by chance. Some patients dislike this, feeling it implies a worrying degree of uncertainty in their cases. Zelen has proposed that patients should be (secretly) randomized to treatments and only *after* this is done invited to accept the chosen treatment without being told of the other treatment(s) under test or of the process of random selection. Zelen procedure enhances recruitment of patients (often a hampering factor), but it is ethically controversial in that patients are kept in ignorance of research procedures and of their right to decline to enter the study (even though the investigator may think that medically this is irrelevant: see **equipoise**). (*MA Zelen*; New England Journal of Medicine 1979;300:1242–1245). (The term *pre-randomization* has been somewhat obscurely applied to this procedure).
- Trials may also be classified as: *explanatory (or fastidious)* – conducted on selected patients to determine the best that the drug can do (i.e. *efficacy*); or *pragmatic (or naturalistic)* – conducted under conditions of ordinary clinical practice (*D Schwartz, R Flamant & J Lellouch*), (i.e. *effectiveness*).
- Rigorously controlled therapeutic trials (above) are difficult to do on the large numbers of patients that are needed for detecting modest but useful effects in serious common diseases. They are also very time-consuming if clinical outcomes (e.g. survival and avoidance of complications) are used as endpoints. The public demand for speed and early access to potentially important new drugs in, for example, AIDS and myocardial infarction, is leading to the performance of randomized or nonrandomized *heterogeneous megatrials*. In these studies there is some sacrifice of scientific rigour (by using **surrogate endpoints** and heterogeneous enrolment), which, it is hoped, is compensated by the enormous number of patients in the trial, e.g. 50000.
- *Small-scale/large-scale trials*: "The reliable detection of moderate differences in major health outcomes that arise as a result of treatment requires large-scale randomized evidence (and the appropriate interpretation of this evidence once it has been generated). This may take the form of a single megatrial or, exceptionally, a **meta-analysis** of many smaller randomized trials may provide worthwhile information. Small or non-randomized studies cannot generally be trusted to distinguish reliably between a moderate benefit, a moderate hazard, and a negligible difference in major outcomes" (*C Baigent*).
- *Cluster trial*: Patients are allocated to receive treatments by groups (e.g. primary care practices) rather than as individuals.

  See **adaptive clinical trial designs, clinical impression, clinical trial, confidentiality, control, double-blind, ethics, equivalence trial, ethics committee, intention to treat, matched pairs, outcomes research, placebo, ran-**

dom, risk, sample size, stratification, seeding trial, statistical significance, uncertainty principle

therapeutic window   (Gr. *therapeuein*, cure; Old Norse *vindr*, wind; *augr*, eye)
- The term applies to a situation where therapeutic effect occurs over a limited range of **dose** or plasma concentration, being absent at both lower and higher concentrations of a drug. It is said to occur with some antidepressants. Loss of effect at higher concentrations may be due to recruitment of low-affinity receptors that were unaffected at lower concentrations.

  See **selectivity**
- The range of doses or plasma concentrations between the **minimum effective dose** and the highest tolerated (the maximal dose that can be given without inducing adverse effects).   See **individual effective dose**

theriac   (Gr. *theriakos*, of wild beasts or venomous reptiles)
- Originally (before the 1st century BCE) a potion intended to protect against the venom of poisonous snakes.
- By the 1st century BCE it was a universal antidote against poisoning.
- By the 17th and 18th centuries CE it was believed to be a **panacea**, i.e. a cure for all ills. Its constitution, a jealously guarded secret, involved an enormous number of heterogeneous items. Many patients recovered from diseases after taking theriac.   See **placebo**, *post hoc ergo propter hoc*

'they', 'them'   (Old Norse *their*, *thein*, people, to mean other than the speaker)
- Used by ignorant and paranoid people to mean unspecified persons or organizations whom or which the speakers do not understand but resent as having power over them, and of whom or which they are afraid, e.g. "if *they* cannot make safe drugs then *they* should not be allowed to make drugs at all" (heard on BBC radio).

thixotropy/-ic   (Gr. *thixis*, touching; *trope*, turning)
- A property of some fluids or gels in which viscosity decreases with speed of movement (rate of shear) in the liquid, i.e. it becomes less viscous if stirred: also, increase of viscosity with time (undisturbed). Tomato ketchup is thixotropic, as those who have shaken an inverted bottle over their food will have discovered to their cost. (*When you shake the ketchup bottle/None will come and then a lot'll.* Anon). Some laboratory media, e.g. starch **gel** for electrophoresis, are thixotropic.

thrombocytopenia   (Gr. *thrombosis*, curdling, clotting; *kutos*, vessel, cell; *penia*, poverty)
- Decreased number of blood platelets (thrombocytes).

thromboxanes   (Gr. *thrombosis*, curdling, clotting)
- Vasoconstrictor and thrombotic products of the **arachidonic acid/cyclo-oxygenase** pathway.

thymoleptic, thymerectic, thymosthenic (Gr. *thymos*, mind; L. *erigere*, to set up; *lepsis*, seizure; *asthenis*, weak)
- Obsolescent terms for mood-elevating and antidepressant actions.

time constant (O. Eng. *tima*, time; L. *constare*, to be steadfast)
- For a process in which a **variable** (e.g., concentration, number of bacteria, voltage) changes exponentially with time, the time required for the value of that variable to change to any given fraction of its starting value (for a decay process) or final value (for an accumulation process) is constant. The *time constant* (τ) for any simple exponential process completely specifies the time course of that process:

$$y_t = y_\infty + [y_0 - y_\infty]e^{-t/\tau}$$

where y_0, y_t and y_∞ are the values of the variable at time zero, time t and infinity respectively, and e is the base of natural (Naperian) logarithms (2.718). The *time constant* is the time taken for the variable to fall to $1/e$ (i.e. 36.79%) of its initial value (for a decay process) or to rise to $1-1/e$ (63.21%) of its final value (for an accumulation process).
- The reciprocal of the time constant is usually described as the **rate constant**. The **half-life** (more correctly *half-time*), or $t_{1/2}$, is the time taken for the variable to reach half its initial value (for a decay process) or half its final value (for an accumulation). This equates to $\log_e 2.0 \times \tau$ which works out to be 0.69315 $\times \tau$.

time trade-off
- "Under the *time trade-off* approach the respondent is asked to consider the relative amounts of time he would be willing to spend in various health states. For example, in order to value a chronic health state, the respondent would be offered a choice of remaining in this state for the rest of his life vs returning to complete health for a shorter period. The amount of time that the individual is willing to 'trade' to return to perfect health can be used to obtain a preference value for the chronic health state. A similar approach can be used to calculate the relative values of temporary health states" (*MF Drummond*).
See **standard gamble, utility measurement**

tincture (L. *tinctus*, to dye)
- Medicinal alcoholic solution (generally of dried plant matter). When mixed with water, ammonia, glycerine, ether, this is reflected in the name, e.g. ammoniated tincture. Tinctures are obsolescent if not obsolete. The most famous tincture is that of opium (*Laudanum*, from L. *laudare*, to praise; or "quite arbitrary" etymology, **OED**), followed by those of iodine and ipecacuanha. The description 'alcoholic solution' is preferred.

TiPS
- *Trends in Pharmacological Sciences*: a monthly review and news journal.
See **review articles**

titrate   (Fr. *titre*, proportions, e.g. of metals in an alloy)
- *In quantitative chemistry*: to add one reagent carefully until a preset condition pertains, e.g. adding an acid to an alkali until a particular pH is reached.
- *In medical practice*: to adjust the dose of a drug in accordance with the subject's response, e.g. blood glucose, blood pressure, leucocytes.

titre/titer   (Fr. *titre*, proportions, e.g. of metals in an alloy)
- Concentration of a substance (usually antibody) in the blood.

t_{max}
- The time from administration of a single dose, or beginning a constant infusion, of a drug to when the concentration reaches its peak or plateau (maximum; usually in blood).   See **plateau principle**

7TM receptors   See **receptors** (*Heptahelical*)

TNF
- Tumour necrosis factor – one of the **cytokines**.

tocolysis/lytic   (Gr. *tokos*, birth; *lusis*, loosen)
- Reduction of uterine contractions, or an agent that does this.

tolerance   (L. *tolerare*, to endure)
- *Acquired*: diminished **sensitivity** to a drug resulting from previous exposure to that drug or a related drug (cross-tolerance).
- *Natural*: the higher end of the normal distribution curve of **individual effective doses**.
- Often confused with **tachyphylaxis**, in which the maximal response declines with no change in **sensitivity**.   See **desensitization**

'tomato effect'   (Nahuatl. *tomatl*; L. *efficere*, to work out)
- The tomato effect occurs when an efficacious treatment for a disease is ignored or rejected because it does not make sense in terms of currently accepted theories of pathology or pharmacology. Tomatoes have, on theoretical grounds (see **theoretician**), passed through several cycles of being deemed a food and a poison. The matter was thought to be settled when in 1820 Robert Gibbon Johnson ate a tomato in public (in Salem, NJ, USA) and survived, although as late as 1896 tomatoes were proposed as a cause of cardiomyopathy. In 1997 there is evidence that a carotenoid (lycopene) in tomatoes (especially if cooked) is an antioxidant that may protect against heart attacks.

tonic   (Gr. *tonos*, tension)
- A medicine supposed to invigorate those who feel the need for it: see **placebo**.
- Continuous maintained tension in a muscle is described as *tonic* activity or *tone*.
- Continuous **endogenous** activity in nerves is also, confusingly, described as tonic activity or tone.   See **constitutive activity**

topical (Gr. *topos*, place)
- Relation to a particular place: application of a drug to a surface (e.g. skin, eye or nasal mucosa) is topical administration.
- Of the moment. Fashions in pharmacology and medicine change.

topology (Gr. *topos*, place; *logy*, subject of study)
- Topology is concerned with geometric factors when an object, e.g. a molecule, undergoes deformation by bending, stretching or twisting.

torture, drugs and (L. *tortura*, twisting)
- Regrettably, drugs have been and are being used for torture, sometimes disguised as 'interrogation' or 'aversion therapy'. Facts are, not surprisingly, hard to obtain, but it seems that suxamethonium, hallucinogens, thiopentone, neuroleptics, amphetamines, apomorphine and cyclophosphamide have been employed to hurt, frighten, confuse or debilitate in such ways as callous ingenuity can devise. When the definition of criminal activity becomes perverted to include social dissent and activities in defense of human liberty, the availability of drugs offers easy opportunity for inhuman behaviour. Such use, and any doctors or scientists or others who engage in it, or who misguidedly allow themselves to believe that it can be in the interest of victims to monitor the activity, must surely be outlawed. See **truth drug**

total quality management (TQM)
- A concept developed in the pharmaceutical industry to implement official requirements for **GMP, GLP, GCP**.

Tower of Babel bias
(The overambitious building of the ancient tower was confounded when God caused the constructors to speak in different languages; the *Bible*: Genesis 11).
- The effect, in **meta-analysis** or **systematic reviews**, of confining the review of literature to studies published in one language, e.g. excluding non-English languages.

toxicity (Gr. *toxicon*, arrow poison, widened to mean any poison)
- Toxic or poisonous quality.
- Capacity to produce an **adverse drug reaction**. See **toxicology**

toxicity tests (Gr. *toxicon*, arrow poison, widened to mean any poison; L. *testum*, earthen pot used in assaying gold)
- Toxicity tests for **medicinal products** in animals (now largely prescribed by official regulatory authorities) must precede the use of a new drug/potential medicine in humans. The objective is to predict the adverse effects likely to occur in humans, and to determine their mechanisms. The different animal tests provide variable levels of prediction. The *European Union* regulations prescribe the following studies:
  1. *Single-dose toxicity* (*acute toxicity*) studies on at least two animal species of known strain.

2. *Repeated-dose toxicity* (*subacute*, generally lasting 2–4 weeks); (*chronic*, or *long-term*, generally lasting 3–6 months); duration depending on the conditions of proposed clinical use; for single-dose use in *humans* an animal test should last 2–4 weeks. Two species of mammal should be used, one a nonrodent.

3. *Fetal toxicity*: administration during pregnancy to at least two animal species.

4. *Reproductive function*: if the results of other tests reveal anything suggestive of harmful effects on progeny, e.g. fertility and peri- and post-natal studies.

5. *Carcinogenicity tests* are essential if the results of long-term toxicological tests have given rise to suspicion, or if the substance has a close chemical analogy to known **carcinogenic** or **co-carcinogenic** compounds, and may be required for medicines "likely to be administered regularly over a prolonged period of a patient's life". The drug is administered for a major proportion of the life of the test animal, e.g. 1.5–2.0 years in the rat.

- Administration by the route that will be used in man *must* be included.
- Toxicity tests for pesticides, industrial chemicals, etc., are adapted appropriately for the manner in which they are used.
- Predictive toxicity tests have been likened to searching for a needle in a haystack; except that it probably is not a needle and it may well not be in the haystack.

toxicokinetics/dynamics (Gr. *toxicon*, arrow poison; *kinein*, to move)
- The **(pharmaco)kinetics/dynamics** in toxicology studies of **xenobiotics** in general, especially of high doses. **See toxicity, toxicity tests**

toxicology (Gr. *toxicon*, arrow poison, widened to mean any poison; *logy*, subject of study)
- Traditionally, toxicology is the science of poisons. Toxicology is now the body of knowledge dealing with all those actions of substances capable of causing adverse effects on living organisms. It therefore includes not only the study of acute effects, but also of the long-term effects (chronic) of low-level exposure to medicines and otherwise useful substances, such as food additives, pesticides or industrial chemicals. Carcinogenic, mutagenic or teratogenic effects, and effects on living creatures in the environment are also considered. The subject is based on the study of mechanisms by which adverse effects are caused, and so draws on the basic sciences of pharmacology, biochemistry and pathology, as well as epidemiology and clinical medicine. The branch that seeks to determine whether chemicals are likely to be toxic is known as *predictive toxicology* (see **toxicity tests**). That branch dealing with detecting and treating human poisoning is *clinical toxicology*. **See poison**

toxin (Gr. *toxicon*, arrow poison, hence any poison)
- *Microbial*: An agent, usually a protein, produced by a microorganism, which is poisonous to the species infected, e.g. tetanus toxin, pertussis toxin. Some toxins, e.g. botulinum toxin, are produced by an organism that does not itself

infect man. Botulinum exotoxin is produced by *Clostridium botulinum* bacilli in meat, fish, etc., and poisons those who consume the contaminated food.

See **drugs as tools** (*Botulinum toxin*)

– *Other naturally-occurring substances*, often **alkaloids**, which are poisonous when introduced into the body, e.g. ricin, a lectin constituent of castor seeds (*Ricinus communis*), normally removed during the making of castor oil.
– A *poisonous derivative* of an agent (natural or synthetic), for example *N*-acetyl-*p*-benzoquinone, a reactive metabolite of paracetamol (acetaminophen) produced when the normal conjugating mechanisms are saturated, as in overdose.

toxophore   (Gr. *toxicon*, arrow poison, widened to mean any poison; *phoros*, a carrier)

– The chemical group, or part of a molecule, that is responsible for causing toxic effects.   See **toxicity, pharmacophore**

tPA
– Tissue plasminogen activator.

tracer dose   See **radioactive labelling**

traditional medicine   (L. *tradere*, to hand on)
– Traditional, or indigenous, medicinal therapeutics has developed since before written history in all societies. It comprises a mass of practices, ranging from worthless to highly effective remedies, e.g. digitalis (England), opium (Middle East), quinine (South America), reserpine (India) and atropine (various countries). It is the task of science to find the gems and to discard the dross, while leaving intact socially valuable supportive aspects of traditional medicine.

See **complementary medicine**

tranquillizer   (L. *tranquillus*, calm, serene)
– A drug that will quieten a patient without notably impairing consciousness (e.g. benzodiazepines – 'minor' tranquillizers; phenothiazines – 'major' tranquillizers). The term **anxiolytic** is preferred for the older term, minor tranquillizer, and **neuroleptic** or **antipsychotic** replaces the term major tranquillizer.

See **sedative**

***trans-/cis-* isomerism**   See ***cis-/trans-* isomerism**

transcription   (L. *trans*, across; *scribere*, to write)
– The process by which the genetic code of bases is copied from DNA to mRNA.

transcytosis   (L. *trans,* across, Gr. k*utos*, cell)
– The slow passage of small particles/large molecules and fluid, across endothelia (blood, lymph) by transport in small vesicles.
– Also know as *cytopempis* (Gr. *kutos,* cell; *pempis*, send through).

transdermal delivery system (L. *trans*, across; Gr. *dermatos*, skin)
- An adhesive device for controlling release of drugs for transfer across the skin; an extended-release formulation; a useful route of administration over prolonged periods which is uninvasive, avoids peaks and troughs of blood concentration and avoids **pre-systemic drug elimination**. Also known as a 'patch'. **Gels** and **ointments** are also used for transdermal absorption; accurate dosing presents obvious problems.

See **iontophoresis, modified-release drug delivery systems**

transducer (L. *trans*, across, through; *ducere*, to lead)
- A device that transforms one sort of energy into another, e.g. a drug or hormone **receptor**; an electronic strain gauge.
- Receptor–effector coupling is known as **transduction**.

transducer ratio See **Black & Leff model**

transduction (L. *trans*, across, through; *ducere*, to lead)
- *In pharmacology*: the process by which occupancy of the receptor by an agonist is converted into a response (i.e. receptor–effector coupling).

See **Black & Leff model**

transfection (L. *trans*, across; *ferre*, to carry)
- Transfer into or infection of a cell with DNA from another cell, and which is followed by replication; a mode of gene transfer.

transformation (L. *trans*, across; *forma*, shape)
- *Of a variable*: A change of the scale on which the **variable** (y) is measured. Transformations such as $\log(y)$, square root(y), $1/y$, **probit**(y) are common examples. Transformations are used, for example:
  - To make a relationship linear.
  - To change the distribution (i.e. make it more nearly a **normal distribution**) of a variable, or to render it **homoscedastic** (i.e. the data points having the same scatter at all points along the curve).
  - To make two curves parallel.
  - To change a scale of time (seconds) to one of frequency (reciprocal seconds), e.g. *Fourier transform* in noise analysis (*JB Fourier*, 1768–1830, mathematician, France).
- Transformation is often needed to analyze data usefully. *There are four reasons for transforming data*:
  1. To arrange that the dispersion of coded observations is similar across all treatments or diagnostic groups – so that changes in **mean** or **median** are not obscured by greater variability in some groups than in others.
  2. To induce normality – because many statistical tests, e.g. **Student's *t*-test**, require that the data are normally distributed. It is better to work with derived observations that have a normal distribution than to use less powerful statistical methods on the untransformed (**skewed**) data.
  3. To produce simple relationships – the eye easily assimilates straight lines but is less good at detecting other patterns, such as quadratic, cubic or

exponential. By transforming one or both of a pair of variables an association can sometimes be presented as linear on the transformed data when it was more complicated on the original observations.

4. So that there is good agreement with biological or physiological principles (*S Gore*).

- *Of an equation*: Devices such as the *Laplace transform* are used to change the form of algebraic equations in order to facilitate their solution (*PS Laplace, 1749–1827, mathematician, France*).
- The process of a cell becoming cancerous.   See **heteroscedasticity**

transgenic animal bioreactors   (L. *trans*, across; *genea*, race; *animalis*, having breath; Gr. *bios*, life, L. *re*, again, *agere*, to do)

- Transgenic animals are creatures into which have been inserted **genes** from another species. For manufacture of **medicinal products** they are usually farm livestock carrying human genes programmed selectively to secrete human therapeutic proteins in their milk. The process has been designated *pharming*. The mammary tissue of the farm livestock used (sheep, cattle, pigs) is enormously more efficient than any engineered bioreactor (tanks containing cell cultures) hitherto made by man.

translation   (L. *trans*, across; *latus*, carry across)

- The process by which the sequence of **bases** in mRNA is read by ribosomes to produce proteins.

translocation   (L. *trans*, across; *locus*, place)

- Translocation is the transposition of a segment of chromosome after a break to another position on the same chromosome, onto another chromosome, or to move within the cell, e.g. from the nucleus to the cytoplasm, or from the cytoplasm to the membrane.

transmitter/neurotransmitter   (L. *trans*, across; *mittere*, to send)

- A chemical stored in nerve endings which is released upon the arrival of sufficient action potentials and which crosses the **synaptic cleft/gap** and activates receptors on the postsynaptic cell membrane. Examples include **acetylcholine, noradrenaline, GABA, glutamate**, glycine, **dopamine, 5-HT**.

transmural stimulation   (L. *trans*, across; *murus*, wall)

- Electrical stimulation of a hollow organ or tissue *in vitro* such that the electric field passes through the wall of the organ (*field stimulation*).
                     See **co-axial stimulation**

transparency   (L. *trans*, across; *parere*, to appear)

- A principle of European Union administrative law under which, to ensure fairness, decisions are required to be made by reference to published criteria that are objective and verifiable and are notified with reasoning sufficient to enable the person affected to test the application of the relevant criteria and exercise whatever appeal rights are available (courtesy *Ian Dodds-Smith*).

The principle is relevant to the operation of medicines regulation, and indeed of **natural justice**.

transport (active)   (L. *trans*, across; *portare*, to carry)
- Movement of molecules across a membrane with ('down') or against ('up') a concentration or electric potential gradient by an energy-requiring process which is saturable and can be inhibited by other molecules.

See **diffusion (facilitated)**

transporter proteins
- Transporters selectively reaccumulate certain released neurotransmitters across membranes into presynaptic terminals and vesicles, aiding termination of synaptic transmission and recycling of neurotransmitters. They are classified by ion dependence (commonly either Na^+ or H^+) and **topology**. Examples are the dopamine transporter and the glutamate transporter. They can be a site for (medicinal) drug action. Most transporters are proteins with 12 membrane-spanning **domains**.

trapezoid rule (linear)   (Gr. *trapeza*, table; L. *regulare*, to regulate)
- Method for estimating the **area under the curve (AUC)** in pharmacokinetics. The method consists of first dividing the drug concentration v. time curve into small segments of time by drawing a series of vertical lines. Straight lines are then drawn joining the concentration at the beginning of each time period to the concentration at the end of each period. This results in numerous trapezia, the areas of each of which can be easily determined using a simple mathematical formula; the AUC is the sum of all these areas. If $AUC_{0-\infty}$ is required, the line joining the last two measured concentrations is extrapolated, producing a triangle the area of which is added to the sum of the areas of the trapezia.

trapping hypothesis   See **ion trapping**

Trendelenburg preparation
- A preparation of guinea-pig isolated ileum in which changes in volume and length are measured simultaneously. The lumen of the segment of ileum is filled with bathing solution, cannulated and connected at the bottom of the bath to a device measuring volume. The upper end of the segment is connected to a device that measures length (or tension). Drugs are added to the fluid bathing the serosal surface of the tissue. In a later modification, drugs can be added to either the serosal bathing fluid or the luminal bathing fluid (*P Trendelenburg*, 1917, pharmacologist, Germany).

triage   (Old Fr. *trier*, to sift, to pick out)
- To sort according to quality or degree of urgency, e.g. to decide which patients are likely to derive great benefit from, and therefore should be accorded priority to receive, an *expensive treatment* or *scarce resource* that cannot be made available to all sufferers.

trimeric proteins/ trimers   (G. *tres*, three; *metron*, measure; *proteios*, primary)
– Proteins composed of three identical (*homotrimeric*) or different (*hetero-trimeric*) subunits. For example, **G-proteins** are trimers.

See **homomeric receptors**

'trip'   (Middle Dutch. *trippen*, skip, hop)
– A drug-induced experience, usually by a hallucinogen (cannabis, lysergide). A trip may be 'good' or 'bad'. Bad trips may often be terminated by diazepam.

triple-blind study
– An extension of double-blind, where there is a committee monitoring results of a **therapeutic trial** and it is kept in ignorance of the identity of treatments.

See **double-blind, single-blind**

trohoc
– **Cohort** spelled backwards.   See **case-control study**

true/truth   (Old Norse *tryggr*, Gothic *triggws*)
– In accordance with fact or reality, not false or erroneous: quality of being true or accurate.
– Popper's notion of 'the truth' is very like this: our concern in the pursuit of knowledge is to get closer and closer to the truth, and we may even know that we have made an advance, but we can never know if we have reached our goal (*K Popper*, 1902–1994, philosopher of science, UK).
– The most we can ever say is that a theory is supported by every observation so far, and yields more, and more precise, predictions than any known alternative. It is still replaceable by a better theory (*B Magee*).
– The strongest argument in favour of the truth of a statement is the failure of competent, energetic efforts to demonstrate its falsehood.
– The grand, and indeed only, character of truth is its capability of enduring the test of universal experience, and coming unchanged out of every possible form of fair discussion (*JFW Herschel*, 1792–1871, astronomer, England).
– "Truth is rarely pure and never simple" (*Oscar Wilde*, 1856–1900, writer, Ireland).
– "Scientists know so much about the natural world by knowing so much about whom they can trust" (*S Shapin*) (see **research misconduct**).
– "Truth is not absolute, but rather a series of working hypotheses that are defined by increasingly rigorous rules; that means that the range of credible heterodoxy steadily diminishes" (*J Maddox*).

See **Bayes' theorem, knowledge, science in pharmacology**

truth drug
– It might be urged that it is justifiable to use drugs to protect society by discovering serious crimes such as murder. There is no such thing as a 'truth drug' in the sense that it guarantees the truth of what the subject says. There al-

ways must be uncertainty of the truth of evidence obtained with drugs, e.g. thiopentone, that cannot be independently confirmed. But accused people, convinced of their own innocence, sometimes volunteer to undergo such tests. The problem of discerning truth from falsehood remains. A truly effective 'truth drug' would disrupt society, public and domestic.

– *In vino veritas*: the truth comes out in wine (*Pliny* the Elder, 23–79 CE, writer, Rome), and so it sometimes may, or may not.   See **torture, drugs and**

tryptophan
– An essential amino acid, precursor of **serotonin** (5-hydroxytryptamine, 5-HT). Some efficacy in the treatment of psychological depression has been shown and it has been widely available by direct sale to the public for self-treatment as a nutritional agent. In 1989 a potentially fatal condition (eosinophilia-myalgia syndrome) was attributed to an impurity apparently introduced by changing the manufacturing technique from simple chemical synthesis to a fermentation process. It was not licensed as a medicine in the USA where most cases occurred.   See **nutra(i)ceutical**

t-test
See **Student's *t*-test**

tubocurarine
See **curare**

tumorigenesis/-ic
(L. *tumor*, swelling; Gr. *gen*, to be produced)
– An unnecessary bastard neologism that is gaining use despite the existence of the euphonious equivalent, **oncogenesis/-ic**; the science of tumours is *oncology*.

tumour promoter
(L. *tumor*, swelling; *pro*, before; *movere*, to move)
– A substance that, although noncarcinogenic itself, induces cancer if applied *after* an **initiator** (subcarcinogenic dose of a known **carcinogen**). The validity of this two-stage theory of carcinogenesis has been subjected to cogent criticism.

turnover time/rate
– Endogenous body substances are maintained at concentrations within a range that varies for each substance (**homeostasis**). But the actual molecules change as a result of dietary intake, of synthesis and of elimination processes, i.e. there is *turnover*. The process also applies to the persistence of drugs in the body, when it is called **mean residence time**.

two-sided test
– A **statistical significance** test in which deviations from the **null hypothesis** in either direction are considered.

Tyndallization
– Fractional sterilization. Used to sterilize microbial culture media, etc. in cases where excessive heat would be detrimental. The heat applied does not kill

spores and so several treatments are applied, between which spores germinate only to be killed during subsequent treatments (after *John Tyndall*, 1820–1893, physicist, Ireland).

tyramine   See **drugs as tools**

U

uncertainty principle (in therapeutic research)
- For ethical reasons, **randomization** can be contemplated only if both doctor and patient feel substantially uncertain as to which trial treatment is best. The uncertainty principle maximises the potential for recruitment within this ethical constraint. Simply stated, the *uncertainty principle* is that:

    "Patients can be entered only if the responsible physician is *substantially uncertain* as to which of the trial treatments would be most appropriate for this particular patient. No patient should be entered if the responsible physician and/or the patient are for any medical or non-medical reason(s) reasonably certain that one of the treatments that might be allocated would be inappropriate (in comparison with some other treatments that could be offered to the patient in the trial or outside it)" (*C Baigent; British Journal of Clinical Pharmacology* 1997;43:349).   See **equipoise**

uncompetitive inhibition/antagonism   (Gr. *an*, not; L. *com*, with; *petere*, seek)
- Form of inhibition in which both the maximal velocity of an enzymatic reaction (V_{max}) or maximal response of an isolated tissue to a drug (E_{max}) and the **dissociation equilibrium constant** (K_m for an enzyme or K_A for a drug) are reduced by the inhibitor/**antagonist**. In enzymology this pattern is shown when the enzyme inhibitor cannot form a complex with the enzyme unless the enzyme is already bound to the substrate. In the double **reciprocal plot** the slope remains constant and the value of the intercept on the y axis ($1/V_{max}$) increases and the value of the intercept on the x axis ($-1/K_m$) decreases with increasing concentration of the antagonist/inhibitor. A rare mechanism of drug action. Uncompetitive antagonism is not the same as **noncompetitive antagonism**, in which the maximum response (E_{max}) is reduced by the antagonist, but the K_A is unaltered. Neither is it appropriate to state that antagonism is uncompetitive if the mechanism simply fails to meet the criteria for **competitive antagonism** (i.e. is not competitive).

unlabeled (off-label) use (of a drug)
- Use of a drug for an unlicensed indication.
- The prescription of a drug for an unlabeled (off-label) indication is entirely proper if the proposed use is based on rational scientific theory, expert medical opinion, or controlled clinical studies. The **FDA** has made it eminently clear that it neither has nor wants the authority to compel physicians to adhere to officially labelled uses, because experience demonstrates that the official label lags behind scientific knowledge and publications. New uses for a drug already on the market are often first discovered through the **serendipitous** observations and therapeutic innovations of physicians (*American Medical Association*: Drug Evaluations).   See **compassionate drug use**

up-regulation and down-regulation (of receptors)   See **receptor**

upside/downside
- *Upside*: potential for advantage or gain.
- *Downside*: potential for disadvantage or loss.

- The terms originated in the 1960s in relation to commercial share prices. They are now used in general **benefit/risk evaluation**.

uricosuric   (Gr. *ouron*, urine, and so uric acid)
- Substance that increases urinary excretion of urate, usually by preventing renal tubular reabsorption.

USAN
- United States Adopted Name.

U-shaped (or J-shaped) curve
- A **frequency distribution** curve that approximates in shape to the letter U (or J). All-cause mortality and alcohol consumption is an example. Non-drinkers have a higher mortality that do light and moderate drinkers, and heavy drinkers have a higher mortality than either group.

USP
- *United States Pharmacopeia.*

utility   (L. *utilis*, use)
- Usefulness.
- The term conveys a balance between therapeutic efficacy and adverse effect. A utility curve may be constructed of the difference between the **weighted** probability of efficacy minus the weighted probability of **toxicity**. It gives some idea of the probability of obtaining efficacy without toxicity. The reason for the weighting of the probability is to emphasize that there is a question of individual judgement as to the relative values of the various measures of efficacy, minor toxicity and major toxicity in reaching a decision (*after Rowland & Tozer*, see Acknowledgements).   See **economics**

utility measurement
- Utility measurement yields a single value for states of health on an interval scale. Usually the scale is standardized so that 'dead' is equal to zero and 'perfect health' is equal to unity. Some states of health have been rated by respondents as being 'worse than death' and are represented by negative values. In North America, three main measurement methods have emerged: the *rating scale*, the **time trade-off** approach and the **standard gamble** (*MF Drummond*).   See **quality of life**

valid   (L. *validus*, strong)
- Sound, defensible, logical, legally acceptable.
- A measurement is *valid* if it measures what it is intended to measure.

valid patient group   See **evaluable patient**

validation (of data, of a test)   (L. *validus*, strong, effective)
- Demonstration that data or a procedure, activity or system are sound and reliable. Neglect of validation procedures is destructive of both research and practice.
- Efforts made to confirm the accuracy, precision, or effectiveness of results (*AR Feinstein*).

Vancouver Group   See **International Committee of Medical Journal Editors**

van der Waals bond   (Middle Eng. *band*, fetter)
- A weak electrostatic attraction between molecules in which the centres of positive and negative charge are separated. Also known as electron correlation attraction (*JD van der Waals*, 1837–1923, physicist, The Netherlands).
                                                          See **hydrophobic bond**

variable   (L. *varius*, changing)
- Having a range of possible values.
- Any quantity that can have different values. In algebra, variables are represented by symbols, most commonly letters of the Roman alphabet, eg. x, y, z.
- Variables may be *continuous* (smooth change with little or no gap between values), or *discrete/discontinuous* (a distinct gap, or **integer**, between values). What is continuous and what is discrete can merge into each other, but the distinction has value as, for example, it is biologically impossible to have a family of 2.4 children (although that statistic is both useful and commonly used in demography, and a change to, say, 2.2, could be a consequence of the use of artificial contraception). Blood pressure and chemical values, and body weight are, for practical purposes, continuous variables, whereas percentage of individuals responding to treatment are discontinuous variables. Variables may also be *dependent* (the variable being investigated or *predicted*) or *independent* (the *predictor* variable; or variable under the control of the investigator).
                  See **variables and analysis of variable, variables (scales for), variate**

variables and analysis of variables   (L. *varius*, changing)
- A variable is a measurable characteristic that will change (vary) between different individuals or in the same individual on different occasions. Variables may be *independent* (e.g. the dose of an administered drug), *dependent* (an outcome of drug administration) or **confounding.**
                                                          See also **variables (scales for)**
- *Multivariable analysis* is part of everyday life, e.g. deciding on a holiday or what to wear when going outdoors; it is a largely unconscious, informal and commonsensical process.

- But the analysis of formal data requires formal procedures:
  - Univariate analysis involves a single variable.
  - Bivariate analysis involves pairs of any two variables.
  - Multivariable (regarding spelling, see *Feinstein*, below) analysis involves three or more variables. There are four principal methods (in health care literature): *linear regression,* **logistic regression analysis,** *proportional hazards analysis (***Cox proportional hazards/regression model***)* and *discriminant function analysis.*
  - Newer methods include recursive partitioning and conjunctive consolidation (after *AR Feinstein*).
- Exposition of all this and much, much, more can be found in *Multivariable analysis: an introduction* by *AR Feinstein* (Yale University Press, 1996). The author, despite the subtitle, *an introduction,* concedes that "the text is not written in the 'pablum [L. *pabulum,* food] for kiddies' approach that is sometimes used to simplify statistical discussions aimed at practitioners in the health sciences".

variables, scales for
- Principal types approximately in order of precision (downwards):
  - *Dimensional scale* (also called *continuous, interval* or *ratio*): the common form of quantitative ranking, either continuous or with an equal interval between adjacent values, e.g. blood pressure, age.
  - *Nominal scale*: categories that cannot be ranked, e.g. sex, diagnosis.
  - *Ordinal scale*: graded categories, e.g. mild, moderate, severe.
  - *Binary scale*: two categories for an attribute, e.g. dead/alive.
  - *Quasi-dimensional scale*, e.g. visual analogue scale.

See **variables and analysis of variables**

variance   (L. *variantia*, difference)
- The square of a **standard deviation**. A measure of **dispersion** with additive properties that are convenient for some statistical manipulations.
- Measure of dispersion obtained by subtracting the **mean** of the squared deviations of the observed values from their mean in a **frequency distribution**.
- The **scatter** of a function in an experiment.   See **covariance**

variate   (L. *variantia*, difference)
- For a quantity that is subject to statistical variation, the individual values obtained when the population is sampled repeatedly are known as *variates*. If the quantity is represented by the symbol x, then the variates may be represented by $x_1, x_2, x_3 \ldots x_n$.

variation coefficient   (L. *variantia*, difference; *co, com/cum, con,* with, together, in common, jointly, equally, reciprocally, mutually; *efficere*, to accomplish)
- The **standard deviation** expressed as a proportion or percentage of the mean. Coefficient of variation = (standard deviation $\div$ mean) $\times$ 100. It is used to compare variabilities of observation.

V_d See **volume of distribution**

vector   (L. *vector*, carrier, traveller, rider)
- *In mathematics*: a quantity having both direction and magnitude.
- *In medicine*: the agency, usually an animal, responsible for carrying an infection from one host to another, e.g. the anopheles mosquito is the vector for malaria.
- *In therapeutics*, using a virus to carry a drug into a target tissue.
                                                        See **targeting of drugs**
- *In genetic engineering*: the agency, usually a virus, by means of which new DNA is introduced into the cells that are being used to **express** the new genes.

vehicle   (L. *vehere*, carry, convey)
- A substance used to facilitate the delivery of a drug (e.g. suspending agents, emulsifying agents).

venom   (L. *venenum*, potion, drug, poison)
- Poisonous fluid produced by an animal and introduced into other animals (victims).
- Many venoms have found uses as pharmacological tools, e.g. black widow spider venom; α- and β-*bungarotoxin* from the venom of the elapid snake *Bungarus multicinctus*; *charybdotoxin* from a scorpion (*Leiurus quinquestriatus*); *apamin* from bee venom.   See **drugs as tools**

Venn diagram
- J Venn (1834–1923) was an English logician who "adopted the diagrammatic method of illustrating propositions by inclusive and exclusive circles" (Dictionary of National Biography). A stained glass window celebrating Venn's circles may be seen in Caius College at Cambridge University, England.

verification/validation of data (regulatory term)   (L. *verus*, true;
                                                        validus, strong; *datum,* thing known)
- The procedures carried out to ensure that the data contained in the final clinical trial report (Final Report) match original observations. These procedures may apply to raw data, hard copy, or electronic case report forms, computer print-outs and statistical analyses and tables (**EC/EU**).

vermifuge   (L. *vermis*, worm; *fugare*, to put to flight)
                                                        See **anthelmintic**

vesicant   (L. *vesica*, bladder, blister)
- An agent that causes blistering, e.g. **mustard gas**.

viable   (L. *vita*, life)
- Capable of maintaining life or development.
- Feasible, practicable.

vinca alkaloids
- **Alkaloids** obtained from the Madagascar periwinkle plant (*Vinca rosea*). They disrupt microtubules in cells and are useful in cancer chemotherapy. The two principal alkaloids are vincristine and vinblastine.

VIP
- Vasoactive intestinal polypeptide.

virus   (L. *virus*, slimy liquid, poison)
- An infective nucleic acid (RNA and DNA) that subverts the synthetic machinery of living cells in such a way that more copies of itself are produced. The nucleic acid normally has a protein capsule.
- "A piece of bad news wrapped up in a protein" (*PB Medawar*, 1915–1987, zoologist/immunologist, Nobel Laureate, UK).
- Unlike bacteria, viruses cannot be grown away from the living cells they infect. It is incorrect to speak of viruses as if they were tiny microorganisms using the cell sap as a culture. A virus's genetic information is encoded in the host nucleic acid, DNA or RNA. For this reason the problems of antiviral chemotherapy differ significantly from those of antibacterial chemotherapy.

visiting fireman (slang)
- An invited visitor to an institution or department, who is famous or notorious (for whatever reasons), who engages in self-promotion at the expense of the feelings and relationships of local staff.
- A hit-and-run visitor.
- A short-term visitor (often self-invited) who leaves behind a trail of destruction.

visual analogue scale   (L. *videre*, to see;
                              Gr. *analogos,* proportionate; L. *scandere*, to climb)
- A simple rating scale for rendering subjective feelings/health states measurable (quantifiable), e.g. intensity of pain, level of mood. A straight graduated line (usually 10 cm) is drawn with its extreme ends labelled with the most and least preferred states (anchor terms), e.g. 'the worst pain I can imagine' and 'no (or almost no) pain'. The choice of anchor terms requires skill; it must suit the topic and the research subjects who mark the line at the point that they judge to be their present state (between the extremes). Thus what is a subjective state is made measurable and statistically analysable.
                                                    See **variables, scales for**

vitamin   (L. *vita*, life; Ger. *amin*, amine)
- An organic substance, essential in small quantities for the maintenance of vital metabolic functions. A micronutrient (in contrast to macronutrients, e.g. carbohydrate, amino acids). Initially the word was spelled *vitamine*, but when it was realized that they were not all amines, the terminal *e* was dropped.

vivisection   (L. *vivus*, living; *secare*, cut)
- The word was introduced in 1707 for the performance of surgery in living ani-

mals for physiological and pathological research. In current usage it embraces all experiments involving living animals, including nonsurgical experiments (and the vast majority of experiments involve no surgery). The evident moral issues are increasingly debated.

V_{max}   See **Michaelis–Menten equation**

voltage clamp   (Named after *Count A Volta*, Italian physicist, 1745–1827; Low Ger. *klamp*, brace, band)
- A method for measuring the electric current that flows across a cell membrane under conditions where the potential difference across the membrane is held constant ('clamped'). It is the basic tool for investigation of excitable membranes (because the time course of events would be distorted by the charge and discharge of membrane capacities if the membrane potential were allowed to vary). The technique allows particular ionic conductances to be studied at a controlled membrane potential. This is important in the investigation of the role of the different conductances and their **modulation** in cell excitability. The technique is also applied to the study of single ion channels in the **patch-clamp** method.

volume of distribution (V_d or V)
- The volume of fluid in which the drug appears to distribute with a concentration equal to that in blood plasma (i.e. as though the body were a single **compartment**):

$$V_d = \frac{\text{(amount of drug in body (i.e. the dose))}}{\text{(concentration of drug in plasma)}}$$

- Because the body is not a single compartment, and because the result of the calculation may be a volume greater than that of the body, it is best to refer to the *apparent* volume of distribution.

volunteer   (L. *voluntas*, will)
- A person who acts of his or her own free will, not constrained or compelled.
- The word is too often used as implying only healthy research subjects. This is undesirable since patients in research are also volunteers, and it is undesirable to imply, even indirectly, that consent might not need to be sought from patients. *Healthy (or non-patient) volunteer* and *patient volunteer* should be used to avoid any misunderstanding. In defining *volunteer* the word human is redundant since it is plain that animals cannot volunteer.
- The term *healthy* does not imply a state of perfect general health, but health in respect of the experiment proposed, e.g. a person with osteoarthritis is deemed a healthy volunteer with regard to a simple pharmacokinetic study.
- Rarely, research is conducted on patients who cannot volunteer, and this can be in their own interest lest they become health orphans; ethical issues are particularly prominent.   See **ethics committee, orphan drug**

warnings to patients   (Old Eng. *warnian*; L. *pati*, suffer)
- Warnings are of two kinds:
  - Those that will affect the patient's decision to accept or reject the treatment.
  - Those that will relate to the safety and efficacy of the treatment once it has begun, e.g. risk of stopping treatment, occurrence of **adverse drug reactions**.
- The doctor's legal **duty of care** includes provision of appropriate warnings.
See liability, negligence

washout period   (Old Eng. *waescan*; *ut*; Gr. *peri*, about; *odos*, way)
- A period between two treatments to allow the effects of the first to dissipate to avoid contamination of the second treatment.   See **carry-over effect**

water solubility   See **hydrophilic, lipid solubility, solubility**

weak/strong   See **strong/weak**

weight   (Old Eng. *wiht*, Old Norse *vett*)
- A measure of heaviness of an object.
- The product of the force of gravity and mass.
- *In statistics*: a measure of the importance, or information content, of an observation, most commonly the reciprocal of its **variance**.

'well established medicinal use'
- This is a term used, but not defined, in a European Community Directive, which allows an *abridged* procedure for licensing of *copies* of 'well established' drugs. A definition might comprise: substantially uncontroversial use in the mainstream of medical practice for some or all of the licensed indications over a substantial period of years, generally at least five. The medicine should have been licensed in at least five countries having regulatory authorities of recognized international credibility, and should have been favourably reviewed in one or more of the various publications devoted to high-quality *consensus reviews* of medicinal products. Such review requires that there is in existence a substantial clinical literature on the drug/medicine.
See abridged application, essential drugs, evidence-based
medicine, generic drugs, regulation (official) of medicines

well-stirred model
- A **pharmacokinetic** model in which instantaneous and complete mixing of a drug within a tissue, e.g. the liver, is assumed (*Rowland & Tozer*, see Acknowledgements).   See **model**

WHO
- World Health Organization.

WHO – ART
- World Health Organization – Adverse Reaction Terminology.

Wilcoxon signed ranks (sum) test
- A paired test (see **Student's *t*-test**) analogous to the unpaired **Wilcoxon two-sample test**. Numerical responses are needed, so that the differences between the responses to two treatments can be found for each individual. These differences are ranked for performance. The test, which is a **randomization test** on ranks, is a *nonparametric* test (see **parametric**).

Wilcoxon two-sample test on ranks
- A significance test in which it is not necessary to assume a particular form of distribution (e.g. **normal**) of the observations, i.e. a *nonparametric* test (see **parametric**). It can be used for non-numerical measurements, which are ranked in order of magnitude, e.g. subjective clinical evaluations such as better, no change, worse: this is a great advantage. It is a type of **randomization test**.

window   See **therapeutic window**

withdrawal syndrome   (Old Eng. *with*, away; Gr. *syn*, with; *dromos*, run)
- Abrupt withdrawal of a drug, especially opioid **analgesics** (see **opiate/opioid**), following prolonged use, may result in physical and/or mental illness, generally characterized by effects opposite to the normal actions of the drug (see **dependence**). A form of withdrawal syndrome, often referred to as *rebound*, may occur in many instances where long-term exposure to a drug has resulted in adaptation of physiological systems (e.g. clonidine use in the treatment of hypertension, and use of a β-adrenoceptor blocker in the treatment of angina pectoris). Gradual withdrawal of a drug avoids or minimizes the **syndrome**.   See **discontinuation syndrome**

within-patient (subject) trial
- A **therapeutic trial**, or other comparative study, in which each subject receives all treatments under test, i.e. subjects act as their own controls.
       See **between-patient trial, carry-over effects, cross-over trial, single-patient clinical trial, Latin square**

women and minorities in large scale clinical trials   (Old Eng. *wifman*, wife of man; L. *minus*, less)
- The USA National Institutes for Health stated in 1993 that any (large, phase III) clinical trial funded by itself, and not ruled exempt by its director, must provide for a valid analysis of gender and racial differences. Although the social intentions of this decision are uncontroversial, scientific, ethical and practical aspects of implementation have aroused debate. In 1997 the **FDA** strengthened its regulations requiring the inclusion of women.
       See **women as subjects in early tests of new drugs, phases of clinical studies of new drugs**

women as subjects in early tests of new drugs   (Old Eng. *wifman*, wife-man; the word *man* was formerly applied to both sexes: *Skeat*. Etymological Dictionary)
- For many years women of 'childbearing potential' have been excluded from

early tests (phase I and early phase II) of new drugs because of fears that they might be, or become, pregnant and bear a deformed child. In 1993 the **FDA** (USA) changed this policy, (1) for scientific reasons (early detection of sex differences can be of value in design of later studies), (2) out of respect for women's 'autonomy and decision-making capacity', and (3) because it is possible to reduce risk of fetal exposure through protocol design. The FDA added that, "Whether removal of the impediments to their participation will increase the number of women in early trials depends partly on drug companies' concerns about liability...If we are to achieve broader participation of women in all phases of clinical trials, legitimate issues such as liability will have to be addressed as part of ongoing dialogue among drug developers, scientists, policy makers, health advocates, and women's groups" (see *RB Merkatz et al.*; Women in clinical trials of new drugs: a change in Food and Drug Administration policy, *New England Journal of Medicine* 1993;329:292). In 1997 the **FDA** extended its authority to require inclusion of women and (ethnic) minorities in all **phases of clinical studies of new drugs.**

xanthine-containing drinks   See **xanthines and methylxanthines**

xanthines and methylxanthines
- Principally **caffeine** and theophylline, which have social and medicinal use. **Tea**, **coffee** and **cola** drinks contain substantial amounts of caffeine, a psychostimulant, probably acting largely by inhibiting the enzyme *phosphodiesterase* which destroys **cyclic-AMP**. It is said that no usable caffeine-containing plant has been discovered in historic times, i.e. all had been discovered and used by prehistoric man. Cocoa contains theobromine and caffeine; it is used to make chocolate (Ancient Mexican *chocolatl*).
  - Quantities (approximate):
  - 1 cup of coffee, caffeine 85 mg
  - 1 cup of tea, caffeine 50 mg
  - 1 bottle (360 ml) cola drink, caffeine 40–50 mg (about half the caffeine is added as pure alkaloid).
- **EU** regulations define decaffeinated coffee (bean) as 0.3% or less of caffeine (normal content 1–2%).

xenobiotic   (Gr. *xenos*, strange, foreign; *bios*, life)
- A substance that is taken into the body but does not enter the pathways of metabolism used to derive energy, or act as a precursor for body constituents.
- A foreign substance.
- Particularly used of environmental contaminants, but including drugs.

xylocholine   See **drugs as tools**

Yates's correction   (*F Yates*, 1902–1994, statistician, UK)
- A device for reducing **bias** when using the continuous **chi-square distribution** for small sample sizes.

yin-yang hypothesis   (Chinese *yin*, dark; *yang*, bright)
- Borrowed from the traditional Chinese: the idea that levels of **cyclic-AMP** and **cyclic-GMP** have opposing intracellular actions, and that cell function is a balance of the levels of these nucleotides relative to one another within the cell. Membrane receptor activation is believed to change the balance of nucleotides and hence cellular function. However, not all cGMP effects are opposed by cAMP (and *vice versa*), e.g. cGMP-gating of retinal cation channels. In Chinese philosophy *Yin* is negative, dark and feminine, and *Yang* is positive, bright and masculine. Their interaction maintains the harmony (if there is harmony) of the universe.

yohimbine   See **drugs as tools**

Z

Zelen randomization   See **therapeutic trial**

zero-order kinetics   (Arabic *sifr*, zero; L. *ordo*, array, degree; Gr. *kinesis*, motion)
- The rate of transfer or metabolism is constant and independent of the amount (concentration) present. It is called *zero*-order because the rate is proportional to the concentration raised to the power of 0. (*Note:* $x^0 = 1.0$ for any value of x.)   See **first-order kinetics, saturation kinetics**

zero-sum   (Arabic, *sifr;* L. *summus*, highest)
- A situation in which gains are equal to losses.   See **benefit/risk evaluation**

zwitterion   (Ger. *Zwitter*, mongrel; Gr. *ion*, going)
- A molecule carrying positively and negatively charged groups, e.g. amino acid.